The *Dai* and the Indigenous

This is a book about the *dai*, or traditional birth practitioner, and her place in the emerging therapeutic domain in colonial and contemporary India.

The book employs a caste-informed feminist reading of the colonial archive against the grain and explores papers by Englishwomen physicians, texts of indigenous medicine and practitioner accounts, administrative documents, public commentaries, and legislative assembly debates from the 19th and early 20th centuries. It also examines contemporary healthcare policy discourse. Using these methodologies, the author traces the production of the *dai* as an unsanitary, unskilled indigenous figure in colonial and nationalist accounts. The book goes on to examine the workings of gender and caste in the setting up of this figure, at first for containment and then for removal from institutionalized healthcare – an exercise that is more or less completed in the present. The author argues that this exercise is part of the refashioning of the indigenous, and of indigenous medicine, throughout this period, into a highly codified domain that centres caste privilege and is supported by global capital networks. In such a refashioning, the *dai* figure is rendered remote not only from the centre of the healthcare apparatus but also from the centre of the contemporary nation. This genealogical tracing of indigenous medicine in Indian contexts, rather than separate histories, is also useful to understand better what is termed the healthcare assemblage today, and this book provides a ground on which this can be done.

Asha Achuthan is presently a faculty member at the Advanced Centre for Women's Studies, Tata Institute of Social Sciences, Mumbai, India. She was initially trained in medicine at Calcutta University and defected to Women's Studies thereafter. She teaches courses on feminist science and technology studies, sexuality and queer studies, and feminist methodology. Her current work explores the contexts of gender and biomedicine, with a focus on feminist epistemological critiques of the same. She has most recently published in the areas of gender diversity in science institutions, feminist standpoint methodologies, interdisciplinarity in higher education, and sexuality and the nation.

Therapeutic Cultures

This interdisciplinary series explores the role which therapeutic discourses and practices play in the organisation of social life, critically addressing the two broad questions of how therapeutic knowledge is popularised beyond academia and mental health care, and how it participates in popular culture, and in institutional structures and processes in government, law, education, media, health, work, family life, public and private policies.

Therapeutic Cultures seeks to address the histories of therapeutic culture and engage with its contemporary manifestations, so welcomes books that examine the transnationalisation of therapeutic discourses and practices and their uses in local institutional settings, as well as studies of the ways in which therapeutic discourses and practices participate in the social organisation of power, and how they become ingrained across a wide array of institutions.

Series Editors

Daniel Nehring, East China University of Science and Technology, China
Ole Jacob Madsen, University of Oslo, Norway
Edgar Cabanas, Universidad Camilo José Cela, Spain
China Mills, University of Sheffield, UK
Dylan Kerrigan, University of the West Indies, Trinidad and Tobago

Titles in this series

Assembling Therapeutics
Cultures, Politics and Materiality
Edited by Suvi Salmenniemi, Johanna Nurmi, Inna Perheentupa and Harley Bergroth

Beyond Therapeutic Culture in Latin America
Hybrid Networks in Argentina and Brazil
Piroska E. Csúri, Mariano B. Plotkin and Nicolás Viotti

The Dai and the Indigenous
Notes on the Appearance and Disappearance of a Figure in the Therapeutics of a Nation
Asha Achuthan

Unruly Subjectivities
Mental Health and Otherness in Immigration, Transsexuality and Drug Use
Ilana Mountian

For more information about this series, please visit: https://www.routledge.com/Therapeutic-Cultures/book-series/TC

The *Dai* and the Indigenous

Notes on the Appearance and Disappearance of a Figure in the Therapeutics of a Nation

Asha Achuthan

Routledge
Taylor & Francis Group

LONDON AND NEW YORK

First published 2025
by Routledge
4 Park Square, Milton Park, Abingdon, Oxon OX14 4RN

and by Routledge
605 Third Avenue, New York, NY 10158

Routledge is an imprint of the Taylor & Francis Group, an informa business

British Library Cataloguing-in-Publication Data
A catalogue record for this book is available from the British Library

ISBN: 9780367424282 (hbk)
ISBN: 9781032859385 (pbk)
ISBN: 9780367824051 (ebk)

DOI: 10.4324/9780367824051

Typeset in Times New Roman
by Deanta Global Publishing Services, Chennai, India

To *Papa*, who believed in me
I wish I had been given the chance to put this in your hands

Contents

Acknowledgements

This book has had some short and some very long histories. My ideas began from conversations with the not-to-be-named *didis* – traditional childbirth practitioners – who confounded my training in paediatric emergencies with their articulations of childbirth practice and who introduced to me alternative models of knowledge and practice. My debt to them remains the highest.

Meeting and being mentored by Prof Shefali Moitra, forever *Shefalidi* to her students, within and outside academia, helped shape my ideas during my MPhil research, where the contemporary livelihoods and knowledge communities that *dais* inhabit became clearer to me. To that amazing presence in my academic journey, I am ever grateful, and one of the persons I secretly wish to impress with this book.

Some parts of the material that have found its way into this book are drawn from my doctoral thesis, and to Prof Tejaswini Niranjana, my uncompromising PhD supervisor, I remain grateful for all the inputs on methodology, clarity of argument, and writing during that time.

A Charles Wallace fellowship at the King's India Institute enabled me to visit the British Library and the Wellcome Trust Library in London and access the archives, where some of the introductory thoughts in this book began. To Richard Alford at Charles Wallace Trust, who introduced me to more scholars in the field than I was then aware of, and to Kriti Kapila at King's India Institute, who kindly listened to my early articulations, I remain thankful. To the wonderful librarians at the British Library, thank you for all the support in finding material and helping navigate the system.

I am also grateful to the Maharashtra State Archives for access to materials there.

China Mills – you are the reason this book has seen the light of day. Your curiosity at the first mention of this work, your interest in envisioning it as part of the *Therapeutic Cultures* series, your incisive yet gentle comments, and your support all the way to the finish line, have felt like I have a true colleague and friend – always a difficult combination. It was in our conversations that I was able to see the power of therapeutic cultures and regimes as a framing argument for the book. Thank you, *bondhu*.

I am grateful to the other series editors who reviewed the idea for the book.

I also owe thanks to Daniel Nehring, who, along with China, as series editors, helped with a great deal of the last-minute bumps during publishing.

I thank all the publishing support at Routledge for helping to see this book to print.

Portions of these arguments were presented at the King's India Institute, at the Tata Institute of Social Sciences, Bombay, and at the Humanizing Birth: Launching Critical Midwifery Studies symposium organized by IIT Bombay and the University of Humanistic Studies, Netherlands. I am grateful to all who responded.

To my people at the Advanced Centre for Women's Studies, TISS, for holding time and space for me, for believing that I must be doing good work(!), thank you. That is you – Bindhu, Sujatha, Sujata, Meena, and Sangita, but also Ilina. Ilina, I think you would have liked what I have tried to do here.

To my students, for the energy they bring to my classroom, for pushing me to think more and better, I continue to be grateful.

To Wandana and Sangita, for looking out for me, for reading and responding to my chapters, and for believing in me, thank you. And to Shilpa, for also reading my chapters and being happy for me!

To KP, for also reading my chapters, for being my home editor, for taking over when I am terror-stricken by proofreading … but more than anything, for being my home – thank you. I would not have gotten here without you. I promise, and threaten, to take over the cooking now.

1   Introduction
The *dai* and the terrain of indigenous practice

Introduction

This book is being written at a time when the subject of its tentative exploration, popularly referred to in northern Indian contexts as the *dai*, is, in part, the site of feminist epistemological concerns around models of knowledge, and, in part, a receding yet extant figure in vulnerable childbirth scenarios. This subject is also notable in her absence from the dominant articulations of a seemingly unified indigenous therapeutics, as available in health planning and systems vocabulary.

In the extensive scholarship on histories of medicine in the subcontinent, the *dai* has not been a prominent or visible figure; while this might have to do with the gendered and institution-centric nature of much of this scholarship, biomedicine has constantly been presented in contest with indigenous systems of medicine, and the *dai* has not been seen as part of either. Feminist historians, philosophers, and anthropologists (Dalmiya, 2002; Dalmiya & Alcoff, 1993; Forbes, 2005; Van Hollen, 2003; Sadgopal, 2009) have, in commenting on reproductive healthcare access and models of knowledge, focussed on the *dai* as offering an alternative epistemological model to the atomistic, technologized biomedical assemblage, and in so doing, sometimes marked her as part of an indigenous way of knowing that is invalidated and marginalized in modern healthcare settings. They have linked this presence to colonial histories of targeting the *dai* figure as an obstacle to institutional childbirth care. Midwifery as practice and the *dai*'s epistemic location, sometimes put together, are seen as offering an alternative model of knowledge – an experiential 'knowing how' rather than a 'knowing that' which is a propositional form of knowing that anchors biomedicine and the dominant sciences (Dalmiya & Alcoff, 1993; Dalmiya, 2002; Achuthan, 2017).

Tracing the changing relationship between the dai and the indigenous

It might be useful, as I begin, to offer some context on the figure of the *dai* and the dynamic set up between the terms 'dai' and 'indigenous' that I will keep returning to. *Dai* is a term extant in most northern Indian languages, to refer to a non-familial birth attendant, who comes in to attend at various points in pregnancy and childbirth. This term has populated the colonial archive as well as the post-independence policy space, and the figure has been the subject of feminist resistances to

DOI: 10.4324/9780367824051-1

biomedical violence in women's reproductive lives. The term has been sometimes replaced by the term 'traditional birth attendant'.

Indigenous as a term has been used at various points in the history of the Indian nation-state. From being a chosen reference point for nationalists in Assembly debates pre-independence, to being a correlate of the 'vernacular' or non-English, to a pejorative or esoteric reference to non-modern systems of healing in early post-independence health policy documents, it now has associations with an apparently pan-Indian 'way of life'. In this framing, indigenous refers to self-sufficient, or *swadeshi* (Longkumer, 2018); the link to histories of the struggle for independence from colonial rule is apparent. It also references, by extension, a homogenous national community. The term has had a fraught usage in therapeutics in colonial India, as I demonstrate in Chapter 3, with heated debates in the Indigenous Drugs Committee over how to classify an indigenous drug. In the debates over training of the *dai* or traditional birth attendant, the term '*bazaar* or indigenous *dai*' is used to largely indicate an untrainable, marginalized-caste woman – the bane of reform efforts. The term has not been used significantly to denote the lives or therapeutic practices of *adivasis*, or primary inhabitants of the land (scheduled tribes in official language) in a manner in which the term is mobilized elsewhere across the world, except in critical scholarship from the margins. Xaxa (1999) opens up the term indigenous in conversation with other terms 'tribe', *adivasi* and 'aborigine', to speak of how an administrative term such as 'scheduled tribe' has been reclaimed by dispossessed people more as a way to claim the natural resources of a land as primary inhabitants than as a claim to being *original* inhabitants.

Terminologies in public health and community medicine have moved, in the present, from 'indigenous systems of medicine and homoeopathy' to Ayush. Although these nominally include a variety of non-biomedical systems of healing, Ayurveda and Yoga occupy centre stage in Ayush. Where visible in contemporary public health literature in the Indian context, the term indigenous has travelled in from global scholarship, sometimes uncritically so. In other words, over time, the term has become the preserve of the nation rather than its margins. To belabour the point, the mainstream today has already replaced 'indigenous' with Indian.

I use, in this book, the unstated tension between the *dai* and what I call the canonical or dominant indigenous, to trace the movement of this figure into and out of the nation's therapeutics. By canonical or dominant, I refer to the homogenized, textual image of an indigenous therapeutics emerging in the 19th century and consolidating in the present, one that claims the status of an alternative singular system rather than an alternative model of knowledge to the biomedical. This means that the system locates itself within and at the heart of the nation – an institutional entity. This also means that the histories of the system and the nation are presented as intertwined and linear rather than scattered. In such a history, I suggest, the *dai* is rendered absent, although she seems to be everywhere present as an obstacle in the state's attempt to institutionalize and locate reproductive care away from communities.

The observations this book offers, therefore, are located in the wedge between what I term the canonical and dominant indigenous, and this *dai* figure. This is a wedge, I suggest, that has not been adequately acknowledged or explored; it is the aspect of the *dai* being ignored in the colonial and in the contemporary periods, in modern institutionalized reproductive healthcare, that has been highlighted in available scholarship. I explore the histories of production of this figure as a recognizable obstacle to maternal welfare, and thus an impediment to progress in community as well as in expert work. I juxtapose this hypervisible caricatured presence in institutionalized childbirth, alongside her absence in other parts of the colonial archive – whether it be the resistant therapeutic indigenous or marginalized community assertions.

I do not, however, see this exercise as a project of recovery of the *dai* in the indigenous canon. Rather, I seek to explore the gradual extrusion of this figure from childbirth scenarios, following the creation of a flat, fairly homogenous *category* of *dai*, in a coming together of institutionalization, health planning, and the rise of the canonical indigenous, focussing on moments from the 19th century to the present. As I demonstrate in exploring the 'women for women' mantra that is ubiquitous in colonial reproductive health framing, the debates around indigenous drugs, the explosion of textuality around indigenous medicine, and the association of indigeneity with nationalism, I see a handing over of the category of the *dai* to institutionalized healthcare – for processing, containment, or dismissal. The impulses for this extrusion operate, I suggest, in different ways across this extended period, mobilizing, at different historical moments, vocabularies of Aryanness and racial strength, caste purity and epistemic authority, modernity, nationalism, capitalist interests, and globally available vocabularies of indigeneity.

This book does not, in exploring this wedge, propose the indigenous as a 'cultural whole' (Sujatha and Abraham, 2012, p. 19). Nor does it offer a pan-India representation of the *dai*; rather, it attempts to identify a few local aspects and explore their implications for the emerging character of the indigenous. It also does not focus on the idea of the indigenous as ex-officio resistant or aim for its epistemic validation, although it does recognize the discourses of resistance within which the indigenous seeks to be placed in nationalist and postcolonial historiography, as I discuss in Chapter 2. Rather, it attempts to open up the multiple meaning frameworks within which 'indigenous' as a term has been placed. In engaging with the lenses of caste and race, which are marked in the characterizations of the indigenous as fixed and universal, and which form very significant reference points for my formulations, I do not treat these as ahistorical or descriptive categories. I attempt to be cognizant of the distance and difference between caste description and caste prejudice then and now – a difference that is not always acknowledged in the histories of medicine, or in reflections on gender and caste in the colony. Marginalized caste status, in particular, has been recognized in some of the scholarship on histories of medicine or the careers of indigenous practitioners, as an identity location. I am interested in understanding how this location is spoken of in colonial administrative accounts – as a found object – as well as nationalist articulations in the 19th and 20th centuries – as either an accepted principle of social organization or a minor attitude among non-moderns, with connections with classificatory governance and the implications for childbirth care organization. I am interested in possible implications that references to caste have *within* the discourse of the time and for the emerging therapeutic discourse. As such, I find useful deployments like Alavi's (2008) that understand these social hierarchies operating through relationships of patronage.

Entry points

Trends in urban development and modernity in India over the past few decades have seen the emergence of living communities labile and fragile in their locations, boundaries, as well as permanence, and some shifts in what might be called traditional caregiving practices following on this. In the case of Bombay (now Mumbai in official documents), displacement of vulnerable people within the city – a direct result of transferable development rights and migration across cities – are both marked by these shifts.[1] For many migrating workers and families in the city of Bombay, this means communal or near-communal residence in very small spaces, sharing linguistic, material, and cultural space with people from other regions, including the idea of the household and who constitutes it. The notions of continuity as well as distinctness – of time, region, and location – that are expected to support traditional practices are also fractured in this scenario.

A somewhat sweeping survey of childbirth practices, a (stereo)typical site for caregiving between women, reveals multiple scenarios in this context. For one, women who have migrated are today often not in a position to revisit their natal homes for traditional childbirth resources. Secondly, and again in the case of Bombay, women in vulnerable communities often access and are considered knowledgeable of the 'indigenous' in terms of healing practices, but such women who had knowledge of traditional plant remedies either no longer have access to them or possibly have access to a different ecology, in a different geographical location, cut through by displacement and urban redevelopment, that will have to be learned all over again. The very understanding of traditional communities (constituted in an admixture of region-locality-language-caste-livelihood-gender), then, also changes and complicates the transmission of several of these practices that are not codified or standardized, where transmission is conventionally expected to be through mother-daughter transactions or among women in a stable community.

In the event, sharing of diverse practices indigenous to multiple regions, as also hybridization of such practices, seems to result among women brought together in the spatially constricted labile communities I referred to above. The value of 'traditional knowledge' or the 'indigenous' as an independent knowledge category in such a scenario is unclear. The *dai*, or the traditional birth attendant as named in policy, appears in these spaces as a fairly low-key, vulnerable figure, in the business of childbirth care/practice but not in great favour. While this may be read as the case of a particular urban metropolitan site where migrant communities are the largest population, other spaces are hardly impervious to analogous impacts of developmental regulation, constricting and fragmented spaces including non-codified knowledges or privatized health care.

This book attempts to understand the distance between these complex, sometimes fragmented realities and shared childbirth care knowledge on the one hand, and the idea of a singular recognizable figure as an exemplar of experiential knowing that critiques of the healthcare assemblage keep returning to on the other. It is also concerned with understanding the place of this singular *dai* figure vis-à-vis recognizably legitimate indigenous traditions. In my earlier research, I have explored experience as a vantage point for knowledge production (Achuthan, 2017), using Dalmiya and Alcoff's (1993) concepts of gender-experiential knowing, collective privacy, and 'knowing how'. I was engaged, there, neither in presenting the *dai* figure as one who could, armed with experience, fracture the narrative of propositional knowledge, nor in tracing organic experiential connections 'among women'. A primary oppositional status or capacity, therefore, was not an easy way to read the situation. Rather, I suggested that in accessing the moments of fracture – moments of incommensurable dialogue or simply disconnection with expert positions – might lie a way to speak of lived experience as aporetic to the available institutional narrative of childbirth care.

In tracing, in this book, the changing meanings as well as value ascribed to experience, community, and the overdone 'women for women' trope in the colonial period, I focus more on the production of the figure of the *dai*. As mentioned above, I trace how this figure, identified in colonial texts as 'indigenous', is extruded from that space, in its nationalist and later consolidations. I suggest that the description of 'the *dai*' today as experienced yet inexpert is a sedimentation of this contradictory history, both in the biomedical assemblage and in anthropological, feminist, and philosophical scholarship.

Leena Abraham presents a sociological account of a related set of circumstances, of the culture and practice of indigenous medicine in an urban metropolitan context like Bombay, in exploring the practice and reception of 'Kerala Ayurveda' among migrant Malayali communities in the city. In an 'interweaving of culture, health and medicine' (2012, p. 187), Abraham speaks of migrant associations like the Kerala *samajams*, constituted during the multiple migrations to Bombay from 'all social classes and communities in Kerala since the 1920s and 1930s' (p. 195), that acted, via Ayurvedic 'dispensaries-cum-pharmacies' (p. 194), as 'micro-institutions' in building a therapeutic indigenous culture that mobilized the migrant regional identity, local Ayurvedic language and vocabulary as distinct from the 'national' or northern Indian, and created a public space that was different from both the state and market within which therapeutic choices could be enacted. Following Abraham, we see how this exercise consolidated regional identity and governance in ways that fracture any notion of a flat national therapeutic indigenism. Cultural and professional identities of the practitioners are often porous in this understanding. Questions of the caste and normatively Hindu character of such seemingly secular associations, while resisted by Abraham, may continue to be relevant, however. It is this normative character that I explore with respect to the indigenous as a route to understanding the exit and re-entry of the *dai* figure in the colonial and present-day periods respectively.

Sujatha V questions the representation of the category 'Indian medicine' as homogeneous, as seen in dualistic representations of Western and non-Western knowledges that also mark distinctions between classical-textual and folk-oral forms. Sujatha draws, in her study of practitioners in coastal Tamil Nādu, a picture of what she terms 'structural pluralism' – a 'pluralism of genres of medical knowledge within a system that emerges from the different cognitive positions of the expert, the semi-professional and the patient/layman' (2007, p. 172). She avers that these positions are 'nodes in a network rather than dichotomous entities' (ibid) and makes a further distinction between 'medical lore' or 'folk knowledge', that is 'built around a set of concepts about the body, health and disease, with certain underlying epistemological principles' and that endures across generations, and 'lay knowledge' that has more to do with individual illness experience.

For my purposes, this scholarship on contemporary indigenous therapeutics offers a few other entry points into this book. For one, it brings into play the sociological, in a space – of scholarship around medicine in India – predominantly occupied by historical and anthropological lenses that I explore in Chapter 2. Second, it speaks of the regular failure of the 'encounter framework' between the West and East that I also explore in detail in Chapter 2, as a lens to understand interfaces of knowledge systems. Third, it presents an uneven and unstable picture of indigenous therapeutics, with a coming into and fading out of view of several 'traditional specialists in health care such as bone setters, *visa vaidyans*, midwives, and practitioners of *marma chikitsa* who belonged to different castes and communities' (Abraham, 2012, p. 190). The 'madrasi doctor' boards that continue to flourish across the Indian cityscape today are another indicator, with these practitioners being accessed for a variety of sexual health, rectal, and related illness conditions occupying taboo bodily regions. The presence of this set of practitioners also challenges stereotypes of rurality as the natural habitat of indigenous therapeutics. Abraham also challenges, through her study of Kerala Ayurveda practitioners in Bombay, the neat dichotomy between institutionalized medicine and its outside; until 2005, she notes, non-institutional practitioners formed at least half of the indigenous practitioners listed in government records. Current studies estimate Ayush practitioners at 0.79 million (Karan et al., 2021).

A more recent shift might be worth speculating on here. In the most recent legislations around indigenous therapeutics, as well as the spectacular symbolism around Ayurveda in the present decade, which I explore in Chapter 6, 'indigenous as wellness' has taken a small step ahead of 'indigenous as medicine'. Sujatha and Abraham (2012), Banerjee (2002, 2004), and others have reflected on the pharmaceutical episteme that the National Policy on Indian systems of Medicine and Homoeopathy 2002 ushered in, or at least consolidated, putting Ayurveda as medicine on the global industrial map. With the newer-yet-old version of Ayurveda, however, local wellness with the 'nationalist touch', to rework Banerjee's phrase, has found a potent connection with global capital. It is in this context, too, that I locate the contemporary policy extrusion of the *dai* figure and the histories of childbirth care associated with this figure that have occupied so much colonial rhetoric. The *dai*, I suggest, is available in an articulation of indigeneity that is neither nationalist nor canonical. The 'common epistemic frame and ... cosmology' that this figure may share with contemporary Ayurveda (Abraham 2012, p. 191) nowhere comes up in current law or policy language, and indeed the commonality is nowhere argued for or acknowledged. While a number of feminist and non-governmental organizations speak of the *dai* within this frame, it remains a ghettoized debate, carrying within it all the shame of the irrational, the under-developed, and the non-modern that the canonical indigenous has long cleansed itself of. I attempt to explore this across the colonial and contemporary in Chapters 4 and 6. I suggest that traces of this might be understood by reading Abraham's text against the grain too. For instance, the Kerala *samajams* that 'give them [Malayalis] a socio-cultural and political identity in the city while at the same time providing them with a collective experience of the social and cultural life that they have left behind' (p. 188) have not been known to speak of the *vaittati* (traditional midwife – the Kerala parallel with the northern Indian *dai*) with the same conviction as the *astavaidyans* (brahman practitioners) who are given the status of experts; her very absence from the study begs this question. This is the wedge I seek to explore and that I mention earlier in this introduction.

Some notes on methodology and frameworks

I use, in this exploration, a combination of methodologies including archival analysis, historical discourse analysis, and critical discourse analysis. In focussing on the period of the 19th to 20th centuries, I have accessed government records including legislative records, parliamentary and committee minutes, communications and bureaucratic dispatches, letters to officials, medical men in the Indian Medical Service (IMS) and the public, and submissions to the government. In addition, print publications that flourished in the period, including medical ready reckoners, Ayurveda texts in translation and commentaries, tracts by native medical men, autobiographical records of prominent women and allopathic practitioners, and home remedy texts in popular circulation, have served as entry points into the archive. Women's and health magazines popular in the period have been another important source.

'Finding' the *dai* in the archive is both easy and challenging. A variety of questions about the manner in which to splice the archive, about the politics of archiving, and about reading the archive with and against the grain come into play in an exercise such as this. At a broader yet related level, a set of lenses and templates in use to chart histories of science and medicine in the subcontinent, to speak of the 'indigenous' or the 'native' sciences or therapeutics, and to engage these in dialogue or conflict are relevant. One of the most enduring and powerful tropes that has been the reference point for this dialogue is that of 'encounter'. This trope, deployed in a range of ways to refer to physical conflict and economic power, to cultural and epistemological systemic engagements across incommensurable landscapes, has been the subject of much critical exploration. While I attempt to review this extensive scholarship in Chapter 2, I reiterate, here, the thickening of borders and boundaries around the indigenous through this history and in a telescoped manner in the contemporary, in the 19th century to the present that is the period of my concern. I am interested in this aspect because it is this process that I see as partially constitutive of the extrusion of the category and the subject position of the *dai*. The incommensurability accorded to the indigenous through this process has been part of theorizations around indigenous 'systems', which then are seen in encounter with Western biomedicine. When the *dai* approaches this incommensurable position, she is treated, somewhat like street practitioners, as a fringe position – illegitimate. It is this unrehabilitated position in both biomedicine and the recalibrated indigenous that I attempt to mark, as I trace both the archival and the contemporary. The critical scholarship around encounter as trope is useful for my purposes in the ways in which it questions the flattening of both biomedicine and the indigenous, but particularly the latter, since this latter today has a new lease of life in the public political life of the nation, and in law and policy around healthcare, as I discuss in detail in Chapter 6.

But my concerns are not only with unpacking the homogenization of the indigenous. The articulation of marginality vis-à-vis the classical indigenous also follows, logically, a parallel flattening. The *dai*, the street practitioner or *fakir*, the *madrasi* doctor, and the woman of the home accessing home remedies are all positioned, in such a flattening, as equidistant from the centre. Following on critiques of centre-periphery models applied to biomedical and indigenous therapeutics (Girija, 2021; Hardiman & Mukharji, 2012), I explore the *unequal* distances of each of these locations from the ever-evolving canonical indigenous. These distances are also related to several other relationships – with the biomedical healthcare assemblage, with global health and wellness vocabulary, with global engagements with what are termed complementary and alternative medicine (CAM), and perhaps most importantly with the reproductive and population health of nations and therefore the investments in control over women's bodies and sexualities. The *dai*, seen as in much more direct conflict with institutionalized childbirth care, as well as with recent corporatized versions of natural childbirth, as also with universally agreed upon midwifery principles seen as commitments to reproductive care made by member states of the UN, is a figure therefore that receives much more attention in terms of the distance that must be kept from her. I trace, in this book, some of this attention, in terms of its continuities and shifts from colonial to contemporary contexts.

I have found broadly useful, for this exercise, post-Marxist positions like Laclau and Mouffe's notion of the complexity of the social, of 'the practice of decentring through antagonism' (1990, p. 40, quoted in Kioupkiolis & Katsambekis, 2016, p. 195); a blurring of the boundedness of political space, in other words. Although Laclau and Mouffe's work is located in the context of contemporary democracies, their argument provides a useful, if unconventional, entry point into the colonial archive. Understanding all objects (including, in our case, the category and name *dai*) as produced in discourse, and the possibility of 'privileged discursive points of … partial fixation, [called] nodal points' (Laclau & Mouffe, 2014, p. 112), the archive may be approached as a temporal articulation of an evolving socio-political field wherein, at different historical moments, different nodal points emerge with

respect to which practitioner-actors, and texts, acquire significance. For my exploration, indigeneity, medicine preparation, imperial vocabulary, corporate pharma-
ceutics, and nationalism, form some of the nodal points around which the discourse
of the time may be articulated.

This brings us to the more familiar critical approaches to archive use. Mike
Featherstone (2006) starts from the idea of the archive as a physical site for the
storage of government records that is inseparable from the act of 'governance of the
territory and population through accumulated information' (2006, p. 591). Further,
'[i]n the 19th century, the archive became seen as the repository of the national
history and national memory' (p. 592), and an attempt 'to "tell history as it was"'
(ibid). Some points relevant to my purposes emerge from Featherstone's formulations. One, the aspect of cataloguing and classification systems that play a role in
the manner in which the archive is spliced by researchers – disciplinary classifications, for instance, that do not encourage interdisciplinary interpretative schemes or
newer questions. Newer or more interesting questions than those asked priorly constitute one of the parameters of validity that Isabelle Stengers and Vinciane Despret
lay down for non-positivist scientific research (Latour, 2004). 'Scientific means
interesting', says Latour, as he lays down Stengers-Despret's recasting of the falsification principle (2004, p. 10). Such newer or interesting questions, it would seem,
could emerge from official archives only by chance, depending 'upon the contingent status of the fragments that found their way into the archive' (Featherstone,
2006, p. 594). It is in this context that Featherstone refers to the work of

> innovatory historians such as Norbert Elias and Michel Foucault, who used
> the British and French national libraries in highly unorthodox ways by read-
> ing seemingly haphazardly 'on the diagonal', across the whole range of arts
> and sciences, centuries and civilizations, so that the unusual juxtapositions
> they arrived at summoned up new lines of thought and possibilities to radi-
> cally re-think and reclassify received wisdom.
>
> (ibid)

Stengers and Despret identify other elements of their definition of falsification,
including '*devise your inquiries so that they maximize the recalcitrance of those
you interrogate*' (Latour, 2004, p. 12, italics in the original). This brings me to the
manner of 'finding' the *dai* in the archive – reading the archive against the grain. I
will, in Chapter 2, explore in some detail this principle of reading against the grain
that Ranajit Guha also proposes in attempting to locate the absent subaltern in the
archive of the nationalist struggle. Here, I suggest the interrogation of the given
and multiply repeated description of the *dai* in the official record, from the point
of view of the absent self-record of the *dai*. I suggest that the 'mimesis imposed'
(Diamond, 2003, p. 113) on this figure that comes to life, in the same form, again
and again in the archive, through this repetition, is the cue to begin such an interrogation, and that is what I seek to do in Chapter 4.

I end this short account of methodological concerns with a focus on the conceptual framework I arrive at in the last chapter of this book, and that I attempt

to develop through the earlier chapters. The biomedical and healthcare assemblage (Rose, 2007), or the medical industrial complex (Hillman et al., 1986; Baru, 2018), have been powerful forms through which to understand the complex webs of power, as also a combination of actors – human, technological, artefactual, and economic, institutional, and epistemic techniques, that produce subjects of health and illness in the contemporary. I suggest that in Indian colonial and postcolonial contexts, indigenous therapeutics, as a heterogeneous, multi-faceted entity, needs to be introduced into this assemblage/complex in order to delineate the picture more fully. Rather than a separate set of histories allocated to indigenous medicine, as Mukharji has pointed out has been the case in India, this means that we need to explore the *manner, rather than the extent*, to which indigenous practitioners, medicinal preparatory modes, texts, language, and vocabulary, engage with those of the biomedical episteme, the pharmaceutical industry, and the institutional sites and structures of institutionalization to produce a discourse within which health-seekers emerge. Focus on the 'extent' has largely been the work of understanding possibilities of integration across medical systems; while this work is valuable, it is not what I focus on in this book. This is the soil within which the broad, porous therapeutic cultures that I speak of at different historical moments also emerge and mutate. I also am able, in this book, to focus more on the assemblage than the soil, while acknowledging their enmeshedness. This is because I am interested in tracing moments of extrusion of the *dai* figure in the construction of this assemblage, through the construction of the *dai* as a category. That is the primary focus of this book.

In speaking of various movements within the assembling of the healthcare apparatus from the colonial period, I put to use a cluster of concepts – classification, segregation, regulation, and professionalization. Each of these terms is put to related but slightly different uses in each of the chapters. Regulation and segregation are the two more primary terms I use, with the others serving as examples of these. The sites I focus on where these processes operate include the dispensary, the text and language, the home, public reform, and, of course, the institution.

Framings of the indigenous

The 'indigenous' as a category has been substituted with a variety of other terms in the particular histories I explore in this book. The 'native', Indian, the local, and the *bazaar* have been some of the terms used in this substitution in colonial accounts; not all of these have been equally in use. Some of these usages are in the context of medicinal products, some to refer to practitioners, and some indicate texts. One of the early usages in the writings of British medical women working in the subcontinent has been the reference to the indigenous or *bazaar dai* – as someone who is 'untrained', part of local oral traditions. In state vocabulary around indigenous drugs, there is a fairly fierce contest on what medicinal drugs may be termed indigenous; George Watt, Reporter on Economic Products and a vocal member of the Indigenous Drugs Committee, at the cusp of the 19th to 20th centuries, insists on the name being limited to drugs *procurable* in the subcontinent *rather than native* or unique to it. Reading between the lines of the minutes of Committee meetings in their historical conjuncture, it is evident that the term is being sought to be divested of any national(ist) underpinnings, their merely economic value being reinforced. While the neutral scientific is offered, in these meetings, as the reference point for all evaluations of indigenous drugs, the workings of imperial power are clear. Similarly, in some of these discussions, as also in the writings by medical women, *bazaar* is an allegory for impure, adulterated, unscientific. It is here that nationalist voices of northern India, including those of medical men, begin to make a claim to indigenous medicine, alongside a demand for vernacular medical education; this is a political claim, but it is one that is intermixed with national aspirations to science and medical education, and a felt need to clarify, literally and figuratively, the definition of indigenous. It is in this process of clarification, then, that classical, yet modern Ayurveda, as Girija refers to it (2021), is born. This clarification is achieved through a series of extrusions – of the *dai*, the *fakir*, several others. This clarification is, as we will see in Chapter 3, a collaborative exercise, with the Englishman of the IMS seeking textuality as a way of purifying the indigenous episteme, and the nationalist seeking classicization while invoking a series of origin myths around race and caste. It is in this collaboration that we might read a consolidation of caste hierarchies and active stigmatizations – including of the *dai* – as well.

Clarification does not occur as a tidal wave or singular process, however. At the same time or even before clarification is being attempted, other nodal points emerge – of indigenous practitioners, supported by new print technologies, putting out eclectic therapeutic texts in large quantities, of caste groups outside of the historically privileged Brahmins participating in and publishing these texts, of large quantities of *gharelu* or *gharoa chikitsa* (home remedies) texts being also authored and printed by non-experts. In both spaces, however, childbirth care emerges through institutional or institutionally supported guides like *Garbharaksha* speaking favourably of a trained *dai* attempting to break into a community space seen as hitherto resistant, or spoken through the voices of male practitioners invoking classical texts and attributing gendered prescriptions and taboos to them.

Somewhere along the way, the term indigenous is substituted by the metaphor of the Indian nation. As I show in Chapter 6, a series of legislations and a discourse gradually shift an imagined spatiality for some kinds of indigenous medicine and practitioners from the remote, rural, multiple, and vulnerable to the singular, central and powerful, national. This is accompanied by a ghettoized, esoteric scholarship focussed on the new 'non-modern'; the term indigenous now undergoes a shift into a different kind of museumized remoteness. The earlier formal political evaluation of the indigenous as inferior, or non-modern, becomes less strident; it persists, however, as an apparently more descriptive term – for the 'tribal hamlet', or the *dai*, among others. These descriptions are none of them at the centre of the nation, although the promise of future inclusion is in place. This might well be an expected moment in a postcolonial juncture where the scientific has been taken in, in an apparently comfortable staging, into the ancient nation, and a new classical identity emerges thereby.

This is also the time when global political vocabulary around indigeneity is at a new high. In this vocabulary, indigeneity is about a relationship with and prior political claim to land; it is an identity that present generations can lay claim to; it is also about an acknowledgement of epistemic communities that have historically been invisibilized. In that sense, indigenous or First Nations peoples are those who have been violently erased in the formation of modern nation-states, while this erasure, as well as the project of assimilation, is today named and challenged (Krakouer et al., 2022; Tomiak, 2016). Global formal institutions, however, continue to mark the indigenous as that or those who must be acknowledged and granted rights by modern nation-states; there is some ambivalence around providing equivalence to indigenous knowledge. Both global institutions and political vocabularies pose a problem for majoritarian visions of indigeneity that do not include the remote, the vulnerable, or the street, because these are the past and present that are sought to be left behind, or repositioned, using the rhetoric of development. As far as therapeutics are concerned, the Indian nation has resolved this by taking in, as I mentioned above, the biomedical into the classical. 'Integration' – a term that comes up repeatedly in policy formulations, as I show in Chapter 6 – is one of the ways in which this is done. Rather than integrating the indigenous into modern healthcare systems, as usually proposed, however, this exercise is done somewhat the other way around, with textual, dominant versions of Ayurveda, for instance, being centred and presented via scientistic vocabulary, thus also referencing the old claim to the nation as the original habitat of modern science. The biomedical is here used as form, with the classical indigenous invoked as content. Corporate wellness vocabulary bears helpful witness to this integration. The *prakriti* questionnaires for wellness in primary health centres recast as Health and Wellness centres that I discuss in Chapter 6, are a good example of this. The remote and the vulnerable are here proposed as docile recipients, not participants or producers of an indigenous episteme. The *bazaar* has been left behind.

Terms

Toggling between the colonial imperial, the nationalist, the majoritarian, and the critical in terms of vocabulary and terminology is a difficult exercise at best. I have tried, in this book, to mark these differences by using critically informed contemporary terminologies when using my own voice, while retaining existing ones to indicate the workings of power in these positions. I use, for instance, the indicators privileged caste or oppressed caste in my analysis, while continuing to use 'upper-caste' or 'lower-caste' when highlighting positions in the discourse. Words like 'native' are used instead of Indian in the same way. This term homogenizes a subcontinent's people, hints at racial inferiority on occasion, and is sometimes claimed in nationalist language as well; those marginalized on grounds of caste, however, are mostly named via their caste-based occupations rather than simply 'natives'. This extends to Adivasi groups, and I attempt to be cognizant of these distinctions in my discussions. This extends to spellings as well – of *purdah* invoking a pronunciation peculiar to the colonial imperial, for instance, instead of *parda* – closer to the 'native' pronunciation. Wherever I use non-English words, I italicize them, unless they are in quotes, where I stay with the text quoted.

Chapters

Chapter 2 approaches the rich scholarship around histories of science and medicine in the subcontinent, attempting to delineate their somewhat divergent methodologies. It explores the historiographic impulses in these histories, tracing internalist, externalist, and 'outside' impulses particularly in the histories of science. The marking of these impulses helps locate the idea of resistance, opposition, or encounter, which becomes the indicator of criticality or counter-hegemony in these histories. Taking on board more recent critical scholarship not actively positioned in the postcolonial framework, particularly with respect to histories of medicine, I attempt to see a more porous, overdetermined character to these histories, and consequently, a less delineable character to indigenous therapeutics. This helps challenge the 'encounter' framework.

This idea of the indigenous I attempt to explore more fully in Chapter 3, shifting focus from the more richly explored analytic of Western medicine as a disaggregated entity in postcolonial scholarship to indigenous therapeutic cultures. For this, I use as sites different forms of medical writing, official debates around indigenous drugs, and debates around the definitions of indigenous in political and therapeutic domains, in the 19th to 20th centuries. Parallelly, in Chapter 4, I explore the emergence of the *dai* figure as a category in the same period, reviled, marked as an obstacle to maternal welfare, and needing the intervention of colonial-imperial medicine to remove her from the privileged-caste home and thus save the woman of that home. I discuss the 'women working for women' framework that informed colonial governance here that affirmed and consolidated both gender and caste segregation as mechanisms of control and regulation. Both in Chapters 3 and 4, I mark the voice of the privileged nationalist medical practitioner, who collaborates with imperial institutions in justifying and activating this removal. I suggest that it is in this time and space that the *bazaar dai* is produced and marked for removal – an exercise that is eventually marked by failure.

Chapter 5 explores the 'zenana' – a category articulated in colonial documents to refer to the segregated space of the home in northern Indian contexts – and the woman of the home vis-à-vis the nation, revisiting some of the rich scholarship around these and bringing into it the Indian woman practitioner newly emerging into and building a relationship with this space. Bringing into conversation discourses of educability and trainability for women in this time helps understand the principle of caste segregation more thoroughly, as I demonstrate through a careful exploration of the privileged-caste woman as educatable and others as trainable. This exploration helps me understand the emerging woman of the nation who is 'socially functional' but biologically non-autonomous (Thirumali 2005, p. 16), thus providing the key to caste endogamy and the structures of marriage and family that emerge in modern India. With the retaining of epistemic authority within the institution alongside the classical indigenous at the centre of the nation now is the core idea of this chapter.

I end the exploration of this book through an examination of more recent discourses around indigenous medicine, through legislative and policy actions. It is here that I identify the production of the contemporary nation within indigenous therapeutics, such that the word 'indigenous' itself is rendered somewhat irrelevant in the therapeutic domain, being replaced by the national. This is a sharp difference, I suggest, from contemporary global discourses around indigeneity as related to primary claims to land or identity; the ancient nation imaged here is different from First Nations, having present and full claim over land, identity, and resources. In the face of this ancient classical nation and its therapeutics, the *dai* figure re-emerges as truly remote, unskilled, and not clearly defined even; not as evil and powerful as early colonial discourse would have us believe. In that sense and in this pallid form, this figure persists, continuing to carry the work of removing pollutants, with no question of epistemic privilege or authority. Removed comprehensively from the centre of the nation, this figure is no longer to be feared, and thus, no longer deserving of institutional attention.

Note

1 As different from earlier responses by the State to people whom it displaced from land they lived on, for infrastructure development for a few, couched in the language of nation-building, such responses took the form of unconditional eviction, or later on, monetary compensation. Transferable development rights in this case simply mean granting of alternative living space, almost always in neighbourhoods not economically commensurate with and usually distant from their pre-displacement localities. For these displaced people, whose livelihood options would be intrinsically linked with place of residence, this usually means a blow to both life and livelihood at the same time. See Bhide (2009), Bhide A. and R. Raj (2016), and Birkinshaw and Harris (2005), for details on the histories of redevelopment following textile mill closures and restrictions on urban land usage in the 1990s in Bombay.

References

Achuthan, A. (2017). Feminism and science: Present-day notes for a feminist standpoint epistemology. In S. Krishna & G. Chadha (Eds.), *Feminists and science: Critiques and changing perspectives in India* (1st ed., Vol. 2, pp. 147–174). New Delhi: SAGE Publications.

Alavi, S. (2008). *Islam and healing: Loss and recovery of an Indo-Muslim medical tradition, 1600–1900*. Hampshire: Palgrave Macmillan.

Alcoff, L., & Dalmiya, V. (1993). Are old wives' tales justified? In L. Alcoff & E. Potter (Eds.), *Feminist epistemologies* (pp. 217–244). New York and London: Routledge.

Banerjee, M. (2002, March 23–29). Public policy and ayurveda: Modernising a great tradition. *Economic and Political Weekly, 37*(12), 1136–1146.

Banerjee, M. (2004, January 3–9). Local knowledge for world market: Globalising Ayurveda. *Economic and Political Weekly, 39*(1), 89–93.

Baru, R. V. (2018). Medical–industrial complex: Trends in corporatization of health services. In P. Prasad & A. Jesani (Eds.), *Equity and access: Health care studies in India* (pp. 75–89). New Delhi: Oxford University Press.

Bhide, A. (2009). Shifting terrains of communities and community organization: Reflections on organizing for housing rights in Mumbai. *Community Development Journal, 44.* 367–381.

Bhide, A., & Raj, R. (2016). *Mumbai in redevelopment mode: Implications for violence and justice.* Mumbai: Centre for Urban Policy and Governance, School of Habitat Studies, Tata Institute of Social Sciences.

Birkinshaw, M., & Harris, V. (2005). The right to the "world class city"? City visions and evictions in Mumbai. *The Urban Reinventors Online Journal, 3*(9).

Dalmiya, V. (2002). Why should a knower care? *Hypatia, 17*(1), 34–52.

Diamond, E. (2003). *Unmaking mimesis: Essays on feminism and theatre*. London and New York: Routledge.

Featherstone, M. (2006). Archive. *Theory, Culture & Society, 23*(2–3), 591–596.

Forbes, G. H. (2005). *Women in colonial India: Essays on politics, medicine, and historiography*. New Delhi: DC Publishers.

Girija, K. P. (2021). *Mapping the history of Ayurveda: Culture, hegemony and the rhetoric of diversity*. London and New York: Routledge.

Hardiman, D., & Mukharji, P. B. (Eds.). (2012). *Medical marginality in South Asia: Situating subaltern therapeutics*. London and New York: Routledge.

Hillman, A. L., Nash, D. B., Kissick, W. L., & Martin III, S. P. (1986). Managing the medical–industrial complex. *New England Journal of Medicine, 315*(8), 511–513.

Karan, A., Negandhi, H., Hussain, S., Zapata, T., Mairembam, D., De Graeve, H., ... Zodpey, S. (2021). Size, composition and distribution of health workforce in India: Why, and where to invest? *Human Resources for Health, 19*(1), 1–14.

Kioupkiolis, A., & Katsambekis, G. (Eds.). (2016). *Radical democracy and collective movements today: The biopolitics of the multitude versus the hegemony of the people*. England: Ashgate.

Krakouer, J., Nakata, S., Beaufils, J., Hunter, S. A., Corrales, T., Morris, H., & Skouteris, H. (2022). Resistance to assimilation: Expanding understandings of first nations cultural connection in child protection and out-of-home care. *Australian Social Work, 76(3)*, 343–357.

Laclau, E., & Mouffe, C. (2014). *Hegemony and socialist strategy: Towards a radical democratic politics* (2nd ed., Vol. 8). London and New York: Verso Books.

Latour, B. (2004). How to talk about the body? The normative dimension of science studies. *Body & Society, 10*(2–3), 205–229.

Longkumer, A. (2018). 'Nagas can't sit lotus style': Baba Ramdev, Patanjali, and Neo-Hindutva. *Contemporary South Asia, 26(4)*, 400–420.

Rose, N. (2007). *The politics of life itself: Biomedicine, power, and subjectivity in the twenty-first century*. Princeton and Oxford: Princeton University Press.

Sadgopal, M. (2009, April 18–24). Can maternity services open up to the indigenous traditions of midwifery? *Economic and Political Weekly, 44*(16), 52–59.

Sujatha, V. (2007). Pluralism in Indian medicine: Medical lore as a genre of medical knowledge. *Contributions to Indian Sociology, 41*(2), 169–202.

Sujatha, V., & Abraham, L. (Eds.). (2012). *Medical pluralism in contemporary India*. New Delhi: Orient Blackswan.

Thirumali, I. (2005). *Marriage, love and caste: Perceptions on Telugu women during the colonial period*. New Delhi: Bibliophile South Asia.

Tomiak, J. (2016). Navigating the contradictions of the shadow state: The assembly of first nations, state funding, and scales of Indigenous resistance. *Studies in Political Economy, 97*(3), 217–233. doi:10.1080/07078552.2016.1249130

Van Hollen, C. (2003). *Birth on the threshold: Childbirth and modernity in South India*. Berkeley, Los Angeles and London: University of California Press.

Xaxa, V. (1999). Tribes as indigenous people of India. *Economic and political weekly*, 3589–3595.

2 Historiographies of science and medicine in India

Introduction

This chapter involves a somewhat extended exploration of histories of science in India, as a means of entering the debate on the hegemonic versus the resistant – which has been popularly read through the framework of 'encounter'. I will, therefore, set down here, in condensed form, the arguments I make. I begin with a recognition, in exploring the different ideological and methodological impulses in histories of science in India, that these histories have been the primary site for an exploration of the colonial relation – a recognition available in the histories themselves. We see in these histories a stepping away from an older explanation of the colonial relation as an encounter and a movement towards both a disaggregation of the actors and providing a more processual account. The most visible end-point in this exercise is, I suggest, the emergence of an expanded hegemonic, made visible through the agency of a resistant insider – variously interpreted as Indian, or indigenous, with the term 'indigenous' having a different resonance from its present global conceptual mappings. The historiographic impulse here is not as focussed on complicating this understanding of the indigenous or its constitutive exclusions, as on a 'studying up' of the hegemonic as an expanded set of actors and spaces. The encounter framework, I suggest, persists here, through the instinctive boundedness and political homogeneity that is retained for the resistant or recalcitrant insider. It is important to complicate this space and position in order to be able to arrive at an understanding of how a figure like the *dai* is marked for extrusion from the category of the indigenous, and that is the rationale I present for this detailed exercise of exploring this historiography.

The histories of science and medicine in India occupy several disciplinary and discursive fields, including orthodox history, mainstream science, alternative models of historiography, and postcolonial theory. The political contexts of these histories have moved across nationalist, Marxist, and liberal terrains, among others. The terminological consensus as well as conflict across these histories on ideas of indigeneity, systems of knowledge, and resistance makes the following understandings of the colonial experience in India dominant – as a binary encounter between formed systems of knowledge of the (broadly) West and its other, with the indigenous other as a homogeneous, identifiable, and ex-officio-resistant form of knowledge. This chapter traces some of the ground covered by histories of science

DOI: 10.4324/9780367824051-2

and medicine in India, as a way of providing context to the trope of the 'native/ indigenous as resistant' as it emerged in these histories in the 19th to mid-20th centuries. This will also involve an examination of the distinction made between indigenous as practice and indigenous as knowledge in these histories. It will pro- vide the ground to then contest the 'encounter' framework as the soil for the emerg- ing language of therapeutics in India. I end the chapter with some questions on the place or absence of the *dai* figure in these histories. Does the tracing of resistance, and the subaltern in these histories, offer scope for a rehabilitation of absent figures like the *dai*? Is it useful, or possible, to offer witness accounts from a different van- tage point than has been hitherto done?

I examine primarily what I term the critical histories, locating them in the con- texts of their production (Iggers and Edward, 2008; Woolf, 2005) and the discursive charting of context and influence that they themselves provide (Mandler, 2004). Iggers and Edward (2008) speak of the institutional frameworks within which his- tory telling develops, the value of reflecting on who writes histories, and the linear view of the past and of progress that are features of modern Western historiography (p. 22). The authors further speak of modern historiography's centring of what is considered the truth and a continuous narrative, as also the emergence of a public and a market for this narrative. With the truth of such narratives being sought increasingly in written rather than oral sources, alongside other modern knowledge systems, then, 'by the early eighteenth century, ... "historical knowledge" as a category' (Woolf, 2005, p. 20) had emerged. Woolf speaks of possible 'indexes of change' that influence the writing of history – 'the emergence of a sense of the past as continuous process and the establishment of the primacy of causal relationships between diachronically contiguous or proximate events' (2005, p. 39). Elsewhere, Woolf also speaks of the 'roles of the nation and nationalism in historical writing' (2006, p. 76), even though Woolf locates this impulse primarily before the 18th century. I suggest that the seeming consensus around this form of history writing is reflected in the national and nationalist histories of science and medicine in India, which continue to be reference points in the later critical histories as well, particu- larly with respect to constructions of an authentic national past and knowledge archive. I will, both in this chapter and the next, attempt to demonstrate how these national and nationalist histories are part of the modern historiographic tradition rather than an inadequate or motivated form as has sometimes been suggested in secular critiques. Using these reflections on the method to explore both the descrip- tive and critical histories of science and medicine in colonial India helps us under- stand the resilience of the 'encounter' frame, as also the idea of the 'indigenous as resistant', that informs, in different ways and to differing extents, each of these histories. I employ this lens to understand the context of these ideas, rather than to dislodge and substitute them with an alternative 'true' history. I do seek, however, in examining the historiographies of this period, to locate more valid accounts. I am interested, however, rather than asking 'how Western' science or medicine actually was, or in asking how local practice re-fashioned that which was received as Western, in tracing the emergence of what I call the 'dominant indigenous' as a distinct and persistent knowledge category/identity, in its complex, layered, and yet identifiable form – a form that has continued its consolidation into the present. It may be time, I suggest, to do this, rather than continue in the exercise of redefining the colonial or the Western.

The contexts and tasks of a history of science and its translation into the metaphor of encounter

The historiographic impulses in the histories of science have been the subject of inquiry almost from the time they began to be written, and in the disciplinary and institutional locations where they were located. I will try to explore these via terminologies used in science studies, frameworks generated to theorize power, and the objects of study chosen in these histories – from the macro structures and institutions to the everyday, micro-events and contexts.

Georges Canguilhem identifies 'three reasons for doing the history of sciences: historical, scientific, and philosophical' (2005, p. 199). The historical reasons are of 'commemorations ... rivalries ... quarrels over priority', the scientific reasons lie in 'looking to the past for an accreditation' (ibid), and the philosophical reason – to have an epistemology emerging from a history of sciences that would be the grounds for a theory of knowledge. Canguilhem goes on to mark proposed methods for the history of sciences – externalist or internalist.

> Externalism is a way of writing the history of sciences by seeing certain events ... as being conditioned by their relation with economic and social interests, with technical demands and practices, with religious or political ideologies. ... Internalism ... consists in thinking that there is no history of sciences unless one places oneself in the very interior of the scientific discipline in order to analyze the methods by which it seeks to satisfy the specific norms which permit it to be defined as science rather than as technology or ideology.
>
> (p. 202)

Steven Shapin, in a 1992 review of the externalist-internalist (sometimes shortened as 'e/i') debate that was the core focus of history of science in the 1960s in Anglo-American contexts, acknowledges its present irrelevance but reminds us of the usefulness of reviewing the directions it has taken, including the institutionalization of 'e/i' as 'boundary-speech'[1] in the discipline, and it is this discussion that I find useful to peg my first questions on the histories of science in India.

Beginning from Merton's evaluation of external factors as only able to influence the 'overall value placed on science in a given setting and the rates at which different scientific foci developed' in societies (Shapin, 1992, pp. 336–337), and not the 'purely scientific' (Merton quoted in Shapin, p. 337), Shapin explores the development and persistence of this position in the history of science, including in the writing of Sarton, Sorokin, and others, all of who casually acknowledged external influence but only as one among many, and not always the most important, in scientific change. Marxist historiography's impact on this debate seems, in Shapin's view, to have been that of a perceived threat to science as a neutral activity and a possible reference to proletarian and material origins of science as a 'denigration' (p. 339). At any rate, with the possibilities of external influence having been deradicalized, an 'eclectic posture' (p. 341) became the go-to position, and the 'e/i discourse was securely institutionalized' in the academic discipline of the history of science by the early 1960s. 'Extreme externalism' (p. 342) had, by this time, been rejected as a possibility.

Shapin goes on to suggest a refocussing, from 'disciplinary purification' post-1970s – what should be an ideal history of science – to 'changing the world' (p. 357), which might have been the initial impulse of the discipline, as it moved between internalism and externalism, for example. I use this very short reflection on a complex debate as a prelude to focussing on the modern histories of science in India, and a position of 'outsideness' they sometimes take – different from but not unrelated to the internalist-externalist debate.

A few more methodological questions on historiographies of science remain before I attempt a conceptual exploration of some of these. Dhruv Raina traces the 'entangled' histories of science and philosophy in India, presenting the comparative method (with the West) as *constitutive* of both these exercises, as well as their interpreters (2012). The premise of the entanglement was the centrality accorded to reason and science as Western in histories of both science and philosophy. Given the normative and dominant status accorded to these core ideas, and their presence as the validation of Western science, attempts to identify, recuperate, or rehabilitate an 'Indian science' or an 'Indian philosophy' invariably fell into the exercise of either offering intuition or spirituality as uniquely Indian counterpoints to reason or claiming reason for itself – in the past or present. My purpose in invoking this argument is to better understand the workings of the encounter framework in both science and medicine in India through an understanding of these histories within the contexts of the comparative. While this idea of encounter has been extensively read into nationalist histories, its shadow can perhaps be extended to postcolonial interpretations as well, and it is to these that I will turn after a brief examination of the former. This latter exercise will involve the delineation of the framework of hybridity and its use in postcolonial circuits to describe Western science as fragmented, thus hegemonic but not completely successful in its dominance, as containing within its dominant self the seeds of resistance. I will also attempt to demonstrate the centring of critique – somewhat akin to Shapin's pointer to 'changing the world' methodologies – in these interpretations. Most importantly, this will necessitate an examination of the claim to difference, which shores up the promise of hybridity as a counter-hegemonic exercise.

Nationalist histories/the nation as history

It is useful to expand the methodological entry point provided by the internalist-externalist debate to understand the contexts and tasks undertaken by histories of science in India. Part of the commitment of these histories has been to critique the hegemony of Western science as a sign of modernity. Depending on their disciplinary locations, historical conjunctures, and ideological obligations, these histories may be seen to demonstrate a primary commitment either to the nation and a civilizational discourse, to history as method, or to science, although these commitments overlap to a certain extent. The most celebrated of the histories of Hindu science written in the colonial period include those written by scientists, among them P.C. Ray's *History Of Hindu Chemistry* (1909), B.N. Seal's *The Positive Sciences of the Ancient Hindus* (1915), *Hindu Achievements in Exact Science* by Benoy Sarkar (1918), and an earlier text – U.C. Dutt's *Materia Medica of the Hindus* (1877). Like other texts that speak of ancient Hindu civilization, these histories use the trope of the decline of an ancient civilization. Mukharji (2009), Kumar (1997, 2006), and Alavi (2008) speak of some of these and other lesser-known histories, like Pramatha Nath Bose's ambivalent survey of scientific articles in the Asiatic Society journals that also attempted to 'situate Hindu science relative to the Western tradition' (Arnold, 2004b, p. 171), which led him to a conclusion about the 'general degeneracy of the Hindus since the thirteenth century' (Bose, quoted in Arnold, p. 172). Interestingly, the internalist histories of science written by scientists in the later period access this trope of decline either superficially and piecemeal, or not at all. But in this very prefatory turn to the past, there would seem to be a turn to civilizational legitimacy, to memory, to past greatness, as Gyan Prakash (1999) notes. B.N. Seal's *The Positive Sciences of the Ancient Hindus* (1915), for instance, is premised on the claiming of science for the Hindu nation, as also the Hindu nation as an influencer of the East as well as West, along with a comparative study of Hindu and Greek science that might, at the very least, yield proof of equal robustness and trajectories (Seal, 1915, p. iv). This idea also seems to have informed texts like *Indian Medicinal Plants* (1918) by K.R. Kirtikar and B.D. Basu, that 'attempted a fresh synthesis of Western materia medica and Ayurvedic botany' (Arnold 2004b p. 175). The language sources and grammar are cited as proof of a robust, exact science here – 'the Sanskrit philosophico-scientific terminology', says Seal, 'however difficult from its technical character, is exceedingly precise, consistent, and expressive' (Seal, 1915, p. iv). P.C. Ray's earlier two-volume *History of Hindu Chemistry* (1909) that focusses on the 'earliest times to the middle of the sixteenth century' (sub-title) too takes this position, seeking to present the 'contributions of the Hindus' (Ray, 1909, vol. I, p. 3), a contribution that could be done justice to only once 'an interpreter who could do full justice' (vol. II, B) could be found – a task that someone like Colebrooke was 'masterly' at but which had yielded only 'fragmentary' results (vol. II, p. B). Ray's two volumes of Hindu Chemistry also, however, do not claim full coverage of the field; the 'Tantric and Iatro-Chemical periods' (vol. I, p. 5) being somewhat under-represented on account of time. Of course, the position of interpreter is claimed by Ray only under the sought tutelage of the celebrated French chemist, M. Berthelot, who appealed to him, states Ray, for information on the origin and contributions of the Hindus to the world of chemistry. Berthelot is eulogized at the start of the text as an undisputed model, to meet whom was akin to a 'pilgrimage' (p. C).

In some sense, then, these nationalist histories, linking universal and civilizational claims, seek to expand the origin stories of positivist science, pegging the claims on certain texts, figures, and authors of the more dominant, accessible, or extant texts of these fields and thus to claim a seat at the table. A pre-emptive argument for the significance of these texts was also using the comparative method. Seal, for instance, in seeking 'a line of communication with the organisations of oriental learning' (quoted in Ray, p. 7), says

> Let us not superciliously dismiss these studies as 'learned lumber'. The Astronomy and Mathematics were not less advanced than those of Tycho Brahe, Cardan and Fermat; the anatomy was equal to Vesalius ... the Grammar ... the most scientific and comprehensive in the world before Bopp, Rask and Grimm.
>
> (Seal, quoted in Ray, vol. I, p. 7)

Comparativeness was also used to retain and claim analogy to terms from Western chemistry; Ray states that his 'study of the original sources has made it clear ... that a "Bhuta" in Hindu Chemistry represents a class of elements composed of similar atoms' (Seal, in Ray, 1909, vol. II, p. H), for instance. Exploring this further with reference to Partha Chatterjee's commentary on modern political thought and the articulation of community (2010), we might see the referencing of 'Hindu' in these histories as a recognizable racial community, but also a scientific one, thus seemingly proposing a continuity of tradition, or an always already modern community, rather than a movement from community to modernity, as Chatterjee suggests was the dominant nationalist narrative. These would, therefore, qualify as revised internalist histories of science, and methodologically part of the modern historiographic impulse traced by Woolf. It is important also to trace one of the later directions taken by national histories of science and medicine – of institutionalized religion and community, and the sharp segregation of Ayurveda and Unani into one or the other of these is an obvious example of this. I will come to this in some more detail later in the chapter.

Post-independence state-supported histories also make reference to or trace continuities with these nationalist histories of science, but in a curiously passing manner, possibly related to the socialist impulse towards centring secular development agendas in the early years of independence. One of the most comprehensive exercises in the 20th century was by the Indian Council of Philosophical Research, in the form of 'History of Science, Philosophy and Culture in Indian Civilization', as part of the Project of History of Indian Science, Philosophy and Culture (PHISPC), a series edited by D.P. Chattopadhyaya. This was a project supported by the erstwhile Ministry of Human Resource Development (now Ministry of Education), although an earlier effort had been made by the Indian National Science Academy (INSA) with UNESCO in 1951. The set of volumes that have emerged from the PHISPC project cover a vast and diverse perspectival terrain, acknowledging history as 'largely a matter of construction' (2011, p. xvi) both in terms of space and time, and yet as 'somewhat like the natural sciences, ... engaged in answering questions and in exploiting relationships of cause and effect between events and developments across time' (ibid).

While some of the work in this project may also be grouped under the commitment to nation with attention to the 'distinction and relation between civilization and culture' (Vol XV, part 4, 2011, p. xvii), with comparison and validation with respect to Western science being one of the tropes (Vol IX, Part I, O.P. Jaggi, 2000), critical genealogical studies of science disciplines and institutions in India have also populated the volumes. Schools of philosophy have been discussed in detail, on the grounds 'partly in terms of its proclaimed unifying character and partly … in terms of the fact that different philosophical systems represent alternative world-views, cultural perspectives, their conflict and mutual assimilation' (ibid, p. xviii). Overall, a movement between comparative and Needhamian historiographic impulses might be seen in the project, with a particular recognition of the 'concrete and particularist' (Vol XV, part 4, 2011, p. xvii) nature of history, as also its non-linearity (Vol XV, part 4, 2011, p. xxiii). This might be said despite the series editor's own claim that its 'scope, continuous character and accent on culture distinguish it from the works … as P.C. Ray, B.N. Seal, Binoy Kumar Sarkar … and also from … Euro-American writers as Lynn Thorndike, George Sarton and Joseph Needham' (p. xviii–xix), as also the claim to be attentive to diverse modes of human experience, including the scientific and the artistic.

A point about commentaries on Indian philosophical traditions may be relevant here. Debiprasad Chattopadhyaya, the Marxist philosopher by the same name as D.P. Chattopadhyaya, has written in some detail on ancient Indian materialism, the possible links of these with older agricultural practices, the contrast with the pastoral lives of early *Vedic* people, the appearance of *Tantrism* and *Sankhya* as two schools that became vehicles for materialism, with *Tantrism* retaining closer links to the proto-materialism of early agriculturalists than the *Sankhya* which became, in Chattopadhyaya's opinion, a veiled form of *Vedanta* – another dominant tradition (1959). Relevant to my purposes, Chattopadhyaya offers an argument for the material basis of philosophy as well as science, for social locatedness, that may find echoes in Sociology of Scientific Knowledge (SSK) scholarship. Implicitly, then, these two philosophers separate into representatives of the idealist and materialist traditions in Indian philosophy, and, following this, to the more and less dominant philosophical traditions. While D.P. Chattopadhyaya's work explores the Vedantic as Indian, Debiprasad Chattopadhyaya is more interested in *Lokayata* – broadly translated as the people's philosophy – grounded in material conditions of living, and following Marxist frameworks, recognizing caste hierarchies, and the suppression and exploitation of early knowledges in the emergence of *Vedic* precolonial societies. Needless to say, this recasting of philosophy as material, as a way of life, and as a space of contestation, had implications for knowledge production in Debiprasad Chattopadhyaya's view. D.P. Chattopadhyaya also spoke of contexts – both historical and social-material – for knowledge production, but the nuances in his writing give the sense of change being introduced via the entry of new cultures like Islamic or European into the Indian, even as the impossibility of sharp boundaries is stressed. I make this point to indicate one of the many ways in which the historical record on an Indian science and knowledge continues to be constructed, and the manner in which extrusions from this record occur.

Critical externalist approaches

The vocabulary of critique had shifted in science studies in Anglo-American spaces in the 1990s, with the emergence of a series of critical histories of science. While the sociologies of scientific knowledge (popularly referred to as SSK), from the 1920s to their heyday in the 1970s across Europe and the United States, spoke of interest groups and the social ethos of science, later ethno-methodologies of the 1980s and 1990s spoke of the multiplicities of actors and networks – human, non-human, and material – within which scientific knowledge is produced. Feminist critiques and epistemologies of science focussed on contexts of knowledge production, tying them to the content produced, called for revision of parameters of validity, a recognition of diversity among knowledge producers, and offered alternative models and grounds of scientific knowledge production. This is the context within which I see a third position emerging – of an 'outside', i.e., a history of science that takes the vantage point of a resistant, refractory perspective – a position outside Western science. In the work of theorists of science in India, like Ashis Nandy, Gyan Prakash, Shiv Visvanathan, and others, the broad impulse of this outsiderness to Western science can be seen, related to the identification of Western science qua knowledge as based in Enlightenment reason. I link the hint at a resistant indigenous in this position.

It is in a movement between externalism and outsideness that I locate what I call the critical histories of science and medicine in India. These histories have swerved between externalist and 'outside' approaches, positions not always clearly demarcated from each other, unlike in Europe and America, where, with a failure of acknowledgement of histories of imperialism and colonialism, externalist histories locate sciences within their local societal contexts, while retaining a historical account of scientific content's development. The critical histories primarily separate from the internalist accounts in a recognition of the differentials of power as constitutive of knowledge and its parameters of validity. Social histories of science and medicine in India, including those by Deepak Kumar, Projit Bihari Mukharji, Seema Alavi, David Arnold, and Samiksha Sehrawat, fit somewhat into this complex description; in addition, some of these social histories focus on micro-contexts, lesser-known texts and figures, recognition of the non-contiguous histories of science and medicine, and step away from Bengal as the chief site of emergence and examination of events in the colonial period. Arnold, who has also contributed to some of the encyclopaedias of science, technology, and medicine in colonial India, and thus been a significant figure shaping the discourse, particularly focusses on some of the links between other sciences and medicine in the subcontinent. Kumar, along with Arnold, was one of the earliest examinations of 'colonial science' as a complex entity, its relationships with colonization itself, and thus an understanding of the phenomenon as 'more than a set of institutions or structures; … an economic as well as a cultural intervention' (1991, 2006, p. 2). Kumar speaks of colonial science as 'inextricably woven into the whole fabric of colonialism' (p. 15) and highlights the repeated affronts to 'native' (a term he takes care to qualify as pejorative colonial terminology rather than an acknowledgement of original claim to the land) capacities, and the active denial of scientific education or recognition of indigenous knowledge, within which he situates the pushback from local practitioners, teachers, and translators, among others. Kumar sees this denial as constitutive of colonial science as well as colonial administrative and economic power; he locates each of the attempts to explore new scientific domains, educate and train 'natives', the hierarchical stratification of such education with simplified courses for 'natives' primarily meant to improve their character, as instrumentally decided within the needs of imperialism, with any success stories of Indian science being read into the script as breakthroughs. Kumar discusses these possibly resistant entities in some detail, as college teachers of mathematics and science in Indian cities in the 1840s, who were also sometimes 'translation-enthusiasts' (Kumar, 2006, p. 61) who spoke of scientific temper and the need for an Indian Bacon, challenged the *puranas* or reinterpreted their sayings, and edited journals that supported these views. Kumar is critical of the Empire's denial of access to rationality and scientificity as either a character trait or a capacity for Indians; while he acknowledges indigenous knowledge systems, his major impulse is towards uncovering evidence of the natural bent and aptitude among natives towards a scientific temper that was actively suppressed in the Raj.[2] Habib and Raina have also noted the overwhelming stress on technical rather than theoretical science education for the 'natives' in colonial policy. It is in this period, however, that Kumar and other social historians note the emergence of national science, with institutions like the Indian Association for the Cultivation of Science set up in 1867. We will come back to this impulse in some detail, but for now, I highlight Kumar's reflection on the Indian claim to science:

> [Mahendralal] Sarkar wanted *pure* science-learning and science-teaching, with reference to the practical applications of science so far only as are naturally and necessarily inferable while carrying on experimental investigations. The object is *not* to drill men in the arts which constitute the manual and the mechanical industries.
>
> (p. 200)

Kumar uses this and numerous other examples to challenge racist stereotypes promoted in the Raj of natives as anti-technology, lacking in initiative or intellectual capacity. In his focus on the everyday teacher-translator, but also on the institutions of science in British India, colonial practices of classification of geographies and populations – in other words, on macro-histories – Kumar attributes to the 'ordinary' native scientist a resistant, insider-outsider stance, one that is committed to both science and the nation's quest for autonomy. In his case, the nation figures the 'people of the nation' left behind by colonial economic and technological exploitation – a position for which he has been accused of 'Marxian deterministic assumptions' (Kumar, 2000, p. 40).

Arnold approaches the history of science in the subcontinent somewhat differently. Starting from a general agreement in critical scholarship on the non-monolithic character of science, although with the 'recognition of the centrality of science to an understanding of the history of India during the period marked by the rise, ascendancy and retreat of British colonialism in South Asia' (2004, p. 2), and the contestations offered by India's pre-existing or independent traditions of knowledge, Arnold goes on to chart, somewhat closer to the spirit of the European externalist tradition than Kumar, the period of the late 19th and early 20th centuries, and the messy field of actors and networks that emerged within. Post-colonial ideas of hegemony as disaggregated, of both Western science needing to be translated into Indian contexts, and of an alternative modernity, also inform his work. Tracing the idea of India as it emerged in Orientalist scholarship – as an ancient and glorious civilization later fallen into decline with caste rigidities and Muslim invasion – and the manner in which this trope becomes the referent for Indian nationalism as well, Arnold explores the material records of the time to suggest alternative possibilities – a more porous engagement with surrounding regions, the possibility of an ecumenical framework for science in India, and most significantly, an interactive rather than a transmission (Basalla) or encounter model to understand engagements with the West. It follows that resistance, or breakthroughs, then, does not suffice here; it is, rather, a method of thick description that is followed in an act of history as ethnography. In fact, Arnold charts the early careers of sciences like botany and geology, for example, as having developed in much more of a learner position with respect to local knowledges. Arnold also speaks of shifting patronage as one factor in the spread of science and medicine in India, thus bringing in not only a multiplicity of actors – elite and subaltern – in relation to Company power, and later, the Crown, thus locating the negotiations in a wider terrain 'of the people' (2004, p. 18), but also opening up the domain of practice in addition to textual knowledge in interpreting these histories. Social histories like those of Kumar, Arnold, and later Mukharji also focussed on the role of dominant social groups that 'resurfaced as agents and interpreters of the new scientific order' (Arnold, 2004b, p. 8). These emerged into newer constellations like the *Bangali bhadralok* – symbols of middle-class educated modernity – that have been much written about in this and other scholarship (Acharya, 1995; Batabyal, 2005, Brown, 1974; Raina & Habib, 1996). Mukharji further recognizes the privileged-caste composition of this elite (Mukharji, 2009). In locating histories of science in the everyday, Arnold and Mukharji also recall Pickering's approach to the practice and culture of science (Pickering, 1993, 2010).

These histories, while broadly fitting the description of the critical externalist, distanced themselves from the idea of colonial power as monolithic or centralized, and of science as flowing from it to the colonies. Rather, Foucauldian ideas of classificatory control and governance were employed to interpret how trigonometric survey tools, for example, served as a mechanism to establish 'a comprehensive network of surveillance and control over the Indian countryside' (Arnold, 2004, p. 40), thus consolidating the idea of science and particularly technology as a tool of governance. A broad look at the conjunction of institutions, disciplinary societies, museums, journals, and, of course, surveys is used in these histories to establish the method of classificatory governance and the emergence of knowledge that could be institutionalized. Further, this delineated power as disaggregated. I will explore this in greater detail in the context of the history of medicine, but it is useful to note here that the postcolonial histories that speak of difference and hybridity find resonance in such an exercise.

The postcolonial impulse

The postcolonial histories are more clearly located from the perspective of an 'outside' than the critical externalist. Most of the work in this field has been located and supported in departments of literature, history, cultural studies, and the 'new humanities' (Gandhi, 1998) which have shown themselves hospitable to a revision of orthodox methodologies. Although the work that appears under the rubric of postcolonial theory remains difficult to draw sharp boundaries around, I am primarily concerned with its influence on histories of science and the nation. The diverse strands of this work have included explorations into the complicated journeys of Western science in the subcontinent, attempting to unpack the idea of a monolithic Western science, as well as the unidirectional notion of its travel and power. There have been different emphases in the scholarship, ranging from a focus on forms of power (Prakash and Haynes 1991; Nandy, 1980, 1995) to a commitment to difference (Chakrabarti, 2004; Prakash, 1999; Nandy, 1980) to relationships between science and the nation, or science and the state. In doing so, it has, in early iterations, looked at histories of institutions and major public figures. This scholarship has also influenced more recent attention to everyday practice and vocabularies as a site of interpretation in social histories, with a focus on everyday technologies, subaltern practitioners, and the vast output of print technology, in association with earlier macro-histories (Mukharji, 2009, 2016; Arnold, 2013). This reflects a growing trend to see power as disaggregated (Foucault, 1979), knowledge as practice (Pickering, 2010), and to write history from the ground up as also from the standpoint of those normatively excluded from both science and history. As we explore some of this scholarship, we will retain an awareness of this but also focus on the vocabularies that persist across this rich and diverse space.

Postcolonial theorizations, in their attention to the 'recalcitrant native', also find an echo in Subaltern Studies critiques of nationalist historiography. Gyan Prakash and Dipesh Chakrabarty, occupying as they do the overlapping terrain of these frameworks, have reflected on these connections between postcolonial theory and Subaltern Studies theorizations (Prakash, 1994, 2010; Chakrabarty, 2000), tracing the original arguments, the movement in Subaltern Studies from subaltern consciousness and politics as an autonomous domain 'at odds with nation and class' (Prakash, 2010, p. 218) to seeing 'subalternity [as] ... constituted by dominant discourses ... [and] a position of critique, as a recalcitrant difference' (p. 219). Thus 'Subaltern Studies could be seen as a "postcolonial" project of writing history' (Chakrabarty, 2000, p. 467), separating itself from 'deterministic, Stalinist readings of Marx' (p. 471), and presenting the peasant, rather than a backward entity, as 'a real contemporary of colonialism and a fundamental part of the modernity that colonial rule gave rise to' (p. 473). This presentation also involved the task of reading the archive against the grain, given the absence of written testimonies or other records that British historians writing Marxist 'histories from below' had access to (Chakrabarty, 2000, p. 468). I will return to this methodological impulse in my attempt to 'find' the *dai* figure, in terms of marking her absence in the archive, as Subaltern Studies scholars have done, or in marking a particular form of naming. But I am interested in tracing what has qualified as resistance within the 'outside' historiographies, and to that end, it is the postcolonial focus on difference and resistance – embodied either in the empirical figure of the subaltern or in the non-modern or differently modern culture of the 'native' that I focus on now. The 'outside' as resistant suggests a boundedness to the hegemonic, a binary relation between the two, and an encounter, and it is this impulse that I am interested in tracing.

Anomalous histories of Western science in India

I discuss, in the next three sub-sections, three major arguments on colonial hegemony that stem from different positions, yet carry a common discontent with explanations of colonialism offered earlier. These include positions on transmission, translation, and hybridity as explanatory models for the travel of Western science. These arguments engage with analyses of hegemony and are interested in identifying the location and content of resistance. They are also interested in investigating the claims to comparativeness that informed scientific work in the colony.

For transmission, against negotiation

I start with Pratik Chakrabarti (2004), who comments on the nature of the relationships between history and science, against existing arguments of Orientalism and its negotiations; he bases this on the framework of hybridity.[3] For Chakrabarti, the object of inquiry is Western science – a science that underwent transformation in its practice and travels in the Indian context, but that was, at the moment of entry, Western science. The task, for him, is to trace the trajectories of this travel – of Western science in modern India – a task that is expected to throw light on the structures of its hegemony in the space of the colonized, through an analysis of 'how its cognitive content was linked to the social and cultural grid of its practice in a colony' (Chakrabarti, 2004, p. 26). As he puts it,

> [s]cience may in a particular location be isomorphic in both structure and form with similar knowledge forms elsewhere, but its essential character lies in its specific manifestations, which are imbricated in the nature of the relationship between the two zones.
>
> (p. 4)

While this might mean, at one level, that the object of inquiry becomes visible only in the moment of its engagement with its other, the study of travel in this case presumes an originary isomorphicity and proposes to chart the cultural specificities of those isomorphic idioms in particular locations. This approach promises to step out of the rational-intuitive binary of West-East relationships that a usual reading of different sciences in different cultures promotes, for such an approach is 'inadequate for understanding the experience of science within the non-West' (p. 3). It also challenges the Needhamian[4] ecumenical view of science as universal end to different paths. It proposes to do this by concentrating on the 'social, political, and cultural spaces within which Western science was *transmitted* and absorbed in the Indian colony' (p. 10, italics mine). It builds these arguments through an examination of the history of the establishment of science institutions, the trajectories of individual scientists, nationalist historiographies, and colonialist accounts of 'native science'. Chakrabarti's work tries to 'locate the links between the social context of science and its cognitive content' (p. 25), and we see here the methodological parallels with sociology of science studies approaches.

Chakrabarti goes on to chart a thick history of what he sees as the subtle shifts from a 'colonial science', to a 'national science' that was not anti-colonialist but aspired to be science, to a 'nationalist science' that made claims to Western standards and eventually proposed original and prior scientific status for itself – a journey best embodied in the delineation of J.C. Bose's personal trajectory as a scientist and then a nationalist. Chakrabarti describes these shifts, tracing the history of institutions like the Bengal Asiatic Society, the Indian Association for the Cultivation of Science (IACS), and the Bose Institute. For Chakrabarti, however, this is not a history that can be traced in isolation in the colony, his definition and articulation of which we will come to later. Going by his thesis of isomorphicity, what is undertaken in 1784 with the establishment of the Asiatic Society by William Jones is the 'quest for "truth"' (p. 30), a quest following on, and in consonance with, the rise of '"truth" in seventeenth-century England' (p. 29) and its associations with science as 'the dominant form of truth' (p. 29). This association 'can be traced to Enlightenment thought, which positioned truth and reality as basic values alongside humanism' (pp. 29–30). What was happening in the colony, then, was the 'obsession to find meaning in a strange and complex world' (p. 31) – namely, the Orient. Here begins Chakrabarti's analysis of the role of the Asiatic Society and his description of 'colonial science' as a pursuit that combined the unique features of marginality (of methods deployed in a space where conventional methods were not feasible), liminality (scientific work being conducted in remote areas), and individual creativity. The scientists in question were 'men of the Empire', often Company officials, working in a 'distant land', separated from the home community. This combination best describes for Chakrabarti the impulse inhering in science 'for colonial investigators [as] the pursuit of intellectual conquests over new territory' (p. 31) – either in the shape of verifiables that confirmed metropolitan hypotheses or as fallibles that forced new hypotheses. It is also 'the journey of scientific wisdom from center to periphery and back, the European study of non-Europe'. As an obvious corollary, this entailed a 'kind of dislocation or disorientation ... [of] European knowledge [that] had to establish itself in a distant land that promised only the unknown and the undefined' (p. 33). And it is also here that Chakrabarti traces what he sees as the fundamental link between Orientalist knowledge and the socio-cultural aspects of scientific research in the colony, in that 'both were attempts by disciplines of European post-Enlightenment epistemology

... to come to terms with the other', as also in that 'both projects [had a] ... critique of Eurocentrism, which of course existed with a typical Orientalist paternalism towards the Orient' (p. 43). Examining work especially in geology and meteorology under the aegis of the Society in this period, Chakrabarti makes a case for this critique having been hosted, articulated, and codified in the Asiatic Society; '[s]cientific works under the Asiatic Society ... [arguing] that the study of nature of Asia would contribute crucially to Europe's understanding of the earth' (p. 44).

What then happened to colonial science as Chakrabarti defines it? What came of its claims to challenge and thereby enrich the European episteme; put differently, what of its critiques of Eurocentrism? In Chakrabarti's analysis, the attempts to answer the second question are more forthcoming. The very vast tracts of land available to geological survey, for example, or the varieties of weather, or the multitude of illnesses, automatically seem to have contributed, in terms of data, enough evidence to confirm or challenge existing metropolitan hypotheses. Rather than extension, diffusion, or simple dislocation of metropolitan science, Chakrabarti sees in the project of colonial science the impulse to come up with new findings that would enrich European science. What is important for him in his analysis of centre-periphery relations is the complicated routes by which peripheral findings influence the centre. While the liminal nature of colonial science allowed the colonial space, in his opinion, to actually function as the true site of flowering of European science,[5] the route back seems arbitrary; at the very least the particular themes on which work in the colony had been undertaken found contingent status at the centre, as he demonstrates in the case of the acceptance among prominent metropolitan physicists of J.H. Pratt's geodetic theory. The possible hybridization through transmission, then, of colonial science, while being more than an extension, needs to be read, apparently, as useful or otherwise in the light of its journeys back, and this is what Chakrabarti attempts to do.

The journey back does not end here, however. The changing relationship that Chakrabarti sees between colonial science and Orientalist knowledge, or between the study of 'nature in Asia' and 'culture in Asia', also impinges upon the fate of science in the colony, although there is sometimes a conflation in his work between Orientalist studies and Orientalist knowledge. Colonial science, as described by him, is at first an enterprise that is, in consonance with its European counterpart, attempting to break from tradition; it is a new science, Baconian in approach, a product of the Enlightenment, and its brief in the colony is to 'make a new and fundamental statement about the natural world in the Orient' (p. 61), as also to reform society. In such a climate, the individual creative colonial scientist, working rigorously amidst deprivation and privation in the colony, was part and parcel of the impulse, indeed its shining example. The divorce that Chakrabarti points to between science and commerce in such a scenario was also destined to contribute to the image of science as disinterested and neutral. But the movement towards professionalization and increasing specialization in European science (a move that was not replicated in the colony where a lot of the work had begun looking esoteric and commercially unviable) transformed the creative colonial scientist into an amateur. As the big picture of colonialism changed from the late 1700s to the mid and late 1800s, as hegemonic associations between the colonial state, commerce, and scientific research strengthened, and as, simultaneously, Orientalist studies consolidated as a discipline in the Asiatic Society and other places, colonial science failed, in Chakrabarti's opinion, in its dream of an alternative centre for science. A universalist position on science that had helped to shape colonial spaces not merely as a happy receptacle but as a happy participant for an enrichment of European *science* did just that – it enriched *European* science, failing to consolidate its critique of Eurocentrism. As colonialism progressed, that mission of enrichment too became a non-reality. In other words, colonialism had frustrated the project of science in the colony.

Post-mid-19th century, however, colonial science attempted a reversal of fortunes. Driven partly by the commercial needs of the colonial state, partly by the logic of science in Europe as a socially useful, practical, need-based enterprise, scientific research from the mid-19th century 'revolved around three contesting points: between applied and pure research; between industrialism and romanticism; and between colonialism and universalism' (p. 99). Chakrabarti's analysis of the last mentioned contestation, between colonialism and universalism, is made through a further study of institutions like the Indian Association for the Cultivation of Science (hereafter IACS) and the Bose Institute, in the context of 'shifts in Indian, British, and international economic trends … the introduction and expansion of railways in India, the growing imbalance of payments of England with other industrialized countries, the First World War, and linkages within scientific research and industrialization' (p. 99). Colonial science was now adopting postures of independence from the metropole, aided by the later scientists' standing in the metropole, as also the administrative changes in the colony – for example 'the "New Industrial Policy" of the Government of India during 1900–20' (p. 105) under Lord Curzon, who insisted that the government encourage free enterprise. This new colonial science still carried the insistence that science 'in India had the same promise as in Europe' (p. 117) but had altered the terms of its relationships with utility and technology as the legitimate handbrothers of science, proposing to 'complete the "economic cycle" … in [and for] India' (p. 119) rather than only use the colony as the source of raw material and ready markets. The argument for applied research in the colony that stemmed from this, however, met with disapproval at the hands of the colonial administration. Rather than read this as a straightforward imperialist position, we would do well to recall that the argument for applied research, by Holland and others, also rested at least partly on the notion of the rich natural resources and the richer skill of ancient India in mining these resources – an argument at least as Orientalist as the opposite one that derided the weak natural world that was the colony, or the accompanying one that described the 'native culture' in similar fashion. It is this situation that Chakrabarti hints at in his delineation of the failure of colonial science. We will see, in the case of colonial medicine, a different trajectory, with conflicts over the definition of 'indigenous' drugs, Watt and others insisting that 'indigenous' should be taken to mean merely produced in the colony rather than discovered in the colony – in a movement perhaps from Orientalist to a more actively imperialist position. But here we are concerned more with the methods undertaken in the histories of science, and I will therefore return to this question later, in the section on histories of medicine in this chapter.

The space evacuated by a failed colonial science gets taken up, in Chakrabarti's analysis, by a national science, and then a nationalist science. Continuing with his theme of isomorphicity, and concentrating on the 'practice of science in a colonial world' (p. 149), Chakrabarti traces the history of the IACS that was established in 1876 with the intent of 'cultivation of and research in science by Indians, [and] ... the popularization of science within the general populace' (p. 150) – a rhetoric of science as modernity and therefore recourse against superstition and ignorance that became a reference point for progressives and reformers. Mahendra Lal Sircar, the founder, proposed science as the guiding spirit for political nationalism, saying that 'the best way, in my humble opinion, to do this [achieve nationhood] is not by platform blustering and newspaper invectives, but by substantial achievement in the field of intellect' (Sircar, 1899, quoted in Chakrabarti 2004, p. 151). This spirit had an epistemic as well as moral component that was seen as essential for fashioning and fostering, in turn, the national character.[6] At the same time, this spirit was said to be alien to the national; if at all there was a greatness and scientificity to India's past, it was certainly not in evidence, the present having been taken over by superstition and institutionalized religion. It was therefore essential to cultivate such a spirit, in the austere mode of Comte's positivism, in order to build a self-reliant national character. The building of this character was associated, in Sircar's mind, with 'man-making', through the physical task of doing, or cultivating, science. The kind of science being spoken of here was pure science, not the technical education that later colonial science had attempted to promote,[7] and the pursuit needed to be free from government. What was the nature of this freedom?

> We should endeavour to carry on the work with our own efforts, unaided by government, perhaps more properly speaking, without seeking its aid. Now this does not mean that we will not accept any aid from that quarter if it comes to us unasked, and unhampered with conditions and restrictions, excepting the all important condition of the continuance of the Association. Let me not be misunderstood. I want freedom for the institution. I want it to be entirely under our own management and control. I want it to be solely native and purely national.
>
> (Sircar, 1876, quoted in Chakrabarti, 2004, p. 162)

A freedom, then, that contributed to self-reliance, that signalled maturity; not an independence that was anti-colonialist in its impulse, a point on which national scientists like Sircar split from 'political nationalists' like Bankim Chandra Chattopadhyay.

But this very alienness of science to the Indian national spirit, and its attachment to the West, while being worthy of emulation, had its problems. A 'Western materialism' in currency after the loss of spirituality[8] was inadequate as a way of life, just as an 'Eastern spirituality' devoid of any material input was. Comte's positivism was therefore to be critiqued, and a judicious mix of Eastern spirituality and Western materialism alone could provide the answer. That Sircar's project of this complicated sharing of the spiritual and material failed to make the grade either in 19th-century Western science or in science as practised in the colony is what Chakrabarti brings to our notice.

By the time of P.C. Ray, C.V. Raman, J.C. Bose, and others, however, science was no longer an alien object to the nation. By Chakrabarti's account, there was by this time a strong reading of ancient Vedic science followed by a break in the Pauranic period when caste rigidities and institutionalized religion took over, and the impulse to construct a monistic worldview in the service of science was in place. Somewhat at odds with Ashis Nandy's psychobiography of J.C. Bose (1995), Chakrabarti poses Bose's journey as the metaphor for this impulse, charting the travel of a scientist coming from the Orient but nonetheless 'heard in the highest institutions of metropolitan science' (p. 185), who turned into a symbol for Indian nationalism, proved that 'Indians could also successfully conduct research in science' (p. 187), and then into a categorical symbol of an 'Indianness' represented in monism.[9] Bose, and others, 'could now play the role of that 'Indian' which the Europeans as well as the nationalists expected him to play' (p. 200).

This understanding of Indianness is, as we can see, in sharp contrast to the *Lokayata* impulse that Debiprasad Chattopadhyaya uses to designate 'the people' – the Indian people. Whether in speaking of power, or of knowledge forms left out of institutions, or of resistant identities, an imagined homogeneous national community continues to be invoked in the nationalist histories as well as in the language of the national men of science. In terms of later projects on philosophy and science, Debiprasad Chattopadhyaya is the odd one out, invoking an actively materialist 'this-worldly' (p. xvii) view, one that is socially situated, and acknowledging his ideological vantage point (Marxist), offering it as historical methodology. It is significant that the social and postcolonial histories of science under discussion do not pick this divergent and fairly visible strand in their analysis; the consequence, for reading the past, understanding the workings of power and exclusion, or reading resistance, is that the space of the 'indigenous' remains less complex and diverse than it needs to be. We will keep this in mind as we look at medical historiographies in the later part of this chapter and the next.

To return to Chakrabarti's analysis, we see that nationalist science could position itself as able to critique the West, not from within European science but from within Hindu or Indian science as the primary system. As Chakrabarti shows in the case of P.C. Ray, once ancient Hindu science could be shown to not only exist but also as prior in antiquity to ancient Greek science (the avowed fountainhead of European science), this case was bolstered in other ways too. It is the essentialization of tradition in these historiographic attempts that Chakrabarti points to, and it is in this pointer that we see the setting up of the encounter, not between two sciences, but between Vedic wisdom and science – an unequal contest that made the space for a nationalist science owing allegiance to the lesser pole of this encounter to now emerge. Chakrabarti puts it thus:

Within both camps, tradition was defined in terms of classical, ancient Vedic wisdom. The debate was on whether it was superior to or parallel with science. It was through such a characterization that the cognitive content of science ultimately came to terms with that 'tradition'. Thus, while science continued to be debated on and rejected in the popular arena, a museumized tradition increasingly posed the lesser threat to its cognitive status. This shaped the course of the 'other' science of Bose which attempted to infuse the two – which he sought to realize through the Bose Institute.

(Chakrabarti, 2004, p. 214)

The Bose Institute, then, was a space that 'would realize the possibilities [both] of science and the regeneration of India' (p. 214). It was through the latter that Bose attempted to do the former. And in Chakrabarti's opinion, it was this pressure of 'Easternness' that 'paralysed him qua scientist' (p. 217).

Chakrabarti ranges his readings against those of Ashis Nandy (1995), Gyan Prakash (1999), and Dhruv Raina (2003), who commit, according to him, the error of concentrating on negotiation as resistance to hegemonic structures of Orientalism and colonialism, and who therefore, in his opinion, present nationalist scientists as resisters, the popular as appropriating and re-defining Western science in the colony (Prakash), and contingent trajectories of science as having a mutative effect on the practice of science itself (Raina). For Chakrabarti, the more important task is to show, for one, that the starting points and agendas for science in the metropole and the colony were the same, or at least analogic. For another, Orientalist knowledge of the 'culture of Asia' and scientific knowledge of the 'nature of Asia' had differing trajectories that converged later, and he is unwilling to consider that the discourse of science in India could be easily understood or subsumed within the discourse of an essentialized cultural difference – a position and a problem that he identifies in 'culturalists' (p. 19) like Nandy and Prakash. It is this failure of subsumption that Chakrabarti sees in all his studies of scientists, institutions, and documents, and it is in their individual and collective attempts at the convergence (of science and culture) that he sees the 'failure' of science in the colony. In seeing such a failure, however, he states that he is not taking the Needhamian ecumenical approach to a history of science but simply doing a reading of the practice vis-à-vis its claims. Chakrabarti expects an avoidance of both these positions – the Needhamian and the cultural essentialist – to guarantee him a better reading of hegemonic Western science as well as its embedded resistances. For him, this understanding of Bhabha's framework of hybridity, where resistance is often at the core of hegemony, is the useful one, as against Prakash and others who have applied it in order to make resistance appear decisive. We will see how, in the medical historiographies, negotiation is seen as evidence of the non-uniformity of Western science or of the unevenness of power. I find Chakrabarti's understanding of hybridity useful; I am more interested, however, in the consolidation of a dominant indigenous in the process of hybridization.

For dislocation, for hybridity, through translation

Science as 'a metaphor for the triumph of universal reason over enchanting myths' (Prakash, 1999, p. 3) may indeed seem the sweeping statement that Chakrabarti bills it, and a readiness to see 'the distorted life of the dominant discourse' (p. 19) may seem a suspicious failure to see the dominance of that discourse. Chakrabarti certainly does introduce a useful ambivalence in approaching even nationalist science in its plural and contradictory moments. Prakash may be read, however, as actually bolstering some of Chakrabarti's arguments, albeit with some differences. He makes a case, for instance, for how nationalists articulated an Indian modernity as '*irreducibly different*, [one whose] modern configuration … must reflect India's *unique and universal* scientific and technological heritage' (Prakash, 1999, p. 7). The pressure for both uniqueness and universality we have already seen in Chakrabarti's reading of P.C. Ray and others; how Prakash differs significantly in his reading of the success of nationalist efforts is to see them as making this call to irreducible difference. To that end, Prakash presents the 19th century as an undivided period, or more precisely, P.C. Ray as the 'dislocated destination' in whom the search for originary antiquity, Hindu science, and universality can be fairly read. In that sense, Chakrabarti's complaint of Prakash's having ignored the 'journey' would stand, and the emergence of difference as a category in this framework would seem to somewhat mimic the idea of the nation as an imagined community.

But what exactly is Prakash doing here? As different from a more visible 'encounter' argument that Kumar makes, but more so against classical readings of colonialism's power as a triumphant single narrative,[10] as well as against the simple counter-argument that 'the reality of heterogeneity explodes the myth of the homogenous nation rooted in archaic Hinduism' (Prakash, 1999, p. 90), Prakash sets out to examine

> the story of the powerful colonial transformation of the elite and an account of the elite's emergence as a force that called into question the terms of colonial dominance. It would be a mistake to characterize science's divided, hybrid authorization as a story of the cultural adaptation of Western knowledge to Indian conditions … To achieve hegemony, science was compelled to disavow dominance; it had to implode prior conceptions of Western and Indian identities and express itself in the media of the Hindu atman. What was remarkable in this process was not the strange content … but the estranged position from which the authority of modern knowledge was enunciated.
>
> (p. 83)

This estranged position is what Prakash identifies as the site of translation – a contingent process. To make this clear, Prakash uses the notion of hybridity, by which he refers to

> the implosion of identities, to the dispersal of their cultural wholeness into liminality and undecidability. Such a notion of a hybrid, non-originary mode of authority is profoundly agonistic and must be distinguished from

the concept and celebration of hybridity as cultural syncretism, mixture, and pluralism. Hybridity, in the sense in which I have used it ... refers to the undoing of dominance that is entailed in dominance's very establishment. It highlights cracks and fissures as necessary features of the image of authority and identifies them as effects of the disturbance in the discourse that the "native" causes. ... Hybridization and translation addressed the relationship between languages and subjects positioned unequally.

(p. 84)

This, for Prakash and others working at postcolonial reconstructions, constituted the primary critique of modernity as originating entirely in the West.

This is exactly what Chakrabarti draws from Bhabha,[11] and his reading of culturalism in Prakash is not in order simply because, among other reasons, it is through the examination of 'science's cultural authority', the process of significations, that Prakash establishes the hybridity argument. He demonstrates the argument in what I will call as hybridity-in-process, and I propose that it is actually this demonstration, rather than culturalism, that may invite further examination.

In his own approving reading of Bhabha, Chakrabarti sees hybridity as a condition where resistance is at the constitutive core of hegemony. His problem is in the apparently self-evident and decisive character of resistance that Prakash gleans from hybridity. I suggest that the problem is not the one of 'syncretism, mixture, and pluralism' that Prakash distances himself from. The problem is that hybridity sees hegemony as fractured rather than monolithic – a useful rendition – but also as pervasive.[12] Following such a reading, Prakash brings in the notion of the colonial state as a governmental one, one that began its work with a pastoral form of power, a

knowledge and discipline of the other ... [that] was positioned as a body of practices to be applied upon an alien territory and population ... [with] the establishment [for instance] of new forms and institutions of medical scrutiny; population statistics, sanitation campaigns, and vaccination drives [that] brought a medicalized body into view.

(p. 10)

Apart from this understanding of governmentality and its relevance to the colonial state, this is where my question to the concept of hybridity lies. In this hybridity-as-process framework logically extended, any counter-hegemonic exercise, however fraught, is problematic, because it is through contingent negotiations, rather than an ideological positioning vis-à-vis power, that the built-in response to hegemony comes. In fact, following Bhabha, hybridity is a thorough and *ongoing* description of reality that actually refrains from formulating a theory of hegemony, and this shows up in Prakash's own difficulty in understanding the process itself as more than 'an unequal positioning'. Prakash sets up a meaning-power coalition in order to insert hybridity into hegemony, talking as he does about the cultural authority of science as his primary concern, but even so, he fails to make clear how the arbitrariness that must necessarily be the character of hybridity finds closure; how the 'native' becomes, each time, the discordant note of dominant discourse. In such a case, the multiple dislocations it shows up fail the implicit promise of the postcolonial that it sets up, of being able to offer a theory of the workings of power *that can suggest a response and an after to it*, commonly named resistance.[13]

There is another related and explicit promise that is not met here. Prakash proposes to challenge, through the hybridity framework, the binaries of East/West and colonizer/colonized; notions of an Indian modernity that flows from the West and that acknowledges the latter as the apparent seat of modernity are unacceptable to him. Instead of the isomorphicity framework that Chakrabarti works with, therefore, Prakash insists on a constitution of Western modernity through empire, although the primary evidence he offers is that of the '*simultaneity* of the formation of Western scientific disciplines and modern imperialism' (p. 12). An Indian modernity, he argues, is constituted through the insertion of discord into the discourse of the West in the colony, and elite nationalists working towards a notion of Hindu science were, in colonialism, the chief proponents. Following on the general theme of hybridity, Prakash is clear that this was not a nationalism that proposed naïve nativism drawing in a linear way upon ancient Vedic science; on the other hand, there is a sense of *repetition rather than return* to classical Vedic science, the attempt being *to access anteriority rather than origin*. While this, like Chakrabarti's reading of early colonial and nationalist challenges to Eurocentrism, contests the conventional geographical anchoring of West/East or colonizer/colonized, the fate of the more ambitious promise – of dismantling the categories or concepts – is somewhat unclear. In the face of this ambiguity, the category 'Western science' continues to attach itself to conventional geographies. Prakash and others attempt to 'show up' Western science against its own claims for what it 'really is' – as constituted through imperial practices – and thereby challenge the self-image of geographical anchoring or homogeneity; this anchoring, nevertheless, is the starting point in their accounts too. The critical outsider position that the postcolonial lens offers, then, to historiographies of science – providing a critique of imperialism, modernity, and science – while a powerful model, leaves something to be desired.

Can there be a Needhamian history of science in India?

For Raina, the 'study of knowledge forms of non-Western societies' (2003, p. 1) was an exercise through which the questions posed from these spaces could be, and were, taken back to interrogate Western science itself. Starting from a critical examination of the earlier view of Western science as the triumphalist narrative that marginalized non-Western knowledges, Raina charts the reflexive turn in the last three decades of the 20th century that inflected the work of history-writing, of the study and representation of the Orient, and of science studies. Parallel to the exercises of internal reflexivity that this engendered, a number of 'reverse commentaries', as Raina puts it, were being put in place – critiques from the vantage point of marginalized 'non-knowledges', critiques of colonialism that displaced the centrality of Europe, and feminist challenges – from within and outside the West – to the Western philosophical canon. 'The dialectic of enlightenment had now moved towards the critique of modernity and its most potent symbol, science' (2003, p. 3).

It is the ways in which this critique of modernity/science developed and inflected the writing of histories of science that are Raina's concern. Raina sees this turn as analogical to the turn toward co-constructivism of scientific knowledge and culture in SSK in the global North, and he hopes to bring the reflexive account to bear on historiographies of natural science in India. Unlike Chakrabarti (who is attempting a social history of science in India) and Prakash (who is attempting to see the cultural hegemony of science), Raina sees himself as providing a 'social epistemology of the science and history archive on India' (p. 1). He concentrates on 'how Indian scientists and historians of science engaged with the sciences of India ... [w]hat ... they inherit[ed] from the Occidental discourse about the Orient and where ... they depart[ed] from the former' (p. 2), trying to trace, in the often insubordinate nationalist writing of the history of science in India, a series of 'idea hybridizations at the periphery' (p. 185) that implied a possible critique of Western science. The value of such an exercise for him is in the 'contest[ation of] the script of science as a cultural universal, ... counterpos[ing] it with a more polycentric model of the growth of several scientific traditions' (p. 10) – a task taken up by postcolonial historiography, which he characterizes against Eurocentric models (p. 12). It is the contextual nature of science that Raina sees as the reason why a social epistemology such as his will be useful in contributing towards a *transformative* critique of science, through a pointer at the relation between context and cognitive content. The breakdown of the 'Big Picture' of science afforded by such approaches, Raina is convinced, will change the way we think about science. In fact, Raina asks the question of connections between cognitive content and social or historical context, in order to answer that in the interests of better science, they may be better seen in conjunction.[14] The exercise will, if we follow his train of argument, also provide tools for 'some version of an ecumenical picture of the advance of science ... a notion of situated universality, while recognizing the possibility that politics intrudes into the process of knowledge production' (pp. 202–203), although he points to problems with the Needhamian ecumenical version. Does this mean that he is sceptical of the possibility of a global narrative for science? His larger project, the history of the history of science, as he puts it, is premised on the belief that both global turns in the sociology and philosophy of the sciences and the very visibility of actors outside the mainstream of science – named alternative, different, or marginal – will alter the course of the history of science as a discipline, weakening its positivist tendencies, strengthening objectivity through inclusion, and producing a more robust global account. The task, for him, is to help this happen.

Postcolonialism, for Raina, constituted, along with multiculturalism, one of the chief external factors that challenged and altered the trajectory of the history of science as a discipline. Flagging post-colonialism as 'an address marking the era after the end of British colonial rule' (p. 197), Raina marks the insubordinate nationalist re-writing of the history of science, and not only of the non-West, as both challenging the Eurocentric impulse of earlier streams and taking up the question of why the scientific revolution failed in India. In either case, 'greater attention came to be placed on the impact of colonialism on the knowledge systems of India, and the institutionalization of modern science in the country' (p. 197). It was in such a setting that issues of transmission – i.e., transmission becoming an *issue* for simple centre-periphery models – begin to occupy centre stage, and we have already seen the breadth and scope of this impulse in the work of Chakrabarti and Prakash. It follows that straightforward models of transmission of Western or modern science, from West to east in a centre-periphery fashion, with the failures being identified as those of inadequate implementation, faced challenges from this space. Basalla's (1967) diffusionist model of transmission would fall in this category.[15] This model was built on the premise that (i) modern science emerged in the nations of Western Europe, (ii) a scientific revolution occurred in these nations in the 17th century, and (iii) modern science subsequently diffused to non-Europe. It outlined three stages in the transmission – stage 1 in which a non-scientific society or nation provided a source for European science, stage 2 in which a colonial science developed in the colonized non-scientific society, and stage 3 in which transplantation of modern science was completed and the struggle to achieve an independent scientific tradition commenced. There was, in this thesis, a certain formulaic attempt to fix the categories of modern science, colonial science, etc., but geographically so. Further, colonial science is an undifferentiated category, even geographically and constituency-wise, unclear on whether it meant settler colonies or non-settler outposts of empire. Raina recognizes this and challenges Basalla's model on this count as on several others, including its failure to recognize the possibility of 'idea hybridizations at the periphery' (p. 185). This model was challenged in its own time too, notably by those subscribing to the 'cultural universal' model of science and from the transmission studies genre itself, but it informed policy and influenced early studies on science and imperialism. With Joseph Needham's work on *Science and Civilization in China* (1978) being taken up by nationalist-Marxist historians, however, the coordinates shifted considerably.[16] Scientific rationality was not seen in this second model as a contribution of Western culture; rather, Needham offered what is called an ecumenical view, advocating the notion of science as a cultural universal.[17] The shift he made was in positing science as *internal to all* civilizations; the task for him then was one of charting ways of doing it 'other' than the Western.[18]

Stepping back a little from the postcolonial reading, we see that the Needhamian tradition itself, working with earlier epistemic definitions of science, ignoring 'those scientific traditions or theories that did not join the streams leading to the growth of scientific knowledge' (Raina, 2003, p. 146), merely looking for 'other' ways in which science was pursued in non-Western civilizations, was still a blow to the earlier Eurocentric models like Basalla's that were clear on the site of origin of science (the nations of Western Europe), and which only needed a theory of travel. As such, the Needhamian model was a rallying point for scholars working within proto-nationalist and nationalist frames in the 1950s; they found in it a useful foil to Eurocentric discourse on science. The Needhamian model gave them 'the opportunity to legitimate modern science culturally within their socio-political orders, to reinvent cognitive connections between the practice of modern science and the cultivation of traditional knowledge' (Raina, 2003, p. 147). The project was taken up by a variety of positions, including nationalists and Marxist historians seeing science as a socially transformative force against obscurantism as well as a tool in the anti-imperialist struggle.

The Marxist attitude to science in India also leaned on another influential thinker who had a different kind of impact on notions of science and, consequently, non-science or 'traditional knowledge' in India – J. D. Bernal. Bernal's *The Social Functions of Science* (1939) and his later *Science in History* (1969), coming out from within classical Marxist historiography, were to be the counterpoint to Needham's ongoing work on the China project and were to become the 'red book' for Left organizations trying to deal with seemingly resistant attitudes to science among the 'masses' in India, as also for science policy. For Bernal, science as a form of knowledge was Western in origin, but he was more interested in the impact of science on history through changes in modes of production, and the possible and desirable impact on culture[19] of a scientific method and temper, than in any ecumenical view that could respond to this. Bernal was not unaware of the histories of imperialism and their implications for the presence of Western science in India, but he saw them as a process in decline, and the spread – or transmission – of science as a greater necessity at a time when '[t]he peoples of Asia and Africa and Central and South America are now entering, not as select elites but as masses, into the effective world of our time' (Bernal, 1969, p. 13). In this form, then, and in the sharp separation from religion, art, and magic, Bernal became the icon for the popular science movements – attacking superstition and promoting experiment – that were a major agenda on the Left of a newly independent nation, as also the frame for policy.[20] For the Left in India, then, both Bernal and Needham became pillars of a Marxist way of thinking about science. As Raina puts it, Needham was the inspiration for the '"high church" of science studies in India ... whilst the "low church" drew capital from the Bernalist one' (Raina, 2003, p. 146). The Needhamian project was what, according to Raina, became the anchor for the theoretical work on the historiography of science in India thereafter, providing the 'master narrative, to be elaborated or subverted, for subsequent research into the history of science of non-Western nations' (Raina, 2003, p. 147).[21] To this end, a comprehensive project to write a history of the sciences was mooted by the Indian National Science Academy (INSA) with UNESCO in 1951. However, as Raina looks at the issues that took up space in the various science journals devoted to ferreting out such a history, what he comes up with are a series of priority disputes, internalist accounts, and studies of ancient texts that took on an antiquarian studies mode, all heavily steeped in scientism, inflected with the burden of nationalist historiography, and caught up in the internalist-externalist divide, while the commitment to the project remained rhetorical. Though there was work by individual historians outside INSA, notably Debiprasad Chattopadhyaya and Abdur Rahman, in the Needhamian frame, they took different directions – excursions into the suppression of materialist traditions by later spiritual tendencies that disallowed the growth of science in India, as I have discussed earlier (Chattopadhyaya, 1959), or a pointer to the Bhakti and Sufi traditions in India not being antithetical to scientific practice or growth (Rahman, 1996, quoted in Raina, 2003, pp. 148–149). An ecumenical history seeking to produce a single or coherent account of the history of science in India had, obviously then, failed, or failed to take off.

Why? In looking for answers, and in a direction away from inadequate research, the following possibilities present themselves. The project, while sensitive to questions of cultural reception, was still definitionally attached to a vision of the 'centrality of modern science in contemporary culture, the founding impulse of the scientific revolution of the 17th century' (Raina, 2003, p. 144). In other words, the Old Big Picture of science,[22] and, in the event of there having been no scientific revolution to speak of in Indian contexts, as well as in the 'failure' of the Needhamian project here, Raina chooses to push the question further, to ask whether there can at all be such a history in India. The causes Raina himself identifies of a technical failure of such a history are of an all-permeating scientism that characterized the post-independent Nehruvian Indian scientific establishment that could not but present contradictions for a Needhamian history, the neutralization of the cultural import of modern science by the first generation of scientist-historians, the presence of other issues like the mode of production debates for the Marxist historians of a newly independent republic, and the amateurish nature of much of the work taken up. It is alongside the note of the 'failure', however, that we could identify the claim to a different and perspectival form of knowing made in this field, rather than a 'different paths to the same goal' approach offered in the Needhamian model. This is a claim that never takes up the classical oppositional posture, however, as Nandy points out. Further, it relies on difference as prior, original. We will keep these features in mind in coming to the case for difference in hybridity.

Raina's commitment to the Needhamian question is an epistemological one. The failure of a Needhamian history in India, he sees, however, not as an epistemological phenomenon but as a socio-political one; the possible solutions he sees require a transcendence of the socio-political contexts he places science within. For him, sociological relativism or contextualism should not presume a concomitant collapse into epistemological relativism, and it is a 'situatedness' that takes cognizance of the socio-political that he is attempting while retaining a commitment to a possible ecumenical account of science. In this sense, the repainting of the Big Picture he suggests leans on an externalist possibility and is not entirely free of the externalist-internalist divide, while the revised historiography he suggests is a liberal one.

In the same light may be seen the relationship between science and politics that Raina, along with Prakash and Chakrabarti, relies on while making his arguments. The political is seen as an intrusion, welcome or otherwise, one that needs to be taken cognizance of for an adequate sociology and history of science. Raina believes that equal attention and inclusion in historiography will help set right the inequalities of positioning of metropolitan science and non-visible knowledges, just as, in his view, increasing visibility has forced attention by histories of science. The march of historiography of science towards democracy, in Raina's scheme, seems as inexorable as it is desirable, with the marginal inevitably finding its way in. This is where I would pose some questions of invisibility and exclusion, as I explore, in later chapters, the production and subsequent erasure of the *dai* figure in histories of medicine in India.

Hybridity and the case for difference

The work done by postcolonials has involved building grounds for a critique of imperial power as exercised through science. The hybridity framework, in this context, offers an examination of the encounter, but also more nuanced grounds for critique. It is not only straightforward theories of dominance but also later articulations of consent generation, like Nandy's 'second colonization' that Prakash, Raina, and Chakrabarti are hoping to nuance through the hybridity framework. Put telegraphically, the hybridity framework might be said to bring in certain attitudes – ambivalence, negotiation, contingency, difference. Ambivalence is the split at the heart of domination. Negotiation is the quality, through positioning, of resistance by the 'native'. Contingency refers to the arbitrariness of the closures offered by this negotiation (so it is not a simple notion of 'interest'), which is why hybridity is posed as process rather than structure. Difference is, or should be, the inability to be captured within structures of sameness. The postcolonial, in robust definition, could be the epistemo-political act of resisting the hegemonic – here the concatenation of contexts and meanings created by colonial domination, imperialism, or in other words, the act of making active difference, and via that, critique and resistance. In that sense, postcolonial histories are interested in taking an 'outsider' position. But does this work enough? As Bhabha himself puts it:

> the site of cultural difference can become the mere phantom of a dire disciplinary struggle in which it has no space or power. Montesquieu's Turkish Despot, Barthes' Japan, Kristeva's China, Derrida's Nambikwara Indians, Lyotard's Cashinahua pagans are part of this strategy of containment where the Other text is forever the exegetical horizon of difference, never the active agent of articulation. The Other is cited, quoted, framed, illuminated, encased in the shot/reverse-shot strategy of a serial Enlightenment. Narrative and the *cultural* politics of difference become the closed circle of interpretation. The Other loses its power to signify, to negate, to initiate its historic desire, to establish its own institutional and oppositional discourse. However impeccably the content of an 'other' culture may be known, however anti-ethnocentrically it is represented, it is its *location* as the closure of grand theories, the demand that, in analytic terms, it be always the good object of knowledge, the docile body of difference, that reproduces a relation of domination and is the most serious indictment of the institutional powers of critical theory.
>
> (Bhabha, 1994, p. 31)

The work in postcolonial theory that has been drafted into histories of science in India has engaged with this problem of the 'docile body of difference', at least in part via the methodologies of reading against the grain in contexts where voices are missing from the written record or are listed in the voice of the dominant. It has also made active difference through the speech of the dominant, as Bhabha also notes (1994, p. 247). I would, here, offer a thin question to the hybridity framework as well as to the position of critique made through the pointer to 'recalcitrant', resistant nativeness in these readings of history. It is here that I would like to briefly recall the Kuhnian notion of the anomaly that is part of normal or paradig-matic science. According to Kuhn, it is the transformation of anomaly to crisis that ultimately challenges the existing paradigm, instigates the work of revolutionary science, and drives the search for an alternative paradigm that can take its place (Kuhn, 1970). While disciplinary exercises in both the physical and social sciences have stressed on the notion of paradigm that Kuhn brings to the fore, it seems to be the work of pointing to the anomaly, and the crisis, that both spaces seem to have actually engaged in. Looking at the histories of science in the Indian context that are driven by a commitment to postcoloniality, I would suggest that the notion of difference is held forth in these as the *anomaly that is expected to do the work of crisis* in the paradigm that is Western science. This is most visible in the resistance-revolution pair of terms that is at work in histories of science and critiques of tech-nology, and I would tentatively suggest that this is the problem with the work that the hybridity framework is put to or expected to support – a pointer to anomaly, which is difference, and the expectation of its always already graduating to crisis, which is revolution.

What is the possible methodological impulse that is visible in these histories? What does the shift from internalist histories of science written by scientists, to externalist histories written by historians without a clear idea of the cognitive content of science, to outside histories that see Western science in conjunction with imperialism and colonialism, entail for a critique of science? What ultimately comes, for instance, of Prakash's suggestion that Vedic science was being accessed as the discontinuous repetition of a past, or of Chakrabarti's analysis of the prior antiquity (to Greek science) of Hindu science that nationalist scientists attempted to access in order to corner universal and good science for themselves? The discon-tinuities between past and present that these readings show up are radical, perhaps, for classical history-writing; for science, a discovery of discontinuities may merely confirm the traditional dynamic picture of science. Which is another reason why the relationship between history and science here remains externalist, just as the early 'influence' models of SSK did; even the contextualism proposed by Raina or the political connection forged by Prakash is more accurately read this way.

The possibility that began with the conventional reading of colonialism as an economic relation, and that Chakrabarti attempts to follow in his tracking of the journey, ultimately becomes an issue of the need to shift from transmission to translation. Translation is also a way to talk about the colonial relation. Translation means, for Prakash, a process by which the colonial idiom expressed itself in the language of the 'subordinated'. Prakash posits translation as an anterior rather than later event to difference, or different languages, as in the constitution of an 'irreduc-ibly different' modernity through the act of translation; further, it is an event made possible in situations of unequal positioning, as in the colonial relation. Similar strands of thought can be found in Chakrabarti too, and this notion ties up with their common ideas about hybridization. In the event, translation is their articulation of mutation rather than preservation of meaning across the colonial relation (sci-ence posing as myth, for instance, in Prakash), leaning heavily on the 'provisional' aspect, offering individual agency, heady in its difficulty of closure.

This provisionality is approached differently by Nandy, who is attentive to the content or vocabulary of what is seen as resistant. Nandy travels, speculatively, through the psyche of the Indian national scientist, not always sure if the case for difference can be made; more importantly, recognizing the possible 'strategic essentialism' in that exercise. Nandy, a psychologist by training, first wrote *Alternative Sciences* on the life histories of two scientists, Jagadis Chandra Bose and Srinavasa Ramanujan, in 1980, exploring the ambivalences towards modern science in their work, and their efforts to answer the questions posed by their own cultural contexts. In Nandy's exploration, however, the separation between the content and context of science was clear. Bose, felt Nandy, 'projected a distinctive concept of science and gave tantalizing clues to the personalized meaning given to science by an Indian scientist' (p. 1). It is in a later, fresh preface to a new edition of the book appearing in 1995 that Nandy takes up 'a position with the victims of modern science outside the perimeters of the "civilized" world', and it is at this juncture that Bose's biophysics in the tradition of Indian science or Ramanujan's mathematical worldview as shaped by indigenous schools of mathematics acquires new significance for Nandy. This is a clear shift, then, from a focus on science as central in these lives, and on these life histories as reflective of 'others' relationship to that centre,[23] to one where the reflections are on difference and are more complicated. Nandy develops this latter strand more intricately in *The Savage Freud* (1995), speaking of a way of accessing the past as a vantage point for a critique of the present.

This is not, however, a shift from a comfortable insiderness in relation to Western science, to a recalcitrant outsideness. In *Alternative Sciences*, Nandy is sceptical of the currency of a particular image of science as an unchanging, impersonal, ahistorical, and acultural 'mass of knowledge' (p. 11) and as 'a problem-solving technology which can cure some of the world's major ills' (p. 10), both among a large section of scientists and the laity, premised on a denial of the cultural and historical roots of Western science. Moving away from such a notion, he builds up a more embattled vision of science and positions Bose as caught up in the

> weary conflicts between the traditions of his society and the traditions of science, between a Westernness associated with the culture of his country's rulers and a Westernness characterizing the ruling culture of modern science, between science as an ideology and science as a gentlemanly hobby.
>
> (p. 2)

He sees Bose's attempt (and subsequent failure) 'as [that of] a creative scientist who hoped to delineate for Indian scientists the outlines of a possible collective identity' (p. 2) through his belief in the autonomy of science itself. Nonetheless, it is in science's 'use as a creative process which allows the scientist and, through him, his society and times to impose a *particular meaning on personal and social existence*' (p. 12), that Nandy sites the project of the book. In other words, the impulse here is towards a re-cognition of science through its individual practitioners. To this effect, Nandy cites Bose's reception by the leading lights of the Western scientific academy – including Einstein and Huxley – as something that can be classified as neither Orientalist nor positivist[24] but as symptomatic of a movement towards a new philosophy of science as a shared environment of discovery, anxieties, and conflicts – a subjective world.

Despite the ambivalences contained in Nandy's formulations on the possibilities offered by a 'creative scientist' for shaping a collective identity for Indian scientists, or in taking the question back home to the West, Nandy is not taking up these histories in the attempt to 'support an alternative Indian model of science' (p. 14) where the referent would continue to be the Occident. Nor is he 'providing a defence for a worldview for those to whom an alien culture, such as the ancient Indian or the modern Chinese, becomes important on ideological grounds' (p. 15). Clearly, Nandy is denying the possibility of an oppositional difference. 'Fortunately', he says,

> in the case of contemporary India, such an inverse relationship between an 'Indian science' and its Western counterparts is difficult to establish. The Indian 'alternative', for even the most ardent alternative-seeker, is impossibly unmanageable. It not only seems a half-dissent, it also seems inefficient, chaotic, abstruse, amorphous, and unsure of itself. Its capacity to become a dedicated opponent or even a counterplayer of any other culture is … much poorer … India's 'dissent', in this limited and peculiar sense, is less controllable.
>
> (p. 15)

He also seems to suggest the impossibility of any 'dissent' being captured or co-opted into the dominant.

We may take issue with this notion of a 'chaotic, amorphous' location. The metaphor of chaos has been too readily used in the language of Empire, associated with representations of 'primitivity'; Arnold speaks of this in some detail in his exploration of how the subcontinent gets marked as tropical (2015). As such, Nandy's claim to an anti-modernity would seem difficult to make in isolation from this stereotype. By the time of *The Savage Freud* (1995), however, Nandy has a clearer sense of what the chaotic, amorphous half-dissents should bring. His

> source of inspiration in this enterprise are those Asian, African and South American intellectuals who, whether they know it or not, are trying to ensure that the pasts and the presents of their cultures do not survive in the interstices of the contemporary world as merely a set of esoterica.
>
> (Nandy, 1995, p. x)

Hence Nandy sees the 'desperate and often-pathetic attempts to return to the past in the Southern world' as a way of discovering 'possible alternative bases for social criticisms of the existing order' (ibid). For Nandy, these bases then become sites from which to take back the question to the West. In a chapter on 'Modern Medicine and its Nonmodern Critics: A Study in Discourse', he takes the reader through three spaces – one, that of what he calls 'occult feminism';

two, Gandhi's experiments with truth; and three, G. Srinivasamurthi's critical response to Western medicine from the perspective of Ayurveda. Occult feminism, which recognized in Western medicine and its cohort with modernity the semantic impoverishment of the feminine body, the inability of modern medicine to treat the patient as a woman of knowledge, and its inability to account for a plurality of bodies, took up on each of these strains to push the limits of the system of modern Western medicine. Gandhi himself, says Nandy, declared that '[m]odern mechanistic civilization [and by extension modern medicine] is a disease because it violates the integrity of the body' (p. 181). *Hind Swaraj*, Gandhi's ideological manifesto, held modern doctors responsible for perpetuating the urban-industrial civilization by 'disconnecting over-consumption from its bodily consequences' (p. 185). In this philosophy, Nandy sees 'a demand for a cognitive resistance to the gross appetite of modern science' (p. 185). And Srinivasamurthi advances a critique of Western medicine from the vantage point of Ayurveda, centring on the

(1) the opposition between external and internal conceptions of disease [in Western medicine and Ayurveda respectively]; (2) the relationship between the disease and the patient [of great prognostic significance in Ayurveda]; and (3) the relationship between clinical and laboratory conceptions of disease [in Ayurveda and Western medicine respectively].

(p. 189)

In another chapter, 'The Savage Freud: The First Non-Western Psychoanalyst and the Politics of Secret Selves in Colonial India', Nandy speaks of Girindrasekhar Bose, the 'father' of psychoanalysis in India, and his identification of the introspectional element of thinking in India as akin to psychology, but sees Bose not so much as identifying it as another method of psychology but as a method shared with the past of a community. Rather than read this 'merely as an expression of nationalism ... [Nandy would suggest that it] be read partly as a statement of intent, a construction of the past *oriented to* a preferred future and serving as a critique of an imperfect present' (p. 143, italics mine).

If Nandy's polemics look to strengthen viable marginal vantage points – 'remembered pasts' – not as romantic utopias but as suitable alternative bases to critique the existing social order as also the dominant categories – development, the nation-state, secularism – from which and into which critique is today allowed and co-opted, Prakash, picking up on some of Nandy's formulations, sees potential in the negotiations between 'colonizer' and 'colonized' that disrupt the very binary oppositions they are meant to suggest. While 'science's history', in his schema, is indeed seen as 'a sign of Indian modernity', his interest is in 'science's cultural authority as the legitimating sign of rationality and progress' (Prakash, 1999, p. 7). This, he says, occurred through the act of translation that

required the displacement of the colonizer/colonized binary and the undoing of the science/ magic opposition. Indians had to be conceded the capacity for understanding if they were to be made into modern subjects, and science had to be performed as magic if it was to establish its authority. The irruption of this dislocation unleashed another, uncertain dynamic of translation, making possible both the indigenization of science and the formation of the Western-educated elite at the borderlines between cultures.

(Prakash, 1999, p. 8)

Prakash is saying that Western science, Western medicine,[25] as knower of the colonized subject, functioned through its very failure to transmit completely its coordinates. Here Prakash could be seen as re-reading as an intended failure of translation, the intended career for science in India (the British administrators' rhetoric of the 'failing of the people'). We could see, with Nandy, in the failure a refusal. Here then lies the tension in the interlocution between Nandy and Prakash. If for Nandy the journey has been one from a personalization of science through (an Indian?) remembered past, to a marginalization or a failure to be captured in science's wondrous grasp, for Prakash it is the very indigenization of science with all its uncertainties, the failure to remain insulated from magic, that laid the foundations for its functionality.

Both Nandy and Prakash bring in the perspective of the indigenous way of knowing as 'outside' or anterior in some way – while Nandy starts from 'The Alien Insiders' to science to arrive in later work at the other end, Prakash sees the production of a hybrid knowledge from the negotiations with Western science during the colonialist and nationalist moments (using, among others, the specific case of Gandhi's responses to technology). Here I reiterate my question on difference. One, if, for the production of an 'irreducibly different modernity' that was constituted of science, a resistant anterior difference needs to be accessed in consolidated form, the only critique that can be made available is resistance by a pre-given community. This is not to deny the possibility of anterior difference but to recognize its givenness and immutability. If, on the other hand, it serves as a vantage point, as in Nandy, or a posterior event, it is still possible to step outside the externalist frame and address the cognitive content of science. These are some of the implications of these historiographies that I flag.

Feminist methodologies and historiographies

I undertook this somewhat detailed reading against the grain of the postcolonial and modernist impulses in historiographies of science, in part to present a distinction between these and other methodologies within which resistance is framed – subaltern consciousness, standpoint, or situatedness, for instance. Standpoint understandings emerge in the context of understanding knowledge as having been historically held within dominant communities seen as legitimate knowledge producers. This knowledge is understood to have been held through the pushing down and out of other knowledge producers, and of models of knowledge other than the positivist. In this framework, knowledge is also seen as tied to lived experience and location, but this connection is denied in normative models. What is termed normative knowledge has been held by socially and historically dominant communities. In this framework, the *dai*, for instance, has historically been excluded from knowledge communities; her caste, race and class locations have been ever-present but unacknowledged aspects of this exclusion. This figure neither inhabits nor appears within the domain of the resistant that any of the historiographies discussed above have detailed. Reading against the grain of the given histories of science, then, would be a next step to explore this absence, taking on board standpoint methodologies. Feminist standpoint theories, in revisiting parameters of knowledge validity, have re-centred lived experience and location, and re-positioned figures like the *dai* in knowledge work (Harding, 2004; Haraway, 2004; Dalmiya & Alcoff, 2013; Dalmiya, 2002). Debiprasad Chattopadhyaya's *Lokayata* (1959) comes close to this form of critique. The Subaltern Studies School, in its earliest work, has presented the subaltern as an autonomous location and voice, distinct from the nationalist aspiration to state power represented by elite nationalists. Other efforts, by feminist historians, for instance, have been to position some of these exclusions and resistances vis-à-vis histories of colonialism (Forbes, 2005; Chawla, 1994; Van Hollen, 2003; Sadgopal, 2009). These have taken different routes, with Geraldine Forbes linking the caste-based stigmatization of the *dai* figure alongside the dominance of the Englishwoman physician who became the primary entrant to the *zenana* (2005), Chawla presenting the *dai* figure as ritual practitioner rather than simply a childbirth attendant (1994), Van Hollen tracing briefly the emergence of the *dai* figure historically (2003), and Sadgopal speaking of the epistemological position denied to the *dai* as knowledge and care practitioner (2009).

We also see other feminist historiographies, like Abha Sur, Neelam Kumar, and Samiksha Sehrawat, for instance, that take up specific methodological questions. Abha Sur (2001) traces a very different history of science in modern India from the ones we have been discussing. Focussing on the careers of known and relatively unknown women in one of the premier physics laboratories in emerging India of the 1930s, Sur explores the 'enabling (and disabling) aspects of culture in the making of women scientists in India' (Sur, 2001, p. 97). Within the colonial relation, the imperatives of nationalism, and the norms of gender and caste, Sur's historiographic impulse focusses not on numbers – a method usually recognized as a marker of exclusion, nor on individual narratives – usually applied to marginal lives but on the social and structural contexts, both local, societal, and national, within which women scientists' lives are scripted. Focussing on collective biographies (p. 97), Sur thus writes a 'local' history of science that has generalizable implications and that presents both a critique of history-writing and of science. Savithri Preetha Nair's recent biographical account of cytogeneticist and ethnobotanist E.K. Janaki Ammal reflects on this same methodological approach, of one such biography being an entry point into the experiences of a collective (2022). Neelam Kumar (2012) locates women's science careers with respect to gender norms in colonial and contemporary India. Samiksha Sehrawat (2014), in looking at medical reproductive care in the colonial period, focusses on institutional segregation as a method of control over populations and, in doing so, traces the state as one of the most significant actors in medical control, and their collaboration with the national elite in this process. Not surprisingly, each of these histories focusses on institutions and the central presence they have in the lives of the marginal. We will see, in Chapter 5, the meanings of these accounts, which occupy interdisciplinary and gender studies domains, but only rarely the domain of histories of science.

I attempt, in this book, to engage in conversation between the extended discussion on colonial power in postcolonial scholarship and this other set of resistance frames, in the context of emerging therapeutic cultures. The difference I make from both these sets of ideas is in seeing the resistant figure, in this case, the *dai*, not as pre-existent but as produced in the collaborative discourse between the colonial and the national(ist). After a brief but hyper-visibilized historical colonial presence, this figure becomes, in the contemporary, suitable for extrusion as part of the consolidation of a dominant indigenous. I trace, in the next chapters, both the hypervisibility and the extrusion.

Re-reading the 'encounter' model and its effects in histories of medicine in India

Histories of science and medicine in India are non-contiguous, particularly in terms of the use of the encounter frame. It is the keen eye brought by some of the histories of medicine in India that question the encounter model – a model that would follow on binaries of West/East, rational/intuitive, science/tradition, and so on. Understanding the archival historical impulse as both wide and narrow, seeking patterns as well as dissonances, particularly in more recent historiographies, we see that the idea of the encounter, even when referenced as a frame, has become increasingly untenable – temporally, in terms of actors and events, or spaces. The nature, scope, and permanence of interventions, too, has been questioned. To restate the framework under question here, I refer to the work of one of these recent historiographies, by Projit Bihari Mukharji, who speaks of the classical 'formulation of colonial medical history in terms of "an encounter" ... a confrontation where two relatively discrete entities meet each other in a zero-sum game for domination' (2009, p. 8), as a lens to interpret what was going on in the 18th to 19th centuries in a complex therapeutic terrain. Mukharji points to the several assumptions here – this metaphor and approach 'stages a complex conflict as a single episode of violent confrontation' (p. 9), it assumes that this confrontation is single or episodic and that the two entities, on a level playing field, are 'relatively well-bounded, internally coherent entities' (p. 9). It also assumes rivalries between discrete systems of knowledge – a language that is not available, as Mukharji avers, till the end of the 1820s. We could see the link between this and the shift from national to nationalist science that Pratik Chakrabarti traces, as also from Orientalist to imperial and colonial impulses. I have, in earlier work, discussed the 'choice between systems' approach that has inflected critiques of Western knowledge, where for instance the critique is posed between Ayurveda or Unani on the one hand and allopathy on the other (Achuthan, 2017). Mukharji argues that the encounter framework has created a bifurcation in studies of medicine in India, resulting in one set that focusses on medicine and public health in the colony, that draws relationships between medicine and colonial hegemony, and another set that explores indigenous medical systems. The travel, reformulation, and rearticulation, of knowledge and categories, have resulted, in Mukharji's estimation, in '"Western" medicine's links with *repressive* dimensions of (colonial and more recently postcolonial) power [being] explored in depth, while its *productive* role in constituting new subjects and subject-positions [being] relatively unexplored' (p. 10). It is in this context that Mukharji follows the work of Stacey Leigh Pigg and others in focussing on histories of travel rather than 'belong[ing] to one culture or another' (ibid). It is also in these contexts that Mukharji proposes a focus on the socially significant identity of the native *daktar* who performed Western medicine, and the histories of nationalization of the body through vernacularizing of Western medicine. Following Foucault, I would insert here a point about power in its productive form being still about control and governance; rather, Foucault rejects the repressive hypothesis in favour of the productive one to understand newer modes of governance (1990). Following the spirit of Mukharji's critique of the encounter model, however, I now examine some of the histories of medicine that inhabit this debate and discourse. I am interested in following what I see as the emergence and consolidation of a dominant indigenous constellation, not necessarily bounded or stable but 'staged' in an encounter framework, to re-use Mukharji's critical term (p. 8). This staging, I suggest, changes in different historical contexts, extruding that which does not fit. But for now, I follow Mukharji's impulse to explore approaches in available histories of medicine that make the encounter model untenable. One is work like Seema Alavi's that speaks of the process of hegemonization as a much more extended exercise than limited to the 1830s that have been marked by Arnold and others, thus focussing on multidirectional processes distributed over several actors and locations. Another is Arnold's own understanding of resistance as constitutive of the hegemonic, rather than a separated action; the overdetermined character of knowledge follows. A third, seen in Arnold, Mukharji, and other historical accounts, is a focus on practice and the everyday that, by its very nature, refuses a static or even stable reading of science or medical knowledge, offering instead a chaotic, unpredictable process. We will look at each of these in some detail here and in the next chapter.

A hierarchical, overdetermined terrain

At the same time that Deepak Kumar spoke of the active co-workings of colonial science and the colonial state, and the consequent pushing down and erasure of native experience or authority, David Arnold seeks to depict the history of colonial medicine and public health as one where resistance is stitched into and centrally constitutive of the directions and shifts in powerful state-centred medical systems (1991, 2004). He suggests at the outset that 'an interactive model might be more appropriate for the colonial period rather than one that depicts either outright confrontation between two intransigent forces or an automatic unassailable Western ascendancy' (2004, p. 9). This does not, of course, take away from the 'political character of science' (2004, p. 14). This interactive model is also explored more in the trajectory of medicine in the subcontinent, in relation to botany and related disciplines. Arnold presents this idea via an examination of the histories of institutionalization and professionalization of state colonial medicine, British medical attitudes towards the textual traditions of Unani and Ayurveda, and towards folk practice, as well as Indian practitioners in the 19th and 20th centuries. Arnold talks of the tying of institutionalized biomedicine to 'military and administrative needs of the colonial state and [with the Indian Medical Service (IMS)] staffed almost exclusively by Europeans' in the mid-19th century (p. 58). This created professional and institutional structures that eventually became the grounds for an emerging public health system (Arnold, 2004, p. 60). Both the character of the IMS and its racial composition changed in the late 19th to early 20th century from being exclusively white European. With medical practice being so tied to the IMS and to Europeans at the time, with this kind of institutionalized professionalization, however, Indians in medicine seemed to have lagged behind Indians in law or government service (p. 65); whether this was on account of indigenous practice having a stronger hold in native communities is an argument we will look at with Alavi's work. Prior to this, the Native Medical Institution (NMI) had been set up in 1822 to provide vernacular medical training to Indians, with the Sanskrit College and the Calcutta Madrasa providing additional training in Ayurveda and Unani, respectively. Arnold observes that with the closure of the NMI in 1835 and its replacement with the Calcutta Medical College (CMC),

> [i]t has been assumed that ... an era of 'peaceful' cooperation and 'friendly' coexistence between the Western and Indian systems [ended] ... and signified the replacement of a benign Orientalist policy of patronising and learning from indigenous medicine by an intolerant Anglicist one, with disastrous consequences for the subsequent history of indigenous medicine.
>
> (p. 62)

He counters this assumption with a tracing of what seems to be a pragmatic rather than ideological policy at work, to render 'cheap but reliable medical aid for Company servants' (p. 62), with Ayurveda and Unani training in the NMI having been only about attracting 'recruits from the *Vaidyas* and other communities with a tradition of medical practice' (p. 63) who, it was thought, would eventually recognize the superiority of Western medicine. Rather than the radical shift it was made out to be, then, institutions like the CMC may have had more continuities of perspective with, than departures from, the NMI. In terms of texts and drugs too, Arnold suggests that the approach of the early British Orientalists was more of an interested though sceptical stance towards a museumized therapeutic culture than a living one; this was partly replicated later in the works of Heyne, Ainslie, and Wilson, who chose to study Ayurvedic texts, seeing them as valuable ancient material that had later fallen prey to religious dogma and thus into decline. The exception was J. Forbes Royle, who made a 'seminal claim for the anteriority of Hindu over Greek and Arabic medicine' (p. 67). Some of this work, like Ainslie's *Materia Indica* (1826), also seemed to take an ecumenical approach, trying to find connections between the medicines of Europe and Asia. Arnold also suggests that British practitioners' attitudes toward Indian practice treated the latter as having practical knowledge, particularly regarding indigenous drugs and diseases particular to Indian contexts. This attitude shifts, says Arnold, by the mid-19th century, to a rejection, indeed a decrial, pointing to the violence and harm caused by indigenous practices, although European medical practices of the time were as violent. By this time, 'scientific pharmacology and the isolation of active chemical ingredients' (p. 69) had also begun to become protocol for European medicine, and we will see this in the workings of the Indigenous Drugs Committee in the next chapter. It is also in the mid-19th century that the idea of India as a 'tropical', physical environment and therefore host to particular kinds of climate, vegetation, disease, and temperament emerged, suggests Arnold; we may see in this both the movement in the English perception of India as Oriental to tropical, as Arnold suggests, and as also empirical grounds for a hierarchical difference, an othering, a building of the idea of India as static resource rather than active agent or knowledge producer. Arnold talks about how this 'made medicine central to the investigation and representation of the Indian environment' (2004, p. 77) and how the 'medical investigation of climate and topography helped fashion a new, more censorious, attitude to India' (p. 78). Arnold's reading, then, also offers some insight into the discourse around race and fitness, with the Empire putting sickliness down to race, and particularly as a way to read illnesses such as malaria as 'emasculating', more so, to read differences 'between the 'manly' and 'martial' races of the north and northwest, and the 'effeminate' Bengalis' (p 79) who were inhabitants of some of the flood-hit and therefore malarial districts of Bengal. This stereotype travelled into Bengali Hindu nationalist discourse, consolidating the bodily threat perceived from the Muslim other, as Arnold's reading suggests:

> In the wake of the census reports of 1891 and 1901, the view became widespread among middle-class Bengali Hindus that theirs was a 'dying race', decimated by malaria, while the Muslims of eastern Bengal, where malaria was less prevalent, continued to multiply.
>
> (p 80)

This is useful to keep in mind as we see the development of the sub-discipline of tropical medicine with its celebrated institutional beginnings in the Calcutta School of Tropical Medicine in 1914, and the manner in which this idea features in the curricula of 'tropical diseases', squarely put down to climatic context, nearly recalling early miasmatic theories (Snowden, 2019), in the discipline of Preventive and Social Medicine later. We may read aspects of scientific racism in this exercise as well. All this of course lays the ground for control over landscape and populations, and the discourse of the civilizing mission, with the 'natives' always falling just short of fitness to self-govern – a discourse that assumes centre stage after the experience of the 1857 revolt or war of independence. Finally, we see Arnold speaking of the conflation of textual traditions like Unani and Ayurveda with folk practices in the decrial of these, the most visible example being the appropriation of the labour of *tikadar* castes into vaccination drives while outlawing their own practice of variolation. In fact, says Arnold, '[t] he Smallpox Commission of 1850, in comparing variolation to *sati* and infanticide, declared that the time had come to suppress 'this murderous trade' (p. 73, quoting from the *Transactions of the Medical and Physical Society of Calcutta,* 1831).

What we see in this historiographical impulse is, for one, a focus on multiple moments – of eclectic practice, pragmatic policy, conflict, interaction, particularly in the attitudes and practices of Indian practitioners like Bhau Daji Lad, who were exemplars of 'interaction and assimilation' (p. 70). This suggests a much more complex history over space and time, one that traces a finally undecided account than an encounter with a clear outcome; and Arnold's history is thus methodologically closer to being a Foucaultian one. Most significantly, it presents the 'encounter' not as a frame but as a developing racial relation between Indian and English practitioners, as also a struggle across caste equations.

About a decade later, Arnold is writing histories of science and medicine in India outside of the institutional, more in terms of negotiated practice in the everyday that offers an expanded history, a framework that culminates in his work on everyday technologies in 2013. While this is an idea that also finds resonance in earlier work by Shiv Visvanathan (2003), the possible difference is in terms of Arnold representing this everyday as a route to refashioning received knowledges, unlike Visvanathan who sees everyday technologies as a form of resistance that emerges in the encounter model. Ideas of hybridity in postcolonial theorizations are definite parallels here, and the focus on 'science as practice and culture', an idea mooted by Andrew Pickering in the science studies field (1993, 2010), alongside the actor-network frameworks proposed by Bruno Latour (2007), is to be seen as at least some of the contexts for these shifts in reading the career of medicine in colonial India. Mark Harrison also speaks of the 'historical contingencies of South Asia' and the need to take these into account when understanding the spread of ideas of public health and western medicine (2009). Mukharji speaks of histories emerging in the late 1990s that presented the state as a more disaggregated entity, through a focus on 'ideas and categories', 'transnational networks', and 'histories of specific institutions and medical projects' (2011, p. 18). This set of histories shifts the idea of colonial medicine from being a monolithic state-centred and controlled project entirely to one that emerged much more via a layered image of the state and the spaces outside of it.

Nationalism and the consolidation of the indigenous practitioner identity

One of the specific pegs on which the encounter gets staged in histories of medicine is the practitioner, and the emergence of this subject vis-à-vis the community, nation, and colonial state is a possibility that Alavi and Mukharji, as also Arnold in different ways, explore in some detail. Medical training as a parameter to validate knowledge, as also protocol to allow entry into practice and service, is something we see most visibly in the colonial period, as Arnold notes, but Mukharji writes in some detail about the dialogue with Western medicine that was in place at least two centuries 'before the term *daktar* emerges as a socially significant identity' (2009, p. 1). In fact, Mukharji's question is of why, well before 'a clearly articulated sense of nationalism has emerged', the native *daktars* show 'sympathy for their fellow countrymen' (2009, p. 22), and he finds an answer in the idea of 'felt community' proposed by Rajat Kanta Ray – 'that predated the nation and continued to exist alongside it' (p. 22). Tracing closely the history of training in Western medicine and employment in civil and military hospitals for the 'natives' in the time of empire, he speaks of the presence of the native trained in some form of Western medicine, at all levels of the medical services since at least 1822, with the setting up of the Native Medical Institution (NMI). As expected, this presence was much more in the lower, lesser paid levels of the services, with racism playing a big role in this disparity (2009, p. 7). One of the outcomes is that a 'homogenized State medicine' (p. 7) was not possible. A question that follows, for my purposes, is of whether regulation at these levels was also poor, so that the native *daktar* also stood in as a representative of indigenous medicine, more reliable than both their Western counterpart or the *Vaidya* or *hakim* on account of being able to evaluate it on the basis of Western-legitimated expert knowledge. While Mukharji is concerned with the social identity of these practitioners, I worry the terms 'indigenous' or 'native' as markers of cultural situatedness, which allow this figure of the *daktar* to legitimately operate at the interface of practices, representing Western medicine within an emerging indigenous system, as also hybridizing the Western. It is this multidirectionality that might recall Raina's definition of a postcolonial theory of transmission of science (Raina, 2003). My concern is with the consolidation of the indigenous in the soil of this transmission, and I find most useful, to my purposes, Mukharji's suggestion of this period as one of the co-emergence of what might be called a medical profession within which practitioners found themselves, the market and advertising for indigenous medicines, a social category of *daktars* who were not necessarily clubbable into Western or native, the conflicts over language, medium of training, and parameters of validation that accompany training, and the coeval role of the colonial state and market in all these. This is one aspect of the emergence of a therapeutic culture that I speak of in this book.

When and with whom was the 'encounter'?

Seema Alavi starts the reading of the 'encounter' from an entirely different vantage point than other scholars in the field – 'the Mughal legacy ... rather than the British colonial frame' (2008, p. 1). Putting together in the same frame of analysis the precolonial and colonial, the national and the communitarian, the practitioner embedded in familial and communitarian soils and the professional outside and above these, and most importantly, bringing into the picture the interface of Mughal traditions and the East India Company as a tentative entity, Alavi is thus an exemplar of acknowledging history-writing as an effect of this vantage point, rather than a description of the entire colonial universe. This attention to the emergence of the Company in 'the huge tide of change in post-Mughal society that had already begun to disembody medical knowledge from the clutches of the royal court' (p. 55) meant that Alavi is able to show how Company rule performed several interventions in the therapeutic cultures of this period. For one, it corralled the hitherto practitioner-focussed Unani learning and practice it encountered into a 'disembodied form of Arabic learning' (p. 55) by the setting up of separate institutions, like the Calcutta Madrasa in 1781, for these. With the active print production of Arabic texts and Arabic translations of European anatomy under the aegis of these institutions, as well as the proletarianization of this knowledge in the 1820s with Urdu and Hindustani becoming the language of texts and instruction, Alavi points to an earlier period of intervention and consequent change than the 1830s that Arnold, Langford, and others have marked as the beginning of the coercive turn with the introduction of English education and the taking over by Western knowledge systems, as also a continuation of this process well into the 1870s and later. Alavi also refers to other work like that of Sivaramakrishnan (2006) who marks a different period, i.e., the 1850s, when indigenous learning, sustained by Sikh ascetics in Punjab, began to dissipate following land reforms. This exercise, at the very least, opens up the process of 'encounter' temporally and, with its focus on western and central parts of the subcontinent and on non-Hindu practices and texts, divides this process as well as the idea of the indigenous, spatially. I will return to this aspect of division; however, Alavi does more in indicating how the 1830s reforms on English education, with the resulting collapse of the Calcutta Madrasa and the NMI, were limited in their impact, having failed to extinguish 'the medical ethos already established via the earlier interaction between the Company and indigenous medical knowledges and linguistic cultures' (p. 56). Rather, as the NMI 'staffers dispersed into the *qasbas* and towns of the North Indian countryside, so did their new ideas and texts. These now became diffused in local society, alongside the flame of Arabic medical learning ignited by the Calcutta Madrasa' (pp. 98–99).

An alternative to this diffusion is available in the closeting of 'discursive techniques' (p. 198), as Alavi states, meant to keep pure and retain control over what was seen as a specialized knowledge system in the mid-19th century, away from colonial authority, with the *hakims* practising these techniques actually being known to refuse public office. These techniques included *darrs* or models of secular instruction borrowed from the late 18th century, and *nusqha navisi* or elaborate handwritten prescriptions, one where the hakim 'entered the cultural world of the patient' (p. 204). The *darr* used learning techniques that placed 'a premium on memory, oratory, writing skills, perpetuation of the name of the *ustaad* (teacher), and of course that of the family name' (p. 198), much like the learning practices of *gurukuls* and Ayurveda, as also training in and separation of musical traditions in northern India. Particularly in the case of Unani, these techniques described an expert model that was both above and alongside the cure-seeker. While British medicine presented itself as class and location neutral, Unani claimed community. Significantly, Unani also claimed the nation, claiming that the *aab-o-hawa* of the patient – the environment, as also the physical climate and the culture – was better understood in Unani, and therefore offered a collaborative healing process with the participation of the patient and *hakim*. This environment, said Unani practitioners, was unknown to the Western systems, which did not have a history in Hindustan. The *Oudh Akhbar* claimed, in 1881, that the 'fight for the cause of Unani mirrored the fight for *mulk* (nation)' (p. 277). We see in Alavi's account of Unani, then, a claim to space, physicality and nation, that appears the most powerful yet, building a cultural nationalist identity and a somewhat ecumenical history of medicine in India, given Unani's claim to both Graeco-Roman philosophy and Islam. This interpretation by Alavi sits in interesting juxtaposition with Arnold's reading of the tropicalization of India performed in the colonialists' vocabulary. We will look more closely at the campaign for professionalization of Unani in *Oudh Akhbar* and other periodicals in the next chapter, but we do see here a proposal for a codified version of indigenous medicine to counter Western medicine, because the 'scientific core of a cleansed Unani' (p. 264), while being closer to the Hindustani *tabiyat* (habitus) could still match the scientific core and antecedents of Western medicine. Muslim reformers like Sir Syed Ahmad Khan (founder of the Aligarh Muslim University) participated in this project of cleansing Unani. Arnold marks, in the case of the other visible textual tradition – Ayurveda – the 'indigenous revival ... seeking to re-establish Ayurveda as the popular and culturally appropriate alternative to allopathy, but also seeking to supplant what were seen as ignorant and superstitious folk practices' (2004, p. 179). The tragedy of the politics of this negotiation remains in the fact that, while all this work is put in by the Muslim public intellectual to mark Hindustan as identity territory, it still becomes abject in the recounting of the nationalist project, and Ayurveda emerges as the nationalist constant. In fact, even after Unani families re-establish control in the early 20th century, these intellectuals are unwilling to participate in the communal atmosphere; although they are called upon to respond to the needs of both *qaum* and *mulk*, they continue to identify Unani as compatible with Hindustan – *mulk* – as locale. This is after the *mulk* and the *qaum* are beginning to be separated in the late 19th century, and 'Unani ... given a new history where its accretive strands, in particular its pre-Islamic Graeco-Hellenic past, and its development in Hindustan, was marginalized and the achievements made in the Islamic classical empires highlighted' (p. 322). A question that emerges here is on the grounds on which each of these textual traditions claims authority. Does Unani make this claim on the grounds of both of similar origins to Western medicine and having a history in Hindustani *tabiyat*, and does Ayurveda need to make its claims stronger by pushing down that which was both the mystical East as well as the folk?

Consolidation, segregation, and the politics of language

It is in the following of the engagement between the Company and the therapeutic cultures it met with (rather than encountered) that some of the consolidation of textual cultures and their consequent separation from their 'chaotic' soil is understood in Alavi's account. Alavi explores this terrain in great detail, tracing first the patronage of madrasa learning by the Company. The Calcutta Madrasa, established in 1781 by Warren Hastings, highlighted Arabic as the universal language of science and medicine, and foregrounded Unani texts in Arabic as authentic textual sources. Between its foundation and the early 19th century, when a medical class was added to earlier taught subjects of mathematics and philosophy, both the ideas of textual learning and of Arabic as its true vehicle were foregrounded. In addition, Muslim students alone, primarily from the traditional elite, were allowed to be educated here. Arabic Unani texts taught in the Calcutta madrasa 'focused on medicine as science rather than comportment' (Alavi, 2008, p. 60) that had been the focus earlier. It is here, then, that we see what the nature of intervention is, what its justificatory claims are, and what its impacts might be. Tytler, the chief medical teacher at the Madrasa, suggests that the indulgence of comportment, a privilege and luxury available only to the elite of the time, was rightly challenged by the introduction of objectivity and distancing from the individual body; this was possible through universal referents to be found in Western medicine that would help 'question the social hierarchies created by Persian medical texts' (p. 60). By social hierarchies, Tytler explicitly names caste, in addition to aristocracy. To his mind, the closest parallel to European medicine was the Arabic Unani texts, and by combining this learning with translated European medical lectures on anatomy, and shifting from manuscript to printed text with the coming and expansion of the printing press in the 1820s, medical knowledge could be demystified and taken out of the patronage and control of wealthy families and individuals, while the hereditary link to Arabic knowledge and texts remained. Tytler, Breton, and others gain, in this stress on anatomy learning, the approbation of the administration in this time; in Tytler's case, the 'governor general appreciated his [Tytler's] efforts to initiate high-caste students towards knowing body anatomy' at Sanskrit College in Calcutta (Alavi, p. 147).

The impulse of codification and classification that has been spoken of as constitutive of/definitional to modern knowledge (Foucault, 1970) is one way to read this intervention – a reading that would make it seem that a textual practice was being selectively supported and promoted, to the detriment of the 'chaos' or heterogeneity (depending on how that was seen) prevailing earlier, in the interests of better control and regulation, in the prevailing climate of scientific universalism, thus installing and making dominant the textual tradition that Orientalists had first encountered. This also opened the door to the inclusion of 'European literature and science [in Arabic]' (p. 58), preferred over Persian and the vernaculars. This is seen as an addition to Hastings' proposal for a cadre of Muslim officers trained in the law and related aspects, in order to help govern newly acquired territory; both needs were fulfilled at the madrasa. Alavi speaks of the manner in which this politics of language shifts, in the later part of the 19th century, with the setting up of the Native Medical Institution and with Tytler's translation monopoly being challenged by Breton, among others. Breton, superintendent in 1825 of the Native Medical Institution set up in 1822, O'Shaughnessy, Trevelyan, and others, began translating European texts into Hindustani, Bengali, and other vernaculars, as also Sanskrit, thus shifting from Arabic-Persian patronage, taking power away, in some sense, from *hakims* and *vaids*, and creating what Alavi terms a new class of

medical or medically aware communities ... [including] the service gentry of
the *qasbas* and towns of Oudh and contiguous areas ... [c]omprising Hindus,
Muslim scribes, accountants, physicians, and a range of literate people ...
[who] looked to the British as their new employers.

(Alavi, p. 153)

Alavi speaks of this shifting patronage, and the emergence of this new community
of practitioners excluded from religious, family, and secular learning traditions,
who, combining Western and Unani, 'took to the vernacular literature as a way of
mobility in a society in which they felt rudderless' (p. 153).

Another shift that follows from Alavi's account of the time of the Calcutta
madrasa is a segregation between Muslim and Hindu students – a segregation
that involves the Company, British medical men seeking an audience, and a set of
gatekeepers from within the indigenous therapeutic community seeking to retain
expert territory. This sharpens already developing demarcations between a Hindu
and Islamic medicine. It is from this history, then, that our understanding of the
communalization of the therapeutic domain, discussed also in Rachel Berger's
account of modern Ayurveda (2013), emerges. Apart from the segregation of textual language that forms one of the grounds for this separation, Alavi also speaks
of the 'British administration of the dispensary [in a mimicking of class, religious
and family lines that were the hallmarks of Unani practice, that] began to change
the social contours of Unani, stamping it with a fresh religious and class profile'
(p. 186). While this profiling was being fashioned by the British to undermine the
grasp of Unani over the populace, taking 'knowledge away from the community to
the laboratory' (p. 186), it of course offered a fresh lease of life to Muslim native
practitioners, who used this space to 'resist colonial medical authority' (p. 186).
We will examine this movement in both Unani and Ayurveda, tied as it is to the
question of text and language, in more detail in Chapter 3; it is the identification of
these as sites in these histories that I mark here.

And yet, Alavi notes that the shift was not really complete, and the texts produced –

neither in their content nor in the way they had been produced – represented
unalloyed European medical science. In fact, ... they were the product of a
truly shared medical knowledge that was as essential for circulation in India
as it was critical for the growth of the profession in Britain. Such vernacular
texts therefore reflected the dilemmas created in the minds of British medics
when balancing the administrative expediencies of empire with the larger
needs of a fast-evolving Western medical science tradition.

(p. 151)

The encounter model, then, continues to be challenged in this reading, with Alavi's
point perhaps being also about the prolonged period over which the loss of power
occurred. Breton's production of lithographic texts still involved an earlier 'public'
with actors like the 'calligrapher, artist, scribe, and elite readers' (p. 80). Both in
the production of these texts and in practice, Breton seemed to be working with a

variety of practitioners – including Muslim *maulvis* and Hindu *pandits* – a heterogenous, porous, collaborative exercise, with also a source of varied employment. Was this engagement opportunistic? Was it a conscious act of knowledge collaboration? Was it an exercise of power? These questions remain somewhat open and unanswered in Alavi's interpretation. In fact, when under the 1830s reforms, the Hindu-Muslim segregation was critiqued, and the NMI and Madrasa education lost backing, with English education being seen as the way to go, the Calcutta madrasa continued to be handled carefully, to appease elite Muslim families, and as Alavi says 'reflected that the medical culture of the period outlived these reforms' (p. 97). It is unclear whether Alavi's pointer here at a plural medical culture that she suggests 'colonialism itself had helped sustain' (p. 205) is adequate, or we are looking at a less coherent or cohesive therapeutic culture, or at the failure of full hegemony. In fact, we might read the 'real' encounter as being with 'back home', as Chakrabarti and others have spoken of in the context of colonial science, in colonial practitioners making the case for colonial medicine as necessary and therefore worthy of funding, as independent, as unique rather than derivative of metropolitan medicine, with the English surgeon as erudite and an author-translator-interpreter of indigenous medical traditions, in contrast to the historical image of the barber-surgeon in England (Singer, 1952). In another reading, Mukharji talks of texts being printed in English for continental audiences and in Bengali for local ones, and this suggests a different trajectory for local language texts that referenced nationalism to compete with the English ones. Ayurveda, while being eulogized in these, was never 'in the market' for the English. Another question, then, to the encounter framework.

Are other readings possible? Was this long period of interventions and an uneven shift of power also pushback against a dominant Mughal culture that was the Company's primary rival – a culture that survived despite its political decline, as Alavi suggests? Was this about prejudice towards native practice, or a challenge to native aristocracy and expert power, and a reaching out to 'the masses' via the creation of fresh gatekeepers? Did the fluid domain of practice work against the consolidation of expert domains, even as professionalization took shape, both in the metropole and the colony? This seems more in evidence in the manner in which dispensaries in the early 19th century were used to provide rough-and-ready training to become a 'native doctor' (Alavi p. 175) – a practice that had gone on informally before, and that gets institutionalized in the 1830s. At any rate, what does seem to happen is the sharpening of distinctions – Unani as Muslim, associated with Arabic and then Urdu vocabulary and *hakim* practitioners, Ayurveda as available in Sanskrit and Devanagiri scripts and the domain of Hindu *pandits*. In other words, a slow transfer of power and an increasingly segregated domain of the indigenous. It is in following through this idea of segregation that this book is located.

In following through on segregation, it is also important to follow through on 'chaos'. As we will see in Chapters 3, 4, and 5, feminist scholars have reported on a variety of strands of culture that get extruded from both private and public spheres in the late 19th and early centuries; *Bottola* medicine is one of them, as Swati Moitra

(2017) and Charu Gupta (2005) report. This genre of print literature, beginning in north Calcutta where the first presses were located, became, in the mid-19th century, a holding space for an oral culture among a communitarian reading public composed primarily of privileged women, who accessed romance and erotic 'low' literature through a network of vendors who entered the *andarmahal*. In contrast, a loose genre of *totkas*, *gharoa chikitsa*, not elevated to the level of science but seen as important translators, if not collaborators, of the authentic indigenous, also emerged. The idea of the quack also features here, not as actor in a plural medical culture but in a market (Mukharji p. 16), and participates in a sense of chaos that informs the therapeutic domain. How this chaos is sifted through, with some actors partially extruded, some appropriated, regulated, and how a canonical indigenous emerges through these processes, are all part of an interpretative historiography, and are some questions I attempt to pose in this book as I try to understand the journey of the *dai*.

Regulation

One of the themes where extended discussions of hegemony are possible is the question of regulation and the role of the colonial state. Arnold and Kumar discuss in some detail the processes of classification, codification, and regulation that take centre stage after 1858 – for example, in the shape of censuses intended to provide 'a convenient digest of information about the Indian empire, its resources, inhabitants and administration' (Arnold 2004b, p. 130). '[T]he Indian census', says Arnold, 'was a central feature of an expanding colonial governmentality' (p 130). While the transition from Company rule to the Crown saw this manner of systematic ordering of population and land information, as Deepak Kumar also focusses on, in the shape of land surveys, physical anthropometry in the gazetteer descriptions of natives, and control within the Asiatic and scientific societies, by the end of the 19th century, this seemed to manifest more and more in the passing of laws on professions like medicine, on the functioning of dispensaries, and related institutional practices. As for indigenous textual traditions like Ayurveda and Unani, Alavi offers the most nuanced account of the relation, recognizing that the *hakims*, for instance, saw value in the institutional network of dispensaries, municipalities, hospitals, and so on, each of which they had a place in, while being able to access a distinct cultural identity and therefore a clientele. From 1912, when registration began to become essential for practice, and when indigenous medicine in dispensaries became illegal, these native practitioners were unhappy, and via the Usman Committee and other committees, negotiated for space within colonial regulation, suggesting that it was the 'chaotic' practices that needed to be brought under surveillance. Regulation, then, may be seen as another mechanism of governmentality, but also one in which indigenous practitioners and their cohorts actively participated, as a route to validation and thus survival.

Conclusion

Following the questions to the encounter model that Mukharji raises, that appear in Alavi's work, and that I develop here, as also the question of whether the interface and engagement was between formed systems or more porous cultures of healing, it is useful to mark a few aspects that may be useful for further exploration. These aspects have to do with a discourse around necessary interventions that the emerging national elite engaged in, in the 19th century. These interventions ranged from the place of women, to religion, to necessary professions, to the role and type of education, to the role of science. It is useful to read some of this discourse in the context of aspirations to modernity. Several of the commentaries on Ayurveda, or on the concern with the reproductive health of women, all written by medical men, that appear in the late 19th and early 20th centuries, indeed some of them beginning earlier, are prefaced with a lament on the sad state of attention paid to womenfolk, or to scientific temper, to ancient knowledge systems, in the country. In addition, we see debates in medical journals like *Bhisak Darpan* in Bengal, run from the 1890s, which saw 'a genuine interest of Bengali *daktars* in intellectually engaging with the indigenous medical traditions' (Mukharji, 2009, p. 96). These were also spaces that saw a certain debating behaviour that might appear as an aspirational sign of civilizational maturity, as also an aspiration to an 'indigenous' intellectual class of men inhabiting the public sphere, in response to the constant judgements on incapacity for self-governance that came from the Raj's administrators. The overwhelmingly Hindu composition of the readership of these journals in Bengal, if seen partly through the language of their writing, the male aspect of this readership as well as its writing, and the gendered occupation of the nationalist and familial spaces by men and women in the profession, with the familialization of the *ledi daktar* (Mukharji, 2011, p. 109), all seem to contribute to the image of segregation that this time overwhelmingly presents. It is some of this, and the putting in place of certain practitioners on the grounds of gender and caste, that I will look at in Chapter 4.

To go back to the question of the encounter, then, we go back to Arnold's point that 'centre-periphery or metropolitan-colonial are a misrepresentation of science's evolution from the seventeenth century onwards' (2004, p. 13). The 'encounter', then, is neither delineable as singular or episodic, as Mukharji puts it. Rather, multiple moments, overdetermined contexts, and multiple interfaces of segregation may be staged as encounters. Putting together what we learn from the detailing of process in these histories of medicine, we see a multilocal science as well as a movement in patronage of practitioners from families and old intellectual elites determined by caste and land hierarchies – hinted at in all these histories – to the colonial state. We see that this is hardly a linear movement and that the political jostling is in fact out of step, often, with the much more disaggregated therapeutic negotiations. We see the pharmaceutical arena becoming the site where the therapeutic negotiations became more visible, sharp, and conflictual, as Alavi, Mukharji, and Arnold all note, and that I will explore in the next chapter. We see, among these histories themselves, a difference in approach to the practitioner, with the native practitioner being seen as both an institutional (Alavi) and a social identity (Mukharji). We also see this time as one that sees as a separation and sharpening of hierarchies between folk and oral practices and textual traditions, as also between textual traditions of Unani and Ayurveda, with the more powerful among these carving sharper boundaries around themselves. Engagements across each of these practices and Western medicine also varied; in the event, a more visible outcome could be a sharpening segregation and conflict 'within' indigenous traditions, accompanied by the stigmatization and exclusion of non-codified practices. For Alavi, this lens, with both the Company and native practitioners as actors, is used to present colonialism as *not* the defining seat of power. In a focus on the late colonial period, Rachel Berger (2013) speaks of a local biopolitics that acts as a determinant of the increasing influence of Ayurveda, in the context of the dyarchy enacted in the 1930s. This making of modern Ayurveda is, I suggest, located in the making of the heterogeneous abject – the subaltern, the non-knowledgeable, the *dai*; and it is in understanding the manner in which that abjectness is refigured, in the form of an unskilled link worker, that the closing arguments of this book are located.

Notes

1 Shapin explains this best when he speaks of 'boundary-speech, including the vocabulary of 'extrinsic/intrinsic', ... as instrumentalities actively used to maintain social and cultural realities, to shift them in some desired direction, to say 'good' and 'bad'. He further traces the 'institutionalization of such speech into allegedly distinct and ideologically charged ways of analysing the nature of science and its mode of change' (1992, pp. 335–336).

2 The education primarily considered essential to improve the character of the native was literary; an interesting throwback to Enlightenment debates around morality, where a prominent counter-Enlightenment thinker like de Bonald commented on the exactitude of the physical sciences without the agency of man that declared their inferiority. For De Bonald, '[i]f modern society were to abandon the natural sciences no noticeable disorder would ensue; if the propagation of the principles of Christian morality with the aid of the social sciences were to cease, however, society would be plunged into moral and political chaos' (de Bonald paraphrased in Lepenies, 1988, p. 11). De Bonald finds an answer to this dilemma in a closer relationship between the literary and scientific disciplines; clearly, here mathematical and scientific disciplines were seen as a non-starter as far as moral development were concerned. This is a useful perspective to possibly situate the motivations, in addition to the need to create a class of Indians educated in English, for the reduced importance of science in educational policy in the Raj till the 1870s, as Kumar notes.

3 I will offer a detailed discussion of the hybridity framework in the latter part of the chapter. For now, it is relevant to state that hybridity spelt, for all parties dissatisfied with earlier explanations of colonialism, a different account of hegemony in general – one where the dominant was not completely triumphant, now or ever, but held resistance embedded in its core. Homi Bhabha, in his *Location of Cultures*, provided a detailed delineation of this framework in 1993, and most postcolonial scholars have since taken from his work.

4 I will provide a detailed picture of the Needhamian account of science in the next section, saying for now that simply put, the Needhamian account proposes a view of the universality of science, arrived at through different routes in different cultures.

5 'Orientalism and liminality suggested to colonial scientists that it was actually in this Indian tropical site that science might attain its true enlightenment' (59).

6 'For that interpretation of national life, past and present, without which the citizen cannot rightly regulate his conduct, the indispensable key is – Science. Alike for the most perfect production and highest enjoyment of art in all its form, the needful preparation is still – Science. And for purposes of discipline – intellectual, moral, religious – the most

efficient study is – Science … Necessary and eternal as are its truths, all science concerns all mankind for all times' (Sircar, 1899, quoted in Chakrabarti, p. 151).

7   'Science had a higher and nobler claim than the narrow, utilitarian, Benthamite one … Do not confound Science with technical education in the industrial arts … let every step of science education be explained by experiments, for science to be effectually learnt should be learnt in the laboratory' (Sircar, 1976, quoted in Chakrabarti, 2004, p. 161).

8   Thus reviving this organic tradition from within the West was part of the picture – work by neo-vitalists like Geddes, etc. would be consonant, in this frame, with Bose's work; by helping '"voiceless" plants speak, Bose appeared to restore the lost mysticism of science, to "humanize" its mechanical worldview' (211). And among the nationalists, there was P.C. Ray who talked of the possibility of a 'civilizational synthesis and the universality of science' (222), further drawing connections between ancient Greece and India.

9   'This also explains Bose's transformation from a physicist in 1896–7, to a plant physiologist, and then to an 'Indian' scientist by the 1900s [who worked on] the demonstration of the universality of irritability in all living tissues' (203–9).

10 'Colonial exploitation as the model for the progress of science, capitalist colonialism as the accumulation of knowledge – such was the representation of history in discourse' (Prakash, 1999, p. 67).

11 '[T]he strength of his ideas lies particularly in their ability to locate a continuous mutation and immanent critique within Orientalist discourse. Thus, resistance can be located within the hegemonic site itself and often unexpectedly at the very core of it. The very enunciation of it as a discourse of power was through dislocations, constant loss, and gain of authority' (Chakrabarti, 2004, p. 241).

12 Using the framework, Prakash presents both colonialism as a discourse that had to present itself from within the particular and that exercised power through such an estrangement, as also nationalism as a fragmented discourse that seeks 'nationness' through rationality and universality yet is disturbed by the unresolved figure of the subaltern.

13 It would be interesting here to note actor-network theories like those of Latour that grapple with a somewhat similar problem – bringing in arbitrariness, but not clear on what provides closure. For Latour, however, hegemony is not the kind of problem Prakash and others set up for themselves, although he does refer to networks of power.

14 '[T]he social theory of science … dissolves the distinction between the social and the cognitive, and retains the possibility of a revolutionary critique and revision of scientific practice. Social epistemology on the other hand entertains the possibility of dialogue between the scientific community and the community of sociologists of science who apparently threaten the former. … The present work does not strictly distinguish between social theory and social epistemology, but since it is positioned as one variant of the post-colonial theory of science, it is programmatically proximate to the social theory of science' (7–8).

15 Historian of science George Basalla, who set out his model in a paper titled 'The Spread of Western Science' (1967–8). The model, being contemporaneous with economic theories of development like Rostow's, offering latecomers like the newly independent nations in the non-West a grid to frame their material, and coming at a time when the optimism residing in science was high, obviously carried legitimacy at the time it was put out (Raina, 2003, p. 179). Basalla's model was also contemporaneous with, and may have drawn from, the centre-periphery model in economics. Centre-periphery is a binary framework used in economics to formulate the linkage between nations. It was presumed that the centre referred to the metropolitan or developed nation states while periphery referred to the underdeveloped countries. The relationship between these was so articulated that the subordination of the periphery was ensured and a flow of surplus value to the centre guaranteed. There are numerous varieties of this model, which was particularly strong among Latin American nations. While Marxists were prominent thinkers

of the centre-periphery models, some non-Marxists too (especially trade theorists who argued that the structure of trade was construed in favour of the centre) were part of it (Chakrabarti & Cullenberg, 2000).

16 Joseph Needham, chemist and historian of science.

17 This refers to 'Needham's idea that the history of science of a region was integrated with its social, environmental, and economic history' (Raina, 2003, p. 148), and further, that 'similar social processes across civilizations either promote or deter the progress of science' (p. 150).

18 Chakrabarti's work too would be reminiscent of this model, and Prakash steps out of it only by befuddling the temporal connection between colonial and nationalist science.

19 Here we find implicit continuities between Bernal and Needham, as also with other historians of science, in whose work science as value-neutral knowledge took the shape of a moral commitment and performed the function of a reaffirmation of the West; a function that seemed to take up on the crisis of humanism resulting from the two world wars. The two projects, then, could be seen as complementing each other in this sense.

20 'Religion is concerned with the preservation of "eternal" truth, while with art it is individual performance ... [t]he scientist, on the other hand, is always deliberately striving to change accepted truth' (43). As such, 'scientific temper' also became the counterpoint to 'culture' and restrictive traditions, seen often as coincidental in these movements.

21 As Raina puts it, Needham was the inspiration for the '"high church" of science studies in India ... whilst the "low church" drew capital from the Bernalist one' (Raina, 2003, p. 146).

22 Where science is born in Western Europe through a scientific revolution.

23 As is evident in the title of the introductory chapter of *Alternative Sciences* – 'Alien Insiders' (italics mine).

24 These scientists were neither 'innocent admirers of Eastern mysticism, nor were they innocent of the philosophical basis of modern science' (13).

25 There is a conflation happening here – between scientific and medical discourse. On the surface, it would seem that the clinical relation itself brings in the element of subjectivity to make for a uniquely individualized discipline. The point could be made that it is a unique 'technology of the self' where practice determines results more than any fixed theory. Foucault has, however (1994), shown beyond reasonable doubt that this *'restraint* of clinical discourse (its rejection of theory, its abandonment of systems, its lack of a philosophy; all so proudly proclaimed by doctors) reflects the non-verbal conditions on the basis of which it can speak: the common structure that carves up and articulates what is seen and what is said'. (xix). In other words, the discourse of medicine, while hardly being a simple confrontation of a gaze and a silent body, neither is a liberal contract between 'one man and another'; it simply sets up the individual in an objective frame.

References

Acharya, P. (1995, April 1). Bengali 'bhadralok' and educational development in 19th century Bengal. *Economic and Political Weekly, 30*(131), 670–673.

Achuthan, A. (2017). *Feminism and science: Present-day notes for a feminist standpoint epistemology* (Vol. 2, pp. 147–174). New Delhi: SAGE Publications.

Alavi, S. (2008). *Islam and healing: Loss and recovery of an Indo-Muslim medical tradition, 1600–1900.* Hampshire: Palgrave Macmillan.

Arnold, D. (2004a). Race, place and bodily difference in early nineteenth-century India. *Historical Research, 77*(196), 254–273.

Arnold, D. (2004b). *Science, technology and medicine in colonial India* (The New Cambridge History of India, Vol. 5). Cambridge: Cambridge University Press.

Arnold, D. (2013). Nehruvian science and postcolonial India. *Isis, 104*(2), 360–370.

Arnold, D. (2015). *The tropics and the traveling gaze: India, landscape, and science, 1800–1856*. Seattle and London: University of Washington Press.

Basalla, G. (1967). The spread of Western science: A three-stage model describes the introduction of modern science into any non-European nation. *Science, 156*(3775), 611–622.

Batabyal, R. (2005, August 27–September 2). Who the 'bhadralok' was. *Economic and Political Weekly, 40*(35), 3834–3836.

Berger, R. (2013). *Ayurveda made modern: Political histories of indigenous medicine in Northern India, 1900–1955*. New York: Palgrave Macmillan.

Bernal, J. D. (1939). *The social function of science*. London: George Routledge & Sons Ltd.

Bernal, J. D. (1969). Science in history: Volume 1. *The emergence of science. Preface to the third edition [1965]*. United Kingdom: Penguin Books.

Bhabha, H. (1994). *The location of culture*. London: Routledge

Brown, J. M. (1974). *The Bengali Bhadralok: An example of competition and collaboration in the nineteenth century* (Doctoral dissertation). Kansas State University.

Canguilhem, G. (2005). The object of the history of sciences. In G. Gutting (Ed.), *Continental philosophy of science* (pp. 198–207). Malden, Oxford and Victoria: Blackwell Publishing.

Chakrabarti, P. (2004). *Western science in modern India: Metropolitan methods, colonial practices*. New Delhi: Permanent Black.

Chakrabarti, A. K., & Cullenberg, S. (2000). *Development and class transition in India: A new perspective*. Department of Economics, University of California, Riverside.

Chakrabarty, D. (2000). A small history of subaltern studies. In H. Schwarz & S. Ray (Eds.), *A companion to postcolonial studies* (pp. 467–485). Malden, Oxford and Victoria: Blackwell Publishers.

Chatterjee, P. (2010). *Empire and nation: Selected essays*. New York: Columbia University Press.

Chattopadhyaya, D. P. (1959). *Lōkayata: A study in ancient Indian materialism*. New Delhi: People's Publishing House.

Chattopadhyaya, D. P. (2011). General introduction. In U. Dasgupta (Ed.), *Science and modern India: An institutional history, C. 1784–1947*. Project of History of Science, Philosophy and Culture in Indian Civilization (PHISPC), Indian Council of Philosophical Research, Vol XV, part 4, New Delhi: Pearson.

Chawla, J. (1994). *Child-bearing and culture: Women centered revisioning of the traditional midwife: The dai as a ritual practitioner*. New Delhi: Indian Social Institute.

Dalmiya, V. (2002). Why should a knower care? *Hypatia, 17*(1), 34–52.

Dalmiya, V., & Alcoff, L. (1993). Are old wives' tales justified? In L. Alcoff & E. Potter (Eds.), *Feminist epistemologies* (pp. 217–244). New York and London: Routledge.

Dutt, U. C. (1877). *The materia medica of the hindus: Compiled from Sanskrit medical works*. Thacker, Spink.

Forbes, G. H. (2005). *Women in colonial India: Essays on politics, medicine, and historiography*. New Delhi: DC Publishers.

Foucault, M. (1970). *The order of things: An archaeology of the human sciences*. London: Tavistock Publications.

Foucault, M. (1979). *Discipline and punish*. New York: Vintage Books.

Foucault, M. (1990). *The history of sexuality: An introduction*. Knopf New York: Doubleday Publishing Group.

Foucault, M. (1994). *The birth of the clinic: An archaeology of medical perception*. New York: Knopf Doubleday Publishing Group.

Gandhi, L. (1998). *Postcolonial theory: A critical introduction*. New South Wales: Columbia University Press.

Gupta, C. (2005). *Sexuality, obscenity, community: Women, Muslims, and the Hindu public in colonial India*. New Delhi: Orient Blackswan.

Haraway, D. J. (2004). *The Haraway Reader*. Routledge: New York and London.

Haraway, D. (2020). Situated knowledges: The science question in feminism and the privilege of partial perspective. In C. R. McCann, E. Ergun & S. K. Kim (Eds.), *Feminist theory reader: Local and global perspectives* (pp. 303–310). United States: Routledge.

Harding, S. G. (Ed.). (2004). *The feminist standpoint theory reader: Intellectual and political controversies*. New York and London: Routledge.

Harrison, M. (2009). Racial Pathologies: Morbid anatomy in British India, 1770–1850. In B. Pati & M. Harrison (Eds.), *The social history of health and medicine in colonial India* (pp. 173–194). London and New York: Routledge.

Iggers, G., & Edward, W. Q. (2008). *A global history of modern historiography*. London and New York: Routledge.

Jaggi, O. P. (2000). *Medicine in India: Modern period*. Project of History of Science, Philosophy and Culture in Indian Civilization (PHISPC), Indian Council of Philosophical Research, Vol IX, Part I. New Delhi: Oxford University Press.

Kuhn, T. S. (1970). *The structure of scientific revolutions* (Vol. 111). Chicago: University of Chicago Press.

Kumar, D. (1991). Colonial science: A look at the Indian experience. In *Science and empire: Essays in the Indian context (1700–1947)* (pp. 6–12). New Delhi: Anamika Prakashan.

Kumar, D. (1997). *Science and the Raj*. New Delhi: Oxford University Press.

Kumar, D. (2000, May–June). Science and society in colonial India: Exploring an agenda. *Social Scientist, 28*(5/6), 24–46.

Kumar, D. (2006). *Science and the Raj: A study of British India*. New Delhi: Oxford University Press.

Kumar, N. (2012). *Gender and science: Studies across cultures*. New Delhi: Foundation Books.

Latour, B. (2007). *Reassembling the social: An introduction to actor-network-theory*. Oxford and New York: Oxford University Press.

Lepenies, W. (1988). *Between literature and science: The rise of sociology* (Vol. 10). Cambridge University Press.

Mandler, P. (2004). The problem with cultural history. *Cultural and Social History, 1*(1), 94–117.

Moitra, S. (2017). Reading together: "Communitarian reading" and women readers in colonial Bengal. *Hypatia, 32*(3), 627–643.

Mukharji, P. B. (2009). *Nationalizing the body: The medical market, print and Daktari Medicine*. London, New York and New Delhi: Anthem Press.

Mukharji, P. B. (2016). *Doctoring traditions: Ayurveda, small technologies, and braided sciences*. Chicago, University of Chicago Press

Nair, S. P. (2022). *Chromosome woman, nomad scientist: EK Janaki Ammal, A life 1897–1984*. London: Routledge India.

Nandy, A. (1980). *Alternative sciences: Creativity and authenticity in two Indian scientists* (No. 4). Mumbai: Allied Publishers.

Nandy, A. (1995). *Alternative sciences: Creativity and authenticity in two Indian scientists* (2nd ed.), Oxford and New York: Oxford University Press.

Nandy, A. (1999). *The Savage Freud: And other essays on possible and retrievable selves*. India, New Delhi: Oxford University Press.

Needham, J. (1978). Address to the opening session of the XV international congress of the history of science, Edinburgh, 11 August 1977. *The British Journal for the History of Science, 11*(2), 103–113.

Needham, J., & Ronan, C. A. (1978). *The shorter science and civilisation in China: Volume 1*. Cambridge: Cambridge University Press.

Pickering, A. (1993). The mangle of practice: Agency and emergence in the sociology of science. *American Journal of Sociology, 99*(3), 559–589.

Pickering, A. (2010a). *The mangle of practice*. Chicago and London: University of Chicago Press.

Pickering, A. (Ed.). (2010b). *Science as practice and culture.* Chicago and London: University of Chicago Press.

Prakash, G. (1994). Subaltern studies as postcolonial criticism. *The American Historical Review, 99*(5), 1475–1490.

Prakash, G. (1999). *Another reason: Science and the imagination of modern India.* Princeton and New Jersey: Princeton University Press.

Prakash, G. (2010). Subaltern studies as postcolonial criticism. In A. Singh & S. Mohapatra (Eds.), *Indian political thought: a reader* (pp. 215–226). London and New York: Routledge.

Prakash, G., & Haynes, D. (Eds.) (1991). *Contesting power: Resistance and everyday social relations in South Asia.* New Delhi: Oxford University Press.

Rahman, A. (1996). Science and social movements: Bhakti and Sufi movements, 10th -18th C. Unpublished Manuscript.

Raina, D. (2003). *Images and contexts: The historiography of science and modernity in India.* New Delhi: Oxford University Press.

Raina, D. (2012). Decolonisation and the entangled histories of science and philosophy in India. *Polish Sociological Review, 178*(2), 187–201.

Raina, D., & Habib, S. I. (1996). The moral legitimation of modern science: Bhadralok reflections on theories of evolution. *Social Studies of Science, 26*(1), 9–42.

Ray, P. C. (1909). *A History of Hindu Chemistry from the Earliest Times to the Middle of the Sixteenth Century, A.D* (Vols. I and II). Calcutta: Williams and Norgate.

Sadgopal, M. (2009, April 18–24). Can maternity services open up to the indigenous traditions of midwifery? *Economic and Political Weekly, 44*(16), 52–59.

Sarkar, B. K. (1918). *Hindu achievements in exact science: A study in the history of scientific development.* Longmans, London: Green and Company.

Seal, B. N. (1915). *The positive sciences of the ancient Hindus.* London: Longmans, Green and Co.

Sehrawat, S. (2014). *Colonial medical care in North India: Gender, state, and society, C. 1830–1920.* New York: Oxford University Press

Shapin, S. (1992). Discipline and bounding: The history and sociology of science as seen through the externalism-internalism debate. *History of Science, 30*(4), 333–369.

Singer, C. (1952). *Technology and history* (L. T. Hobhouse Memorial Trust Lecture No. 21). London: Oxford University Press.

Sivaramakrishnan, K. (2006). Old potions, new bottles: Recasting indigenous medicine in colonial Punjab (1850–1945). *New Perspectives in South Asian History* (Vol.12). Hyderabad: Orient Longman.

Snowden, F. M. (2019). *Epidemics and society: From the black death to the present.* New Haven and London: Yale University Press.

Sur, A. (2001). Dispersed radiance: Women scientists in CV Raman's laboratory. *Meridians: Feminism, Race, Transnationalism, 1*(2), 95–127.

Van Hollen, C. (2003). *Birth on the threshold: Childbirth and modernity in South India.* Berkeley, Los Angeles and London: University of California Press.

Visvanathan, S. (2003). Progress and violence. In A. Lightman, D. Sarewitz, & C. Desser (Eds.), *Living with the genie: Essays on technology and the quest for human mastery* (pp. 157–180). Washington: Island Press.

Woolf, D. (2006). Of nations, nationalism, and national identity: Reflections on the historiographic organisation of the past. In Q. E. Wang & F. L. Fillafer (Eds.), *The many faces of clio: Cross-cultural approaches to historiography, essays in honor of George G. Iggers.* New York and Oxford: Berghahn Books.

Woolf, D. R. (2005). From hystories to the historical: five transitions in thinking about the past, 1500–1700. *Huntington Library Quarterly, 68*(1–2), 33–70.

3 Revisiting the clinical encounter I

Sites and meanings of an emerging indigenous therapeutics

Introduction

I focussed in Chapter 2 on how scholars of science and medicine have, while marking the 19th century as significant for Western science and medicine in India, spoken of this presence as neither a one-way imperialist exercise nor a simple clash of civilizations. Somewhat less visible in the dominant scholarship, but discussed nonetheless, has been the recognition that what is called the colonial encounter needs to be located both spatially and temporally, and that, in addition to the experience of institutions in the 19th century, there are negotiations that occupy a variety of spaces outside the expert domain (Bala, 2019); that the consolidation of indigenous therapeutic language occurs in the public sphere (Gupta, 2005); that the very idea, borders and boundaries, of the expert domain as the core of the therapeutic space, in fact, emerges and consolidates during this century in India. What has also been partly missing is an attention to the conflicts and negotiations in a somewhat messy discourse around the indigenous (Girija, 2017), and on the ways in which these ultimately transition, alongside institutionalized biomedicine, into a dominant indigenous and its excluded others. In fact, Mukharji (2009) observes that the scholarship around the indigenous and the Western in histories of medicine have existed as two fairly independent strands, thus consolidating the spirit of an encounter or at least the notion of two, independent, systems.

I focus in this chapter on broadly four kinds of medical writing that relate to or prescribe childbirth, located at the interface of the institution and its outside, that emerge in the 19th century and the early part of the next in the subcontinent. I focus on these texts partly because of their ubiquity in the archive, and therefore their possible volume in circulation during the period. I also see these texts as occupying a quasi-expert domain, one that emerges after the advent of vernacular presses in the early 1800s (Ghosh, 2006) as a marker of an early claim to expert therapeutics intertwined with populist nationalism, with Western medical vocabulary woven with perhaps a newly 'indigenous' vocabulary through experimental forms of writing. Examining both the authorship and content of these texts, and the debates around language, clinical and therapeutic validity as well as origin, this chapter attempts to delineate some of the contexts of emergence of modern therapeutic language in the Indian context. In so doing, I also re-examine the nature of what has been termed the colonial encounter, suggesting that the conflicts listed under

DOI: 10.4324/9780367824051-3

the label were not necessarily fought entirely on clinical expert domain or within or at the margins of the institution but in a far more disaggregated space of old and newly emerging livelihoods, language, community, and changing systems of patronage, outside the institution. While some of this argument has been explored in earlier scholarship, I hope to supplement this with a closer look at the texts I mention, as also to offer newer perspectives through these in tracing the emergence of a language of the therapeutic, where institutionalization seems to be claiming both the indigenous and Western. This will also mean an exploration of the exercises of vernacularization in this period. I also read the texts of one kind or another in the context of medical publishing in the 19th century across the subcontinent. The texts I examine are by no means a comprehensive reflection of the discourse of the period; however, I explore them chiefly as a way to revisit some of the claims made around the encounter. I also focus, in later sections of the chapter, on the indigenous drugs debate as it played out at the cusp of the 19th to 20th centuries and the native dispensaries as another site where 'native' medicine interacts and flourishes alongside British medicine. Both of these connect developments in the institution with those in the formal and informal political domain, and I try to trace an indigenous therapeutic public sphere through them.

Reading text and context

There is a wealth of scholarship that has read 'indigenous medicine' in the period I am exploring. Poonam Bala stays with the category 'indigenous' to speak of the emergence and 'place of indigenous healers' (2019, p. 1) in spaces under colonial rule and also of the rise of indigenous elites like the Parsi community in Bombay and the *bhadralok* in Bengal, who in different ways, responded to the prospects for Western medical education brought in by the Empire. While the Parsis were great patrons of English medical education, Bala suggests that the *bhadralok* became a source of nationalist resistance, particularly through the promotion of indigenous medicine. Bala points to events between 1905 and 1909, with 'repeated calls for maintaining synonymity between the national movement and cultural revivalism' (2012, p. 5), that bring this about, resulting in the emergence of a 'new medico-cultural identity for Indian medicine' in the 19th and early 20th centuries (p. 1). This is also in the context of the increasing withdrawal of government support for indigenous practice and education in the second half of the 19th century (Bala, 2009), a policy that sharpens in the first decades of the 20th century, with *shifakhanas* and Ayurvedic dispensaries being declared illegal, and practitioners like the *dai* being forced into training or deemed unfit, as we will see in the next chapter. Other scholarship takes a methodologically different approach, seeing colonial effects or negotiations in a more layered manner; it follows that the category 'indigenous' becomes more difficult to define here. Mukharji focusses, for example, in his account of Ayurveda, on 'individual biographies to build a historico-sociological map ... of the social groupings of the actors engaged in the transformation of Ayurveda at the cusp of the nineteenth and twentieth centuries' (2016, p. 37) in Bengal, in an act of 'thick contextualization' (p. 36). Kavita Sivaramakrishnan

looks at the case of colonial Punjab, where the interaction between colonial stric-
tures and physician networks results not in a straightforward indigenous Hindu-
dominant Ayurveda but in a variety of effects, including a community of Sikh
practitioner networks who attempt to formulate a *Desi Baidik* (Sivaramakrishnan,
2006). Jean Langford, in her anthropological work, speaks of the emergence of
modern Ayurveda as a system through the extrusion of earlier categorizations that
failed to offer closure (2002). Yet other scholarship has focussed on Ayurveda's
travel into modernity using these same texts (Berger, 2013). We have discussed
Alavi's work on Unani in the previous chapter, where the temporal location of the
encounter, the actors involved, and the effects, all seem different depending on the
entry point she makes. Each of these exercises provides explanatory clusters for
the print literature of this period. This differential splicing of the available archive
has been part of the interpretative exercise, too, and I will attempt to read both with
and against the grain, to mark not only presences but absences in the archive and its
previous readings. I heed here the methodological warning in Mukharji's and other
scholarship, which warns against an ambition to generalize about or 'find' specific
moments of emergence for what seems to be, for example, contemporary-dominant
Ayurveda as a 'Hindu science' – an ambition that in today's authoritarian climate
nearly seems urgent and necessary. I do, however, attempt to see what the absences
and presences, and the text, may have to say to the general.

As I read some of the archived texts for this and later chapters, positing them
alongside the secondary scholarship, I am aware that these are located in northern
Indian contexts, primarily in languages now recognizable as Bangla and Hindi.
These are also not necessarily representative of these contexts. I do not attempt,
therefore, to make generalizable claims from them; rather, I read these as a way to
unpack existing generalizations, or, in some cases, link with available analyses in
the scholarship.

What I attempt here is to cite and understand the texts in question as extra-
institutional and explore their relationship to the institution, as well as to multiple
events that consolidate therapeutic work in the period in question. As such, I draw
from frameworks of critical discourse analysis to see some of the overlaps and
interlocutions across what are called systems of medicine. In reading against the
grain, I see the performance and emergence of what I call a canonical indigenous
in the vocabulary of 'systems', and the erasures performed in this emergence. The
texture and language of each of these texts, the passing references, become vital
to delineating these movements. I do, however, find valuable the splicing of the
archive that the previous scholarship has done and attempt to engage with them
during the course of these explorations.

Texts and the institution of a therapeutic language and space

The available scholarship has classified texts of the 19th to 20th centuries and earlier in several ways. Gupta (2005) identifies 'instruction manuals, dialogues with
Western medicine, cookery books, popular pamphlets, advertisements, popular
magazines' (p. 21). Berger (2013) looks at

three specific genres of writing ... [in order to] evaluate the ways in which medical discussions pervaded the field. Firstly, ... formalized, Ayurvedic writing, aimed at an audience specifically and primarily interested in consuming this information. Secondly, ... *Grhinis*, or domestic guides, and other writing aimed at women and dealing with the household. Finally, ... discussions of medicine, gender and the body in popular advertising.

(p. 76)

Berger also talks of three kinds of Ayurvedic texts – the medical pamphlet, the text book [both formal and for literate audiences], and a third – it is unclear if these are the home guides. Exercising caution against 'finding' pre-existing groupings of literature in the archive, I engage in an interpretative exercise with the following broad classification I apply to texts that float up from the archive – an Ayurveda made easy text, a therapeutic ready reckoner for the public, a reform-oriented text, and texts specifically approaching childbirth practice – all at the cusp of the 19th to 20th centuries.

Ayurveda made easy

In 1891, a text titled *Susruta Sanhita*, presented as *Bhashanuvaad* (translated into Hindi), was published from Lucknow at the Munshi Naval Kishore press. It speaks of Susruta as the legendary and reputed Vaidyak who is followed and revered by all Vaids and 'itar purush' (mean men – a metaphor for castes considered inferior) alike and as a text that is considered equal to the Vedas, and therefore a text that must be available as a ready reckoner to all practitioners and even 'lesser' men. The text has been, on account of being in Sanskrit, hitherto '*sarvasadharan ko alabhya*' – unavailable to the general public, and this translation is advertised as filling that gap, as also being different from other compilations in circulation. The name of the translator, Pandit Ravidatt Vaid, is inserted on the cover page after an ode to the publisher for having spared no expense to make the text available to the *sarvasadharan*. Munshi Naval Kishore, the publisher, is also praised for his *Svadeshta* – nationalist – attachment to his people. The text also begins with a list of other Vaidyak books of this kind, including the 'last word' on *Vaidyak shiksha*, detailing of disease and treatments, methods of acquiring and administering drugs, compilations from Charaka, Susruta, Lolimbaraj, and other Sanskrit texts, translated into *sugam aajmaye hue nuskhe* – home remedies presented in an accessible fashion. Pandit Radhakrishn, Shankar Prasad, Pandit Keshav Prasad, and his son Nayansukh are some of the authors cited. There is a common thread of lucidity of text that is advertised here, and a particularly attractive form – of *chhand* or *doha* (verse) – that is offered as a common format. The text itself is sectioned into *Adhyays* or chapters, focussing, among others, on *garbhavakranti*, *garbhavyakaran*, and *garbhini vyakaran* (description/discussion of pregnancy, the womb, the pregnant woman), where mention of the preferred kind of woman as *dai* in the *sutika griha* also comes up.

In 1900, another text called *Aushadhikriya*, the 31st in a series titled *Aryabhishek*, priced at four annas, was put out by a Bombay printer, with an ode to Charaka, the legendary surgeon, on its cover. The text itself was bilingually structured into Sanskrit and Hindi, with verses from the *Charaka Samhita*, an older/ancient text often attributed to Charaka, being followed by explanatory paragraphs in Hindi. This text has, among others, sections on conception, pregnancy, and childbirth, and explains how conception occurs, the mood to be induced for sexual relations[1] or conception,[2] foetal personhood and presumed character of the infant-to-be-born, care during pregnancy, how the gender of the infant may be predicted, when to expect disability, the process of childbirth, and so on. There is mention of the *dai* here too, in prescriptions for the *aturghar* or *sutika griha* (the birthing room) in preparation for childbirth. The stated reference for these prescriptions is the text of the Atharva Veda – one among a collection of texts referred to as a source of knowledge or 'manuals of rituals and commentaries on these' (Thapar, 2002, p. 132), written during the pre-Aryan and Aryan period, to which contemporary Hinduism is said to owe formal allegiance (Chattopadhyaya, 1992, 7th edition). Also referred are the prescriptions for attendance during childbirth – by older women of the household, those who have experienced multiple childbirths, those who are favourably disposed towards the woman in labour, and *brahmans* (those deemed the highest, priestly caste). Prescriptions for particular movements for the woman in difficult labour are presented over alternative strategies prescribed in other texts.

In 1901, another text – '*The Ayurvedic system of Medicine, or, an exposition, in English, of Hindu Medicine as occurring in Charaka, Susruta, Bagbhata, and other authoritative works, ancient and modern, in Sanskrit*', authored by Kabiraj Nagendra Nath Sen Gupta, was published by Keval Ram Chatterjee at the Nagendra Printing Works of Lower Chitpur Road, Calcutta, running into three editions till 1907. Nagendranath, who at different points signs off as Nagendranath Sen or Nagendranath Sen Gupta, describes himself on the cover page as Vernacular Licentiate in midwifery and surgery, as a member of several societies in Paris and London, as also author of several texts on medicine, *kabiraji*, and a teacher and examiner of 'Hindu Medicine'. The text begins by tracing the origin of the Hindu nation's attention to medicine and disease to the by-then fragmented and not fully available Atharva Veda. Sen Gupta says this is followed by Punarvasu of the 'race of Atri', and his six disciples; he infers that the available treatises in question-and-answer form were arranged by Agnivesa, and put together by Charaka. These texts are considered as a resource not only of therapeutics but of several other subjects, including 'predestinarianism and its bearing on disease and treatment, the nature of the Soul, what is meant by its birth, rebirth, and Emancipation' (p. iii), and so on – 'the method of the Rishis' (ibid), as Sen Gupta goes on to say. This method may not pay 'much attention to rigid principles of classification' (p. iii), and Bacon is actually invoked to indicate that knowledge may not necessarily be augmented by 'peremptory reduction ... into arts and methods' (p. iiii). Nagendranath goes on to talk of Susruta, the other famed surgeon, 'pupil of Divodasa ... who was believed to have been an incarnation of ... Dhanwantari, who had discovered the elixir that prevents death' (p. v), and makes particular mention of Midwifery as a department where apparently the world had not progressed beyond what this text carries.

Nagendranath, who adopts the honorific *Kabiraj*, or *Vaidya shastri*, on different occasions, has already been a prolific writer; Bangla (*Baidyak Shiksha*, 1900) and Hindi texts on the same material, making the same claims, are available under his authorship prior to this. Compilations in his name are also available, including revised editions of his works in the present. As late as 1960, for example, several years after the 1901 English text, we find a text in Hindi, the *Vaidyak Shiksha*, claiming the legacies of Charaka, Susruta, Vagbhatta, and several others, in a first edition priced at two rupees and naming Sen Gupta as the compiler. In this text, which offers itself as a practitioner's guide, however, a variety of Western classifications is in place – of types of pulse, for instance, with the English terms written in *Devanagari* script. This text goes on to detail manifestations and treatment of ailments, including *streerog* (diseases of women – implied as reproductive), of pregnancy, labour, childbirth, and infancy, with references in English script and terminology. There are detailed illustrations, in addition, on female reproductive anatomy. In these and the directive sections on breastfeeding, infant care, and care during pregnancy, the content begins to look more and more like the Western medical text, with surgical procedures for extracting the foetus in stillbirth like craniotomy, perforators, etc., detailed. Many of the additional directives – on remedies and modes of treatment, like *maalish* (massage) or *kadha* (decoctions for throat and respiratory ailments), for instance – are attributed to the Ayurvedic original. There is, in fact, a near-defensive detailing of precautions and remedies that are presented as *indigenous* expert advice, accompanied by a clear stating of differences yet core similarities between Hindu and Western medicine in understanding reproductive systems (p. 714). In the 1907 edition, Nagendranath states clearly that while 'thousands of years ago the Rishis studied almost all the plants that flourish in this country of continental proportions and discovered their medicinal properties … names they have given to many plants bespeak their principal characteristics' (1907, p. i); he goes on to detail this manner of naming through examples, 'there is poetry … in some of the names' (ibid), and thus 'Sanskrit nomenclature … is … a study for poets and scientists as well' (ii). This is a claim seeking to compensate, somewhat diffidently or tangentially, perhaps, for the acknowledged absence of botanical classificatory systems in 'Hindu medicine'. His text seems offered in subtle competition with the Western; Nagendranath Sen Gupta acknowledges Roxburgh and U.C. Dutt as the tall heroes of botany but expresses amazement that even these comprehensive texts have not achieved a full list of plants, so that '[w]e have been able to give the names of several plants which escaped the searching eyes of the great botanists of the west' (iii). The Western world is the stated audience for Nagendranath; his 'object is to place before the English-speaking world, and particularly before physicians and surgeons practising the western method of Medicine, the knowledge which the Rishis had of disease and its cure' (xviii).

Mukharji (2016) traces Nagendranath to one of three families that attained stature as Ayurvedic practitioners in Bengal, and in so doing, comments on the hereditary as well as perhaps exclusive feature of the occupation. Nagendranath's writing is clear enough on this; he talks in detail about the manner in which the teaching of Hindu medicine is familial or quasi-familial and therefore non-commercial, about therefore a 'few families of great reputation' being the case in Bengal, and positions himself as an author-practitioner within one of those. He also makes the case for the Vaidyas being the legitimate caste location for this occupation, often, by substitution, marking them as Brahmins, although that substitution has historically been a fraught one.[3] Through each of these borders and boundaries that Nagendranath draws for the practitioner, he also elevates them above the 'person of ordinary understanding ... [who] is not fit to receive the highly philosophical ideas of Godhead which the Vedanta inculcates' (p. xiv). In so doing, he seems to declare allegiance to the philosophical and not the religious meanings of 'Hindu', albeit an idealist and not materialist approach. He also marks the contexts of severely reduced patronage within which practitioners operate. It is within these constraints and contexts, then, and particular to Bengal, that Nagendranath builds the picture of early Hindu medicine, where the non-mention of opium is used to antedate the text to 'Mussalman' entry, and the detailing of diseases such as syphilis – marked as *Firangi roga* – associated with the entry of the Portuguese; an implicit association of 'outsider' presence and moral pollution seems in place here. A different set of claims is made with respect to British medicine, both through a declared familiarity with the language and through an active discussion of how Ayurvedic texts have alternate strategies to Western botanical classifications. Borders with Western medicine, then, are more porous than with others; the persuasion here being more in the nature of seeking equivalence through analogy than active difference. Whether this is a fresh argument for patronage is unclear. In looking at the popular texts in the next section, we will see if extra-institutional claims vary from this stance.

The practitioner as expert is at the centre of this *system* that is Hindu medicine for this author. There are, Nagendranath says, no colleges or hospitals for this learning; the teacher-student bond, built through blood and residential disciplehood, becomes the site of learning. From the lecture hall, to notes prepared across generations of students, to the patients whose bedside becomes the teaching space, to sourcing of and preparation of medicines, he builds a scaffolding of texts (Vedas), practitioners (Vaidya men), and tenets; thus, a *formal field of knowledge* is always already in place. There are criteria for who can become practitioners and authors of medical texts. There is thus a claim to non-institutional, experiential, yet exclusive and authoritative learning – for the positioning of this practitioner-as-expert. There is the building of a therapeutic vocabulary that claims both distinctness from and validity with respect to Western scientific criteria. There is, in addition, the invocation of this therapeutics as a *civilizational* discourse, so that, by being attentive to the legacies handed down by the Rishis, one finds a fountain of knowledge and detail more extensive than a Roxburgh, a Dr. Wise, or a U.C. Dutt – all named in the text – can hope to be. In placing the comparison in the past, Nagendranath Sen Gupta has converted it into a no-contest, an established superiority.

Everything that follows, then, consolidates this idea of an expert therapeutics with protocols and patterns. If Charaka's work is seen to be presented in eight volumes, Susruta's work seems to have the same pattern. *Kaya-chikitsakas* (physicians of the body) and *Salya-chikitsakas* (surgeons), with subgroups, have apparently been in existence even before these indeterminately dated texts. Those that followed did more to elucidate these texts than criticize them. In examining the theories of health and disease, Nagendranath advances, through comparison with Western scientific theories, the value and scientificity of the principles of disease in Hindu medicine, while indicating that the words used – *vata*/wind, *pitta*/bile and phlegm – may well be mistaken for their common-use meanings, a mistake to be laid at the door of the later 'framers of the Hindu system of medicine' (p. xxiv). Disease classifications – of mind and body, accidental and constitutional, and other lenses – are offered by Nagendranath, with a great deal of stress on causal explanations as available in the originary texts. Hindu medicines are also presented through various grids of classification attributed to Charaka and Susruta, as mineral, vegetable, and animal. Latin names of caustics are provided; measures indicated; 'indigenous' plants outside of Western pharmacopoeia are listed in the vernacular, while indigenous drug types – *Kacahara, Jwarahara, Trishnanigrahana*, for example – are written in English. Mukharji has spoken of the exotics discourse that *daktari* practitioners accessed in the early 1900s (2009, pp. 103–104); we see both this and the civilizational discourse I spoke of above at work here, alongside the equivalence-through-analogy impulse. In Nagendranath Sen Gupta's second volume, each 'Hindu medicine' is listed in Sanskrit but written in English script, the plants recognized in Western pharmacopoeia named in Latin, local, or indigenous use plants named in English, with attention to the Sanskrit and vernacular names being put in for the benefit of Indian students in the third volume. Directives for taking the medicine, which must be sourced in pure form and from the right sources, are often accompanied by additional directives relating to feeding of Brahmans or particular behaviours and sometimes are accompanied by the promise of male children, for instance. As far as diseases of women are concerned, puerperal diseases and 'Grahani' (1901, p. 754, in modern Ayurveda used to indicate gastro-intestinal disease) form the bulk of the ailments discussed, with additional benefits towards 'digestive fire' (ibid), and beauty (Pancha jiraka Guda ... 'helps the growth of the bosoms of women and makes their eyes as broad as lotus leaves', p. 752), being offered.[4]

My key focus here is on the attempt to seek equivalence, and the manner in which Hindu medicine as an identity is produced within this map. In fact, the very act of textualizing might be seen here as a source of equivalence. We see, through each of the micro-textual moves, the drawing of the borders and boundaries of legitimate practice, and that is why we take such a close look at the text. The naming of drug effects mentioned above is also a building into the episteme of practices, with a reiterative referencing of ancient texts and names. This writing is most confident when naming medicinal plants, modes of extraction, preparation, and administration of drugs. Later texts consolidate this, and it is in them that difference rather than equivalence becomes the strategy. My point in focussing on this time and texts, then, is also to open up, as Arnold and other scholars have, the notion of the 'colonial encounter' across historical time. This engagement will, as we will see in the popular text, open up across space too.

A great deal of space is devoted in the text to describing the processes of drug preparation, to be done by hand and basic technologies, and although the text is entirely directive and prescriptive, practice is brought alive, refocussed, again and again, on the practitioner. While the attempt at standardizing through weights and measures continues, the subtext of the 'good practitioner' is built up. With the paeans to method and classification in Hindu medicine, are also highlighted the tropes of harmony, knowledge of scriptures, knowledge of methods of drug preparation and administration, experience, and 'devotedness to the patient' (xxviii); and yet again, the 'physician [as] ... the chief cause' in treatment. The idea of the expert-practitioner, in possession of exclusive textual knowledge and skills, at the centre of a well-organized system, the product of a centuries-old civilization, is thus strengthened. Several added claims emerge through Nagendranath's and other texts. One is that of Bengal being the primary seat of some of these early texts. *Iti Bangiyah*, says Nagendranath, 'occurs more frequently than *Iti Pratichyah*' (1901, p. viii). We will see, in the next section, how this focus is both the entry and undoing of attempts to canonize Ayurveda, where the practitioner-as-expert is primary, but who can also be imitated.

Why, then, did Hindu medicine not flourish, on par with Western? Having established the credentials for an indigenous, codified system, with institutional analogs to the Western in the form of residential disciplehood, Nagendranath is able to mark the reasons for its non-dominance clearly. He cites the severely reduced patronage within which practitioners operate, resulting in an inability to procure material and prepare medicines, even for the poor, the 'course of national charity having been diverted under the influence of Western ideas' (xvi). Students are unable to access enough books, as non-Vaidyas or Englishmen alleged; although Nagendranath attributes this to the unwillingness of Brahmans to transmit knowledge to 'unfit' students, he does not take the next analytical step of marking this as control, rather interpreting it as a means of retaining the purity and standard of the knowledge. 'The fact is', he says, 'printing was unknown to the Hindus' (xiii), so that students had to copy out passages for themselves. Brahmans may have believed that the transfer of such knowledge through sale would result in its 'vanishing'. But the real worry is the prospect of knowledge transfer to persons 'of ordinary understanding', and Nagendranath goes on to justify the control of texts by Vaidya men since 'ordinary' persons were not 'fit to receive highly philosophical ideas of Godhead' (xiv) that might even lead him to 'abandon his old faith without being able to ... comprehend the higher truths of religion ... [in] such a work' (ibid). There is ample reference to what we know today to be caste practices of purity and pollution, alongside a bit of a nod to the language of public health. Components identified as necessary to drug preparation are listed as not to be ship-borne salt, for instance,[5] while *ghee* prescribed for some remedies must always be 'vaccine ghee', milk used must be vaccine milk – the possible reference here being to pasteurization. The 'quack' is also named in a note of desperation here as having 'set themselves up as healers ... without having read a page of the ancient or the modern treatises on Hindu Medicine' (xvi). And yet, there is, he says, a critical mass of 'duly qualified practitioners' (ibid). Another cause of ineffectiveness and consequent lack of faith in Ayurveda, says Nagendranath, would be that 'medicinal herbs and plants and roots should generally be obtained from the Himavat mountains ... this important direction is not … attended to' (ii, preface to the second volume, 1906), resulting in adulterated and ineffective preparations. This again can be kept in check by the hereditary tradition of learning, which follows not only textual directives but the practice of preceptorial mentorship. Mukharji traces the mechanisms of preceptorial kinship – the *guru-shishya parampara* or residential disciplehood – that operate through a 'reduced diversity of opinion within the preceptorial lineage', as also providing 'a handy constituency that could be readily mobilized in the cause of particular modernizing projects … [like] the Astanga Ayurveda College' (2009, p. 59). This form of kinship, then, is one of the ways in which legitimate practitioner identity and consensus within the community are generated through to the 20th century.

Extensive sections on *streerog*, *garbharaksha*, and *sutika* are available in all these texts. We will examine, in the next two chapters, the links with the ideas of womanhood, motherhood, and the nation that these texts also seem to feed into, and the extensive secondary literature on the subject, but it is useful here to explore the subjectivity of the male expert-practitioners as they speak on 'diseases of women' in the late 19th and early 20th centuries. Diseases of organs are listed with their vernacular/Sanskrit and English names – the equivalence principle. In juxtaposing these prescriptions with sexuality writings by men-*kabirajes* in this period, we see that, different from discourses in the late colonial period that focus almost exclusively on men and anxieties around masculinity (Botre & Haynes, 2017), here the entire focus is on women's bodies, conception, pregnancy, and childbirth. In the spirit of the other portions of the text, this writing too distinguishes itself from Western medical texts while at the same time mobilizing some of their language. It might be worthwhile to consider whether this had something to do with the colonial focus on women's status and childbirth, peaking around the time of the Lady Dufferin Fund and other schemes beginning in the late 1880s, evidence for which is to be found in the literature and government records of the time. While that discourse on maternal well-being develops in relation to these schemes, the texts I mention here seem to focus on the caste location, character of the *'dhatri'/dai*, as also the need for good women, healthy, fertile women, young women without overly sagging breasts, as wet-nurses, with these prescriptions on preferred bodies – open to the eye of the male physician – presented as a marker of good character. Alongside these, a focus on the lying-in room (p. 452), or the time of delivery 'from the ninth to the twelfth month' (p. 447) – as Western clinical diagnostic and intervention details – continues.

At the cusp of the 19th to 20th centuries, then, which is also the period of transition from Company to the Crown following the first war of independence in 1857, and with the advent of print technology in the colony, we see some manifestations of a discourse emerging around Ayurveda, in central, western, and eastern parts of the colony, that place the text at the centre of knowledge, the privileged-caste practitioner as the valid claimant and interpreter of the text, and the ancient Hindu past as a valid source for the practice. Hindu medicine reiteratively becomes a common-sense reference point in these texts. While codification is not complete, textuality is stressed. Both the mother and the *dai* figure appear through this male privileged-caste practitioner's gaze; the *dai* cannot be recognized as a practitioner in this framework. We have seen, in Chapter 2, in Seema Alavi's detailed exploration of the career of Unani during and after the early engagements between the Company and the Mughal empire, the Unani author-practitioner in contest with the British medical officer-author-teacher in the Calcutta Madrasa, with the latter proposing an order to the chaotic Unani world prior; the availability of Unani texts in Arabic rather than Persian being seen as a way to undermine social hierarchies and the control by a few families over the practice. Alavi discusses in depth the contests over language in this time in the therapeutic domain – Arabic and later Urdu as a carrier language for Western medical knowledge as languages of choice pushed by the administration. Breton, Superintendent of the Native Medical Institution set up in 1822, and Tytler, who taught medicine at the Calcutta Madrasa, disagree over whether Sanskrit or Arabic should be the language in which medicine was to be taught to the 'natives', and interacting with the *pandits* and the *hakims* respectively in the race to publish texts. The picture changes with the 1830s reforms in education and medical education, with the NMI being abolished, the setting up of the Calcutta Medical College in 1835, and the declaration of indigenous systems as unrecognized. It is in this context as well that the texts in this section need to be placed.

Scholarship around gender and nationalism has spoken of the links between nationalism, masculinity, and the private sphere as the site of spirituality and freedom and therefore control (Gupta, 2005; Chatterjee, 2019) in the colonial period. Uma Chakravarti (1989) has spoken of the caste-based nature of this control. I suggest that the period represented in the texts I have examined in this section seems to present a less consolidated picture – more in the nature of a claim to knowledge status than a position on gendering of the public-private dichotomy or the control over women. This allows for the idea of the encounter to be split temporally, as I have suggested earlier. We will see, in Chapter 4, if this ambivalence moves towards a more consolidated position vis-à-vis government policies on childbirth reform and the defunding of indigenous medical practice in later decades.

The Vaidyaksaar, or the ready reckoner

Texts representing *mananusar*, or 'as per', one or the other reputed physician, and following the legacies of various canonical texts, put out by authors/compilers taking the humble stance of bringing to the public, have been in circulation through the middle to late 19th century. One such text is the *Vaidyaksaar*, and the compiler Hiralal Mulazim Manve, in 1867, claiming to have put together the remedies as per one Janab Machhu Khan Sahib – the title Mulazim translating roughly into vassal or servant. It is offered 'merely' as a practitioner's guide and takes its legitimacy from the canon it seeks to represent. It offers remedies for feared miscarriages as well as methods for *garbha girana* (those seeking abortion).

Home remedies

A series of texts bringing together Ayurvedic and homoeopathic remedies, for and usable by women of the household, are also to be seen in the first decade or so of the 20th century in Bengal. I will explore, in Chapter 5, the place of women of the home as healers and the role of these texts in that discourse, but here I am more focussed on the texts themselves. *Homoeopathic mate streerog chikitsa,*[6] from Batokrishno Pal and Company, family owners of The Great Homoeopathic Hall, in 1924, is one of them. The text states, in its preface, that Hindu women are by nature *lajjasheela* (modest); they cannot submit to male or even modern educated women physicians, or the use of instruments. A book of this kind, presented in lucid language for practitioners, students, women of the family, or patients, therefore, is welcome. It is advertised as offering the same kinds of help that *Saral grihochikitsa* – another popular publication from the same company – did. Declaring an increased popularity for homoeopathy after a period of eclipse, its value for the laity, and even among educated women, the text goes on to list various diseases related to menstruation, as also details on anatomy and physiology. Advice relating to examination and treatments, as also prescriptions for married women, difficulties of labour and their remedies, are available. In this text too, like the avowedly more rigorous texts, disease terminologies are available in both English and Bangla scripts and languages. A unique feature of this text is that even some Bangla words that might be outside common usage are explained in common-use language. While the treatments for most of the illnesses described are homoeopathic drugs, the text has sections titled *Susruta mat* or *Charaka mat* (directives as per Susruta or Charaka) for employment of *Stanyadayini* (wet-nurses) and nurses for the infant (*Dhatri*) – of the same or *kulin* (of high birth) caste; these are to be young, of presentable features, of medium build, having firm breasts, having living children, of good character, selfless, among other directives. It is unclear whether this prescription is meant to keep infant nursing outside of livelihood options; if, in that case, this practice existed. Disease principles of *Vata-pitta,* typically considered the domain of Ayurveda, are also discussed in passing. Guidelines by one Dr. Fisher on the preferred disposition of an employed wet-nurse are also listed in both Bangla and English, as also the need for surveillance on her, and the preference for familiars for this. Here there is no debate on what is indigenous, rather the concern is as to what is accessible, and a related need for a public understanding of disease outside the expert domain. These texts provide a leaching of terminology outside the expert space, literally into the extended space of the household. Shinjini Das, in tracing the career of homoeopathy in colonial India, speaks of '[h]omoeopathic medicine's intimate entanglement with the institution of "family" in Bengal' (2019, p. 6) and the manner in which this was intertwined intimately with the market and production of vernacular texts by family firms. Das also goes on to explore homoeopathy's specific claim to an 'egalitarian medicine' (p. 9). Some of this claim to egalitarianism or proletarianization of medicine is visible through the tracing of the trajectories of publishers of the ready reckoner texts/ sellers of the drugs themselves; Batokrishno Pal, for example, is described in his biographies as a *Sadhu* (saint or ascetic) – one who left behind his family's occupation to enter pharmacy and set up The Great Homoeopathic Hall, and thus contributed to the 'improvement of the Bengalis' (Das, 2019, p. 58) who were otherwise seen as failures at business ventures and thus at nation-building. Figures like Pal had also broken into the Brahmin monopoly over textual knowledge production. Mukharji, writing on the indigenous drugs debate and the erasure of 'feminine medico-botanical knowledge' under the realm of the maternal (Mukharji, 2009, p. 208), details this. With the introduction of genres of '"Garhosthyo Chikitsha" (Family Medicine), "Bonoushodhi" (Herbal Medicine) and "Totka" (Simples)' (p. 207) into vernacular writing on medicine, and the symbolic elevation of women of the home as practitioners of this art, Mukharji reflects on how their labour is erased; we may read this as a drafting into the normative feminine. The 'subaltern now emerged as the threatening figure of the illiterate cheat, who through either knavery or ignorance became a threat to life itself' (p. 208), Mukharji finds. We might bring in the caste location of those designated in this manner who were sellers of some of these remedies in the open markets and designated as quacks; we will follow this further in Chapter 6. We will also see, in Chapter 4, the figure of the *dai* who occupies exactly this space while not even being listed under the dubious category of quack practitioner. We see, here, however, a public vocabulary of therapeutics that is eclectic, with homoeopathy occupying a large space in home remedies, but the writing also making connections with canonical Ayurvedic texts and their simplified expositions. Are these to be read as constituting an extra-institutional space? Do they represent a messy space of encounter where borders and boundaries between so-called systems or disciplines are impossible? Or do they contribute to a rising discourse of unmarked Hindu privileged-caste indigeneity that consolidates in the first decades of the 20th century? I suggest that the space occupied by this ready reckoner, in the mid-19th century, to perhaps differing degrees in Bengal and central and western India, becomes part of an emerging public discourse around therapeutics that is more significant for its *extrusion* – of practitioners from the oppressed castes, of nomadic tribe women and men plant collectors and sellers, the women who attended childbirth in privileged-caste homes – *than its emphases,* or rather that the emphases are linked to the extrusions. These are aspects of an emerging governmental practice. I will focus on the extrusion of the *dai* figure in the next chapter as a way to illustrate this. Meanwhile, the locations of Munshi Nawal Kishore, Batokrishno Pal, and other publishers, well connected to both the colonial government and the nationalist elite at the cusp of the 19th to 20th centuries, allow us to see these non-expert texts, rather than extra-institutional, as newer sites of institutionalization, thus complicating the analytic of difference or resistance that might be applied in a simple encounter frame.

Approaching midwifery

While titles like *Prasuti tattva,*[7] *Prasuti Mongol,*[8] and *Prasuti Sulabh*[9] are present in large numbers from and earlier than the 16th century, the decade of the 1920s seems, for our purposes and with respect to the questions I ask here, to be the period that sees an explosion of vernacular language texts around childbirth, alongside women's magazines of the time. The Dufferin Fund exercises have also, by then, plateaued, failing to generate enough of a critical mass of trained *dais* to make a difference to the terrible conditions of childbirth that missionaries, administrators, and Englishwomen physicians have lamented since the mid-1700s, that needed to be set right through English intervention. The Medical Registration Act has meanwhile been passed, and the indigenous dispensaries have been declared invalid. While causal associations are not useful, one wonders at the volume of literature of different kinds generated, carrying prescriptions on good care during pregnancy and childbirth, that reproduce the very injunctions of these administrators and physicians, while claiming indigenous tradition as the source, during this period.

These texts range from those written by Indian men trained in Western medicine across the subcontinent and abroad, others taking the ready reckoner approach, and some advocating for employing trained *dais* and improving conditions of childbirth. One such text is by Major Hasan Sohrawardy, MD, FRCS, in 1925, titled *Prasuti o Sishu Mongol.*[10] The cover illustration is of a mother and a male-bodied child, but it is the dedication on the second page that locates the text – a photograph of the Countess of Lytton, the 'patroness and founder of "Bengal Baby week"'. Ambalika Guha (2018), Sujata Mukherjee (2001), and others have written on the discourse around good motherhood and baby shows that emerged during the early 20th century in British India, with particular reference to Bengal, but we are concerned about the commentary on therapeutic language emerging here. Sohrawardy is a senior grade medical officer of the Railways, and a member of the Red Cross and St John's Ambulance Association, among others. The book is a version of his speech in English at the 1920 *Swasthya O Sishu-Mongol Prodorshani*[11] at Calcutta, which had earlier been published and distributed in hospitals by the health minister Sir Surendranath Bandyopadhyay, and caters to a felt need to improve the health of pregnant women through further dissemination of the ideas in Bangla, in lucid and common-use language. As such, this text falls within the category of a coffee table book by a professional. It is authoritative, yet benevolent, not authoritarian. The chief addressees are nationalist men in the public sphere, while other professionals and the public at large are encouraged to acknowledge the gravity of the situation. Sohrawardy begins by marking the moment as a crisis, indicating that the rate at which infant mortality is increasing will ensure the extinction of the Bangali race. He speaks of the impossibility of a successful fight for *swaraj*, if merely resolutions for freedom were pushed for, without the physical health and strength required for it being worked towards. He cites the situation of more than half of young men applying for military service being declared unfit, on account of poor nutrition or health in infancy. He seems to suggest, perhaps to an elite audience resistant to focussing on those marginalized, that unless the health of farmers and labourers, in abject poverty and therefore ill-health, is attended to, neither will the labourer be productive nor will the race and by extension the nation thrive. He urges a non-reliance on government resources alone, and a non-partisan approach at such a *time of crisis,* calling this true patriotism since it is the present children and youth who will constitute the future of Bharat. Like every text of this time, he bemoans cultural and social ignorance and the evil of superstition that is a cause of the crisis. He talks about the following causes for childbirth morbidity and death: women who do not do housework when pregnant, thus distancing themselves from the activities that God intended for them; the failure to have nourishing food during pregnancy; the problem of untouchability that induces the choice of the darkest and dirtiest room for *atur* or childbirth, leading to puerperal fever and neonatal tetanus. He further laments the belief in *bhut-pret* (ghosts, spirits) that endorse such a dark room for the woman in labour, and, of course, the presence of an unsanitary *dhatri* – usually a *chamar*, *hauri*, *dosad*, *dom* or other lower-caste woman – whose apparently smelly bodies, copper or brass jewellery, and uncut, dirty nails, are a ready source of infection. The reference to nails has also appeared in the *Susruta Samhita*. In addition, he condemns the Hindu Vaidyas who feel that attending to sores, surgery, etc. is beneath them and that midwifery is for these lower-caste untouchable women, who have a good time fleecing the countrymen. Among Muslims, says Sohrawardy, untouchability was not a practice in the Middle Ages, when midwives and surgeons achieved great fame using Arab, Parsi, Greek, or Afghani methods; with the adoption of untouchability in the contemporary, however, he laments that these communities too have met with the same fate. Other problems he names are overall poverty and an unwillingness to submit to male doctors or go to hospitals. As Sohrawardy goes on to reiterate the lack of hygiene and the notoriously unclean habits of the *dai* women, he also realizes that they cannot immediately be got rid of and therefore must somehow be forced into some semblance of protocol through training. In time, as poor widows and others from upper-caste homes are trained, he suggests, these naturally unclean lower-caste women can be got rid of.

Sohrawardy speaks of his advice to the Bengal Rural Medical Service on mobilizing the resources of private practitioners, 'lady doctors', and *dhatri* who would, for a fee, attend to diseases like malaria, kala azar, cholera, etc., afflicting the poor for a monthly sum. He talks about the difficulties of finding lady doctors or 'pass kora dai' (trained *dais*) in remote rural areas, or even such professionals who the poor could afford. He proposes the setting up of centres where uneducated *dais* could be trained in the basics and given a stipend to encourage them to participate. He speaks of, as part of training, kitting up the *dais* with soap, etc., and in addition running awareness campaigns by educated men, peer-munshis, and pundits – men trusted by the people. He has detailed instructions on the setting up of the *aturghar* (lying-in room) – airy and with light, new mattresses, the regulation oilcloths and tincture iodine, sterilized cord-cutting thread, eyedrops for the newborn, and goes to some lengths to make the connections between maternal and infant health, the oxygenation via cord blood before cutting of the umbilical cord, etc. Sohrawardy does not, of course, fail to talk about the virtues and need for good housekeeping in order to make sure of a conducive environment in which future nation-builders can be reared. These are accompanied by exhortations to allow women to exercise in enclosed gardens instead of keeping them in *purdah*, referring to western regions of the country where the practice of sleeping in the open air on terraces has actually been found to make them stronger.[12] Sohrawardy's is one of the fewer texts that take on the additional task of speaking for women in Muslim communities, and while he talks of a hoary past where these communities were well-known in medical work, and of free Muslim countries where women move freely in the public domain, he bemoans the borrowing of untouchability practices from Hindus and the subsequent morbidity faced by Muslim women in childbirth. In speaking of *swaraj*, the book offers ways to save future mothers and children, hoping that the cries of these hapless women and infants have reached the hearts of all thinking men. A modern, aware, masculine Muslim public sphere is also the space where Sohrawardy's voice is located.

Another text of the time is *Prasuti o Paricharja*, by Dr. Bamandas Mukhopadhyay, formerly of Eden Hospital and Chittaranjan Seva Sadan (both reputed for obstetrics and paediatrics respectively, and public hospitals later), in 1926. This text begins with multiple invocations to the Goddess Durga, to the author's mother, to all mothers as powerful and producers of powerful sons who will return the lost *gaurav* (honour) of Bharat. The author, while thanking his medical teachers, also quotes the Arya Veda to emphasize the importance of adequate care and the value of *pathya*, i.e., prescriptions for diet and lifestyle practice, over and above that of medication. Like other texts of the time, the author bemoans poverty and *kusanskar* (superstitions) for the condition of mothers but also focusses on the *lajjasheela* (modest) character of the Bharatiya woman, her hesitation to share her troubles even with her husband, an argument reminiscent of the ones early Christian missionaries were making when speaking of the status of Indian women's health.

A third text of this time, titled *Prasuti Tattva* (The Facts of Pregnancy) in Bangla, 1929, authored by Sri Jamini Sen, priced at Rs. 3, is somewhat unique inasmuch as its chief addressees are the *Dhatris* – identified as those who receive the newborn and bring it to the mother, and acknowledged as a traditional and hereditary occupation whose responsibilities have become more onerous in the context of modernity where 'natural' childbirth is more difficult owing to changing and sedentary lifestyles among women. As such, this is more in the form of a reference text for a trained *dhatri* that also puts on her the onus of improving the maternal health of the nation's women (p. 4). Starting with a listing of the signs of pregnancy, changes in various organs during pregnancy, determinations of the time of delivery, all using biomedical language, lessons in anatomy, puerperal diseases, and interventions including douches, principles of forceps delivery, are included; the text reads like a primer in all these aspects.

Hygiene, purity, and the extrusion of the dai from the nationalist indigenous

The position of *daktars*/Indian allopathic practitioners in these texts offers an interesting entry point, revealing some common trends, as well as overlaps with popular texts on home remedies, and even with texts claiming to merely be translations of the Ayurvedic canon. For one, almost the entirety of the text in some cases, or a greater percentage in others, is given over to exhortations around hygiene. In texts like Sohrawardy's, these place the cause of almost all diseases at the door of the dirt that is apparently the embodiment of lower-caste *dais* who are constantly in the *aturghar*, their vain attachments to copper or brass ornaments that are never removed or cleaned, their overgrown nails, and their clothes. These women are alternately described as reformable or as a lost cause, and the source of shame for an otherwise effective indigenous practice. In other texts, poverty and middle-class ignorance alongside superstition regarding the evil influence of light in the *aturghar* are, for instance, cited as the rationale for poor birth conditions. Puerperal fever, neonatal tetanus, and tuberculosis are the diseases cited as the most common causes of morbidity and mortality in the *aturghar* – all preventable through obser-vance of hygiene. There is also some detailing of pathology, bacteriology, and pro-cesses of sterilization, and sterilization is the other big trope around which purity is built – for legitimate agents of childbirth, drug preparers, and their administration. It is the manner in which this idea of hygiene is articulated, how it is linked with untouchability practices, and how it becomes an overwhelming metaphor, that we are concerned with here. So we see Sohrawardy's disgust at the 'smelly clothes' and 'unclean bodies' of the *neech jaati asprashya* (the mean-caste untouchable) women in the *aturghar*, who are held responsible for neonatal tetanus (p. 3). We also see, across texts, the common substitution of the terms *apobitra* (impure) and *aporishkar* (unclean) (Bamandas Mukhopadhyay, 1926, p. 40); we see purity pre-sented as hygiene. We will see later in the chapter the uncanny overlaps with insti-tutional language and practitioner location, where concerns over caste and race overlap.

The responsibility for poor hygiene is shared across the rich and *bhadralok* classes (*Prasuti o Paricharja*) and the poor (*Prasuti o sishu mongol*). While pov-erty is seen as the soil of superstition that keeps the *aturghar* in the dark and the seat of diseases, *bhadralok* households are also held to fail that newborn son who should have been the favourite of the family, instead letting him fall into the hands of the *asprishya* women. The question, then, is whether the consolidation of hard caste boundaries happens in this domain – of the nationalist *bhadralok* household.

It is here, too, that the *dai* as an identity category gets defined more exactly. Whether it is *Prasuti Tattva* that speaks of earlier usages and roots of the term *Dhatri* as someone who holds the infant at birth, Bamandas' *Prasuti o Paricharja* text that names the *aturer jhee* – the associate of the *Dhatri* who is present for labour, Sohrawardy's later text that refers to the *asprashya* women, or the Ayurvedic texts-in-translation that refer to women attendants responsible for care work in the *sutika griha*, the group of women who attend the delivery, cut the cord, come in for breastfeeding, or do post-natal chores around the mother, while referred to separately, begin to coalesce into the *Dhatri, dai*. The *aturer jhee* (literally, servant woman of the *aturghar*) is different from the *shikhito dhatri* – the trained *dhatri* – who knows to maintain hygiene. The *aturer jhee* is usually ignorant, unsanitary, of *neech jati* – as expected. The devil of her identity is in the details – her attach-ment to brass jewellery being an indicator of her non-upper-caste and therefore non-gold-wearing status, her uncut nails as a metaphor for her lack of grooming being an indicator of her caste location, again. And in crafting her, as a single individual, within the realm of abject domestic labour, she is written out of respect-able indigenous knowledge communities. This location also qualifies her as part of nationalist shame. The women of the nation have now effectively been betrayed, and not by the men; to the colonizer as addressee, this is the nationalist resolution of the women's question.

It is useful to see here that once this impurity is marked as the source of disease or of error in therapeutic work, and purity located in the hoary past and its legendary preceptors, the origin story is re-presented rather than challenged, so that a reversal of custom is no longer a necessity; recovery of a lost one is. The cleansing and consolidation of caste barriers that follows is now a logical extension, and one whose onus lies on the educated *bhadralok* men.

Tradition is also being both bounded and defended in this exercise. Authors of midwifery texts speak of appropriate clothing for women in the interests of good childbirth outcomes. Here, modernity, spoken of as wealth and the aping of Western customs, is seen as coming in the way of 'natural' feminine functions like childbirth; refusal to do even 'light housework' during pregnancy, superstition, wearing corsets and other tight Western women's clothing, high heels, and so on, are part of the ills of modernity. A brief perusal of the rapidly changing lifestyles of wealthier women in cities like Bombay and Calcutta at the time, available in other commentaries and writings, is indicative of the fears of mobility and public presence of women, following educational reforms and political participation that accompany these statements; and while we see a consensus around shifting of the goalposts of tradition in addressing untouchability under the rubric of hygiene or in decrying another trope called 'superstition', we also see the consolidation of boundaries between the public and domestic realms through these prescriptions. I will pick up this thread in greater detail in Chapter 5.

The last aspect of purity/hygiene that I would like to discuss here is the aspect of accuracy in drug preparation. Through the different varieties of texts, there are not only repeated prescriptions on measures of materials to be used in drug preparation, exhortations on the need to source these materials in the pure form, and to follow exact procedures for preparation, but these exhortations are also referenced to account for the therapeutic failure of some of these preparations. Nagendranath Sen Gupta's insistence on the need to source plant roots from the Himavat mountains for purity is a case in point. While these rigid prescriptions may be understood as centring the practitioner and preceptor, as I have suggested earlier, and as a way of seeking equivalence through a reference to rigorous methods of drug preparation, the lens of purity returns here. This will have implications, as we will see, for determinations of what constitutes a medicinal plant, what is the right drug, who may be equipped to treat, and which practices are therefore valid. The indigenous drugs committee and its career is a key actor in this drama.

Language, tonality, and textual form

Projit Bihari Mukharji, in speaking of braided sciences (2016), deploys Monica Juneja's use of the term 'braided' (2012) to challenge earlier formulations of hybridity that operate with an acknowledgement of essentialized parent sites of knowledge. He uses the metaphor of braiding to speak of a weaving and emergence of language, knowledge, and traditions that are constantly dynamic. In the context of language, Mukharji remarks on the modernization process for Ayurveda being partly reliant on the 'braiding [of] Sanskritic and European (accessed mostly through English) sciences' (p. 43). Considering that most of those listed as physicians in the period in Bengal – the specific case he examines – knew neither of these languages, the modernization exercise was controlled by 'a tiny, relatively privileged and closely knit elite group of urban physicians' (p. 44). For my purposes, braiding offers a useful lens to understand the form of these texts. I understand braiding here in two senses. The verse form within the Ayurveda made easy texts, divided across Sanskrit and Devanagari, both recall the format of the origin texts being invoked, and open it up for consumption, thus bringing together knowledge and language. Other forms of what might be called braiding also show up, with the location being invoked or slipping in through dialect use. The dialogic form, used in *Garbharaksha* – what I call the reform text – does a job of braiding biomedical, social reform, and domestic vocabulary, almost creating an appearance of a proto-community medicine text, while located in common-use language of the region.

While there are several such texts in circulation in this period and later, with invocations and authorship distributed widely across the named originators of the practice, it is the form, language, and tone that I am concerned with here. The form of the text, in particular, the Hindi or Bangla in use, straddles common-use language, drawing into it recognizably Ayurvedic jargon from the canonical text. It is not just jargon, but Ayurveda's explanations of causes that are present, so that there is an expressed familiarity with jargon, and through jargon, a claim to expertise. The explainer paragraphs, titled as *arth* (meaning), while using this jargon as reference, are a mixture of Sanskrit terms and *bolti bhasha* or common-use language, not the sanitized privileged-caste language of officialdom. Rachel Berger, in her account of Ayurveda in modern India, also speaks of this coupling of the Sanskrit and Hindi, of this as having 'the effect of rooting claims to knowledge within a learned framework, where authors could lay claim to the authority of the Sanskrit texts through the deployment of it as form, while repositioning meaning as something communicated through the colloquial vernacular' (Berger, 2013, p. 83). We see, in looking at the ready reckoner texts as well as those on home remedies, some other reflections of this engagement with codified systems. We see, for example, the use of allopathic medical terminology in English, sometimes written in the Bangla or Devanagari/Hindi script, in both the ready reckoners and the guide books like *Prasuti tattva* for *dais*, with the latter almost like English medicine written in Bangla, with illustrations of the human skeleton, detailed descriptions of anatomical structures named in English, as well as of physiology. We see a performative familiarity with an alien language and episteme, while already embedding the author-practitioner self within a locally enacted one, thus an extended claim to expertise and patronage.

A focus on measures, a reference to lineage, and most significantly, a prescriptiveness pervades these texts. The prescriptions are located not only in the private or domestic sphere but extend to ritual conditions that are to be fulfilled in order to be blessed with *uttam putra* (good sons), with detailed instructions on medicinal plants involved in rituals for such sons. The woman who is *kalahkaarini* (a troublemaker), *vyavaysheela* (non-virtuous), *abhidhya*, or *amarshini*, among others, will have stillborn or otherwise disabled, fearful children (*Aushadhikriya*, p. 575). *Mahagunvale putra* (exceptionally gifted sons) will result if brahmans and the gods are propitiated (*Susruta Samhita bhashanuvaad*, p. 281). *Napunsak* or *hijra* offspring, or a girl child, are expected to result out of a failure to meet directives. In doing so, these writer-practitioners declare themselves collaborators and mediators of the textual knowledge/power emanating from the Vedas and also establish themselves at the top of the local hierarchy. A declared interlocutor, for instance, is the old wives' tale; the text actively picks up common sense around pregnancy and challenges it with canonical prescription – '*streeyan kaha karti hain ... par bhagvan atreya is baat ko sveekar nahin karte hain*'.[13] We see, then, that injunctions towards good motherhood, drawn from an earlier text, pervade writing and translations meant for indigenous male medical practitioners in a later period. A closeness to ritual canons is established here; while the earlier texts stay with these, and with gender-related prescriptions in that regard, the later texts that draw civilizational and racial rationales from these also seek to actively identify and discard elements seen as polluting in order to claim autonomy and consolidate difference. Separating the much-spoken of decade of the 1920s from the ones preceding it as the historical moments producing these texts, but also seeing them in continuity, is useful for this exercise.

Women and medical writing

Women as socially aware participants of reform

What of women as author-practitioners, or addressee subjects, of indigenous medical writing in this extended period? At around the same time that we see the Ayurveda made easy texts and ready reckoners, an 1892 text titled *Garbharaksha-athahidayatnama-daiyanali*, written in narrative dialogic form as a conversation among women, and focussing on the value of having a trained *dai* for childbirth in the home, was published. Broadly attaching itself to the institutional discourse around training for *dai* women, and thus to textual midwifery, but also speaking the language of social reform, and doing that within the domestic sphere, this text, published from Delhi, endorses the value of a trained *dai*, makes her the legitimate advocate of hygiene practices, and takes on questions of son preference, caste discrimination, and community othering, thus setting itself apart from other texts of the time, while using, like other texts, scientific vocabulary to challenge superstition. It tackles a series of stereotypes and myths – around the *dai*, the quack or *nawaqif hakim* (ignorant *hakim*). It takes on board the value of training and links with institutionalized Western medicine, and yet enters into the text, approvingly, several plant remedies for conditions like *dast* or *kabz* (diarrhoea or constipation). It asks for the rejection of practices like *jhad-phoonk* (exorcism) in favour of medical, biological explanations and treatment for experiences of possession that are sometimes associated with pregnancy. It would seem that this text participates in the creation of something like a medically aware community that Alavi speaks of in the Unani context – in this case a medically aware private sphere. While written in *Devanagari* script, it adopts a combination of a Persian vocabulary with several words translated into more shared Hindustani within the text and establishes a Muslim domestic sphere or *zenana* as its participant audience. As such, it sits alongside some of the reform literature produced by men around care of women in pregnancy and childbirth, but spoken in the woman's voice, and in a dialogic, shared knowledge context. Whether this can evoke notions of collective privacy – a knowledge generated from shared birthing experiences that is unavailable to men (Alcoff & Dalmiya, 1993) – or whether they stay with the idea of women's responsibilities, is unclear.

We might mark a text of this nature within some general as well as specific contexts. This is the decade when the Dufferin Fund, the Victoria Memorial Scholarship Fund, and some other private funds have begun to be set up. The lament about the untrained *dai* has travelled from missionary accounts and English medical women in the colony into this time. Apart from these, a language of social reform particularly targeted at the Muslim women's domestic sphere had been taking shape in late 19th century elite North India, focussed primarily on 'literacy, home economics, and "orthodox" practices', as Faisal Fatehali Devji puts it (2018, p. 22). Some of these concerns find an echo in this text, with a focus on the need for education for women; at the same time, a common critique of the *zenana* woman corrupted by modernity, proving too lazy for even light household work during pregnancy, is visible. In other ways, it is almost in the genre of a training and social advocacy manual, centred on Sahbo, the locally acclaimed dai, who is *telan* by *jaat* (believed to be artisan caste converts to Islam). On being asked about her caste status, however, the interlocutor asks, 'why go by caste, as she is far better than "ashrafs"' (the nobility); the implication being that her marginal caste location need not diminish the quality of her work. The text also indicates that she is trained and that there is a need for books that describe and help prepare for pregnancy. There is a reference to publications that abound in the period, responding to this need. There is a reference to a need for education for women or educated women. Needs of the birthing room are spelt out; the self-preparations to be taken by the *dai* – changing of clothes, cutting of nails, and so on – like other texts of the time, which are also referenced. In some senses, then, this is a training manual, although some of the instructions are over-cautious, while some give the *dai* more control and capacity than the trainings would claim, even asking for extra digits to be cut at birth by the *dai*, for example. Further manoeuvres like instructions on correcting breech presentations – even vaginally – are gone through, and in parts, the text goes into detailed descriptions of anatomy. It also, however, endorses more recognizably indigenous practices, like putting the mother's hair into her mouth to induce vomiting so that the cervix dilates, or the preference for ipecacuana vs ergot of rye to induce labour. For childcare, the use of indigenous remedies, alongside *angrezi dava* (English medicine), is discussed, with references to availability in *shafakhanas* or English dispensaries. There is advice on preparing, mixing, and keeping some of these at home, including *castel, tarpin*, caustic, *saunf* water, *vynamapika, cajupat* oil, compound chalk powder, and clark ether.[14] This is, then, a somewhat idiosyncratic text, focussed on

pregnancy and childbirth, giving voice to the *dai*, mobilizing the language of training, of *angrezi dava* as well as the *shifakhana*, with home remedies piggybacking
on biomedical vocabulary.

Who does *Garbharaksha* address? In its form, its participants, its script and
language, it stands quite apart from most of the other writings of this time. It is
addressed to women of the home – mostly Muslim but also perhaps to a more heterogeneous group; its attempts to provide more Sanskrit-origin synonyms to many
of its technical terms may be to address a broader group or to enact the earlier-
mentioned performative familiarity with a language becoming associated with textual expertise. This familiarity may also be part of an address to *dais*-in-training. It
brings on board the English *davakhana* as the primary standard but also as foreign,
however present in the landscape. It speaks boldly of more familiar therapeutic
materials while adopting and appropriating hitherto unknown chemicals with the
confidence and authority of a secure practitioner. This audience, while seemingly
financially comfortable, is not necessarily the nationalist elite, yet it is a participant
in the language of reform. It takes on the reform of the *jacchakhana* (birthing
room), and by extension the *zenana*, and therefore the lives of women. It operates
in a climate where the *dai* is a familiar household name, as also a heterogeneous
group comprising good and bad practitioners. And in so doing, it announces a cop-
ing with a rapidly changing landscape of therapeutics.

Women writing

The authorship of *Garbharaksha* is unclear, unlike its addresses being clearly
women of the household. What of writers among women? Charu Gupta speaks of
Yashoda Devi – a seemingly canonical figure in the world of 'women's diseases'
in Allahabad of the early 1900s, opening her own clinic and pharmacy in the
first decade, and branches later, editing several journals, *Stri Chikitsak*[15] being the
most widely read of them between 1913 and 1938, and a vast number of books.
While the commentaries on sexuality and masculinity that Yashoda Devi made
and their significance for 'women of the nation' will be looked at in Chapter 5, it
is useful to see here the voice of a woman author-practitioner who is active at the
same time as the male practitioners, in the United Provinces region, who is claiming space within the specific domain of 'female diseases' and childbirth, who is
able to access the print boom and 'the complicated politics of Hindi-language
scientific writing' (Berger, 2013, p. 97), and who has knowledge of the textual
canon that is being mediated by the male practitioners. Being born into a family of practitioners may have provided an entry point, but Yashoda Devi, while
initially ghettoized into the women's disease domain, definitely deploys the same
techniques of mediation of biomedical vocabulary that the male practitioners did.
That she also seemed to have a professional and 'well-organised network' (Gupta,
2005, p. 28) that helped sell her preparations in pharmacies, respond to a wide
variety of letters, thus utilizing the advantages of print, and set up multiple clinics,
presents her as both unique and of the time. Interestingly, while the male practitioners pronounced on mothers, *dais* and women in childbirth, Yashoda Devi

seems to have done this as also comment on the dangers of non-reproductive desire among men. The other woman visible in history who seems to speak this language is Dr Muthulakshmi Reddy, and we will try to explore her work – on masculinities required for the nation – also in Chapter 5. The question that the available accounts of this history leave unanswered is of conversations or engagements between, say, a Yashoda Devi and a Sahbo. Were these subject positions as widely separated as they appear, or appear to become, later? Was a Yashoda Devi, as here seems to be the case, more self-identified as a general expert practitioner than as ghettoized into the treatment of diseases of women? Was there a jostling for space between a Sahbo and practitioners like Yashoda Devi, or later, a Haimabati Sen?

The Indigenous drugs cacophony of India

It is useful to locate the texts discussed above alongside other therapeutic interventions at the turn of the century. Before the appearance of the 'Ayurvedic text explained' that I describe, the central Indigenous Drugs Committee was formed in 1896; this Committee began to determine which of the medicinal plants in use by indigenous practitioners were useful and will be allowed into official pharmacopoeias. This is also just prior to the amendment of the Bombay Medical Act of 1912 that set down protocols for the practice of non-allopathic medicine within and outside institutions. Several reputed Ayurvedic pharmacies were being shut down at this time; legislative assembly debates during the period were witness to pleas by Hindu nationalist leaders like Madan Mohan Malaviya for indigenous medicine in the form of Ayurveda, Unani, and Siddha to be taught to 'native' physicians. I will, in this section, attempt to delineate some of the positions emerging in this fractious debate.

Early attempts at institutionalization

About 20 years before the constitution of the Indigenous Drugs Committee, Kanai Lall Dey, one of the members of the committee, had already put out a volume on *The Indigenous Drugs of India* in 1867, listing medicines in common use 'among the natives of India', as also all Native drugs which are named in the British pharmacopoeia. The volume was meant for distribution among medical practitioners. Much in the tradition of the texts discussed earlier in this chapter, it begins from a stated position of humility – that it has nothing original to add to several well-known texts like Shaughnessy's Bengal Dispensary, Waring's Therapeutics, or Drury's Useful Plants of India, but for a few observations regarding new or differing properties that the author is able to offer. The point of the volume, says Dey, is 'the substitution, as far as possible, of cheap Native Drugs for costly English Medicines' (p ii). Dey offers his own experience as primary evidence of their efficacy and therapeutic value and refers to his contributions to the *Indian Medical Gazette* and the International Exhibition of Drugs in London in 1862 as proof of his scientific credibility. It is not clear whether the native medicines thus described focus on one or another sort of illness, although varieties of digestive-related prep-arations, fever preparations, and massage oils feature as well-proven sources of relief.

An important aspect of the format of this volume is the mention of techni-cal as well as vernacular names of these drugs – a feature that disappears in a later edition of this volume 29 years later, in 1896, by which time the work of the Indigenous Drugs Committee is in full swing. This later edition, which reflects the regulations in place in British India much more clearly, is presented as revised and entirely re-written, thus effectively rendering the earlier edition invalid; it is written with William Mair of the Pharmaceutical Society of Great Britain, with a preface by George Watt, Honorary Secretary of the Indigenous Drugs Committee (and Reporter on Economic Products) and in charge of sourcing indigenous drugs for hospital use throughout this period.

The preface by George Watt positions Dey's work within the pupilage of the 'great masters' – the English practitioners – and within the context of the teaching of 'European medical science' (p. vii) in India, alongside his contemporaries U.C. Dutt and Moodeen Sheriff, who published *The Materia Medica of the Hindus* in 1877 and the *Supplement to the Pharmacopoeia of India* in 1869. It is still presented as a 'hand-book', not superseding 'the great works that have appeared recently' (viii), like *The Pharmacographia Indica* of Dymock, Warden, and Hooper pub-lished in 1893; yet it is considered suitable as a textbook for students. Dey is com-mended for recognizing that 'Indigenous drugs' as a term must refer to those drugs *procurable* in India rather than *native* to it, and therefore to be deployed more pragmatically, focussing on what is efficacious rather than what is cheap – a shift from Dey's earlier position on efficacy as well as cost. Many of those drugs called indigenous are redescribed here as introduced and naturalized drugs. Somewhere in between the lines, we also see a redefinition of efficacy of these indigenous drugs as a stand-in – '[t]he few that are good are neglected ... because [of] the cry for imported drugs and European pharmacy' (ix). This is significant because we see the same logic functioning in the deployment of *dais* later and in independent India – as deemed fitting to (merely) fill a resource gap among less-valued populations or marginal groups. Of course, experience is allowed, where knowledge is not. Arnold has discussed the multiple positions on 'subaltern science' (2006, p. 176), particularly botany, and indigenous medicine in scholarship on histories of science and medicine; while some of this scholarship attributes an active constitutive role to Western science 'from the sixteenth century' (p. 177), some speak of hybrid knowledges, and others of '"epistemological violence" directed against indigenous norms and systems of knowledge' (ibid). Nandy, Visvanathan, Prakash, and femi-nist theorists have reiterated this point about epistemological violence. While this scholarship is focussed on the asymmetry, I am interested in the reference points of pharmaceutical therapeutics at this point. We see, in this text, the re-assertion of European terms of scientific validity but also a toning down of any civilizational advantage, race-based claims, or nationalist rhetoric that is evident in the texts discussed earlier. This is a time when a critical mass of Indian practitioners of biomedicine is also available.

In the prefatory memoir by William Mair, we see Dey's gratitude for recognition by the government as pharmacologist – he was elected the only Honorary member from India to the Pharmaceutical Society of Great Britain. He was later given the title of *Rai Bahadur* in 1872, and several other memberships, and therefore a place, however subordinate, in metropolitan science, with religious and caste dogma from his own culture being responsible for holding him back from physically entering the metropole (the fear of the 'black water' crossing, p. xvii). We also see a listing of Dey's many efforts to take the indigenous drugs discourse to various exhibitions and hospitals of the Bengal and Indian Medical Service, which 'has perhaps been all too little made use of' [xvi]; an indication, perhaps, of the constant and fraught nature of his negotiations around the need for this work. We will see this more starkly in the minutes of the meetings of the Indigenous Drugs Committee. Also available in the record of Dey's professional life in the prefatory memoir is gratitude for patronage by princely families for whom he is a medical advisor. While he self-professes his 'Brahaminical faith' (p. xix–x), he also considers 'true religion' to not be conservative but to be found in knowledge, education, and demeanour. Dey is said to have made several suggestions on indigenous drug development as part of his membership of various societies including the Indian Medical Congress; this included the need for medicinal plant farms, a drug emporium, and stocks of indigenous drugs at Medical Store depots for trial and report. It is in the context of these suggestions that he locates the appointment of the Indigenous Drugs Committee, consisting of himself, Dr. George King, Dr. J.F.P. McConnell, Dr. C.J.H. Warden, and Dr. George Watt, to each of whom he also acknowledges the text. All of these achievements, it is useful to note, are seen as contributing to India's economic progress and not as a record of its civilizational greatness.

Some of the conflicts reflected in the functioning of the Indigenous Drugs Committee are visible in this text. The *Pharmacopoeia of India* (1868), a competing text, comes up for severe chastisement for being 'obsolete' and 'neither an official nor a legal standard' (p. xxi), in addition to 'classical' but 'inaccessible' (ibid) texts like the *Dictionary of the Economic Products of India* (Watt, 1890), and the *Pharmacographia Indica*. This volume, then, presents itself, instead of these, as a 'convenient manual' (xxi), much like the earlier edition. A manual, moreover, that fulfils an economic rather than a scientific function, and one in which vernacular names are listed in English with no effort to use popular language descriptions. The nomenclatural shift is the single most significant shift in this edition, with the classical names at the top as 'most universal', the *Flora of British India* being the reference point for these, followed by the popular English name (as different from the popular Bengali name in the earlier edition), and then the popular names in Hindi and other vernaculars, and an appendix with 'pharmaceutical processes for the efficient exhibition of the medicinal products' (xxiv). We might read these as a practice of museumization and marginalization, apart from these 'objects' being put in a permanent state of investigation. At this point, however, the purpose of exhibition was essentially of introducing into classificatory practice these plants, presenting them in their 'natural' state, and this is a way to read Dey's taxonomical efforts.

Several preparations are also no longer present in this edition, partly to remove much that is 'primitive, empirical and irrational' (xxiii), and several included that are cultivated species. The descriptions are much longer, with a focus on habitat, on parts which have the active principles, and discussions of usage – by *hakims*, for instance.

While Dey is ready to give up on a civilizational meaning of the category indigenous, he also calls attention, in the first chapters, to the physicians of the Puranic era and the detailed prescriptions and rigor of preparation of medicines during this time, although he states that it was only since Sir William Jones and later that scientific arrangements of this material were possible. He goes on to at one point mildly chastise the government of India for not taking into account any but one 'country medicine' – *chiretta* – in stocking medical stores in hospitals. It is also here that he cites the value of vernacular names and the 'professional castes who deal in these substances, the *Musheras* of Central and Upper India, the low caste *Maules, Bediyas, Bagdis, Kaibartas, Pods, Chandals, Kaoras*, and *Karangas* of Bengal and the *Chandras, Bhils*, and *Gamtas* of Bombay' (p. xxxiii). William Jones himself is quoted as having followed this practice, and the practicality of it in identifying and sourcing plants is what Dey stresses. The civilizational 'past', it would seem, is a metaphor for that which is lost rather than a present-day competitor; experience is what can safely be granted to the present.

As is evident in all the descriptions, the economic potential of the indigenously sourced drug or medicinal plant is the ultimate turning of the scale – the prospect of an industry which, like in the case of cinchona, would result in presence in European, Australian, and American markets, particularly given the low costs of labour and ampleness of the plants. Dey lists the drugs which might be added to the export market in this context – 'Belladonna, hyoscyamus, taraxacum, podophyllum, jalap, asafoetida, cassia pods, cardamoms, kurchi, gurjun, chaulmugra and nim oils, ispaghul' (xxxvii). The chance of these finding their way into an Imperial Pharmacopoeia is stressed.

Closer to Dey's older edition, Pandurang Gopal publishes, in 1874, a Catalogue of Drugs indigenous to the Bombay Presidency, with the difference, however, that it is 'arranged according to "Drury's Useful Plants of India"', presented by a pharmacologist, refers to his own clinical experience, and is accommodating of the local in more ways than one. Gopal offers this work in the spirit of identifying drugs and names specific to the part of India he is writing from and also in bringing attention to the 'habitat of the drug we use and [the need to] try more than one specimen of each' (p. 4) – a factor that later gets taken up in the deliberations of the Indigenous Drugs Committee in determining pharmacological characteristics of each, and that Arnold has spoken of in his articulation of the tropicalizing of India. Along with local language names – an 'index of Marathi names of indigenous drugs' (p. 7), for instance – there is attention to the parts of the plant to be used, preparations, and dosages, commentaries on preparations available in the *bazaar*, and includes some drugs like *Bael* that are already in the British Pharmacopoeia. Drugs that are reputed or 'much lauded by Waids' (p. 12) are listed, as also those of doubtful value that require more investigation. The 'root of *gymnema sylvestre* and *ophioxylon serpentinum'*, for instance, are suggested as likely to 'prove equal to *ipecacuanha* in efficacy', but are expected to require longer investigation, since the 'progress of inquiry is necessarily always slow', therefore the 'present experience of such drugs ... should not hinder us from giving them further trial' (p. 4). Sanskrit works and 'old Hindoo physicians' (p. 27) are also referred to in detailing some drugs. While some of the local knowledge spoken of includes drugs like *Chota chand* that is used *'to promote delivery in tedious cases, acting upon the uterine system in the same manner as ergot of rye'* (p. 21, author's italics to indicate that the drug has been proved trustworthy through sufficient use), there is no mention of *dais* or women attending childbirth who may be aware of or using these.

The interface – or the institutionalized indigenous: regulate, standardize

The Central Indigenous Drugs Committee first met at the Office of the Medical Depot, Calcutta, on 3 January 1896, after the government asked for a consideration of the practicality and utility of the following – 'encouraging the systematic cultivation of medicinal plants indigenous to India; encouraging the increased use in Medical Depots of drugs of known therapeutic value; sanctioning the manufacture of stable preparations of certain drugs in the Depots' (Central Indigenous Drugs Committee, p. 109). The Committee included Brigade-Surgeon-Lieutenant-Colonel G. King, F.P. McConnell, C.J. Warden, Rai Bahadur Kanny Lall Dey,[16] and George Watt, several of these members being of the IMS, and the first two members being from the Army. Berger (2013) has argued that the Committee was locating its work in the larger discourse of public health and that its impacts may be seen in the later collectivization by elite practitioners to protect their livelihood, the emergence of these practitioners as authors, and the reversal of roles where 'native' doctors could be taught indigenous medicine. I focus more on the interface that this Committee occupies, between the physicality of the medical institution being consolidated at this time, and the messy, murky outside. I suggest that the Committee is as representative of the Orientalist imperialist positions on the dark continent as it is of the negotiations being produced at the staged border between the two. One of the first discussions, about 'drugs of known therapeutic value', is really about who could arbitrate on therapeutic value, and the decision to restrict the inquiry to recommendations for better preparations of indigenous drugs. The resolution of the dilemma was, for the Committee, to contain the 'complex and ... extensive ... assemblage of drugs' in prescriptions by native practitioners so that 'convenient preparations made upon some definite standard', made available to some of the larger hospitals, would help to *generate* new information 'as to their value or otherwise' (Report, Proceedings of the First Meeting, January 3rd, 1896, p. 2). It is useful, then, to see this exercise as an effort at pharmaceutical regulation that works in sync with commerce that also begins to erode and displace earlier forms of therapeutic authority, replacing them with medically trained Indian elites who may directly claim knowledge of and contact with those deemed plant collectors.

It is also in this first meeting that Kanny Lall Dey seeks to claim authority over the field of indigenous knowledge, dismissing the name of a Kabiraj mentioned by

McConnell who might be summoned before the Committee to discuss the drugs they use, and offering to bring others who were more esteemed in the field. A figure like Kanai Lall Dey emerges as the symbol and symptom of the interface, seeking entry into the institution, via status as the legitimate translator-mediator of what of the outside may be validated. A constant tension is evident in the minutes of the Committee's deliberations, around suggestions made by Dey, questioning, implicitly, his legitimacy as authoritative spokesperson for indigenous therapeutics, as also his evaluative capacities; racial loyalties and national belonging are also perhaps in play here, as Nandy suggests in reference to J.C. Bose (1980). Among the many proceedings of the Committee that evidence this is a discussion regarding drugs for particular diseases, like bowel complaints. Here Dey's recommendation on *Mocharas* gum as an effective remedy for dysentery is dismissed by Watt in his role as botanist, physician, and reporter on economic botany, and consequently by the Committee, in favour of Watt's own list of *Bel* fruit, *Kurchi* bark, and *Akanda* root-bark, and Dey's recommendation of a trial for *Thol-kuri* as antipyretic is only listed as a dissenting note (Proceedings of the Third Meeting, 28 January 1896, p. 14).

The Committee went on to involve Surgeon-Major J. Parker, the Medical Storekeeper, Bombay, for information on drug acquisitions like *Kino* (the resin of *Pterocarpus marsupium*) from the forest department, and the purity of these preparations, accompanying this with detailed descriptions of the 'Kurumbers' (a community listed under tribes who have been early inhabitants of Western India) who collect these, and diagrammatic descriptions of their modes of collection (Lieutenant-Colonel J. Parker, 21 February 1896). Watt reminded the Committee of the potential for trade that this preparation offered, considering that the prices were about half of what would be involved in importing the compound. Thus begins a series of practices whereby, while the British Pharmacopoeia remains the reference point, preparations from the Indian Pharmacopoeia, like Indian opium, are brought on to the page; the fact that Indian opium seems to yield over 70%, while the imported opium listed in the British Pharmacopoeia yields 50%, however, is not accorded official sanction in a framework that claims to validate only that which is scientific according to standards of the metropole.

Another aspect of the discussions around specific preparations was the actual lack of experience, either on the part of Dey or any of the other practitioners in the Committee, on use of these drugs. Bound to and believers in allopathic systems as these men were, the possibility of using indigenous drugs remained academic at best, and regulatory in real time, resulting in the dismissal of all but a very few of the ones under consideration. This comes up again in the context of re-evaluations by the Committee of several medicinal plants like *Bel* that are already listed, prompting a decision to omit a sentence from the Introductory that states that those drugs from the Indian Pharmacopoeia that have already found their way into the British Pharmacopoeia be not considered for discussion (Proceedings of the Seventh Meeting, 17 April 1897, p. 26) – a justification of the Committee's use, labour, and time. The experience that was granted some merit was of letters received from outside the Committee. One was from a Mr Amulya Charan Basu, considered to have practical knowledge in the use of indigenous drugs, and whose suggestions were printed in the Appendix. Again, procurability and the argument of at least some of the drugs proposed by native practitioners being 'exotics' introduced into India rather than indigenous, come up again, particularly in the context of listing. Other factors, like the failure of work at the local or provincial committee levels, or the degree of autonomy of the Committee with respect to the government, also play a role in the outcome of these debates and conflicts. Meanwhile, after Dey's death on 16 August 1899, Rai Chuni Lal Bose Bahadur, Chemical Examiner and Assistant Professor of Chemistry at Medical College, takes his place on the Committee.

One of the results of the constitution of the Committee is the setting up of local sub-committees to assist in the production of an Indian Pharmacopoeia, 'to obtain local aid and knowledge' (Report, Proceedings of the Seventh Meeting, p. 25), while ensuring uniformity of procedure in evaluating such knowledge through supervision by the Central Committee. Physiological investigations into drug actions begin to take a back seat in this exercise, which prefers to be guided by the evaluation of drug use effects. There is also, at about the time of the eighth meeting in April 1897, a suggestion to give publicity to the workings of the Committee with a view to inviting private organizational and individual support. Drugs decided for feedback from local committees include *podophyllum, calotropis, picorrhiza, alstonia,* and *adhatoda.*

As we follow the composition of the Committee, we see the induction of Surgeon-Major D. Prain, Superintendent of the Royal Botanic Gardens at Howrah, in April 1898. While the meetings have, by this time, drastically reduced in frequency, and many of the local committees are not offering any suggestions for new drugs to be included, there is also some new trade in recently introduced names like *Podophyllum emodi,* although this root was not yet in the British Pharmacopoeia. The other drug much discussed was the *Indian Squill* (Mukharji, 2008). And it is here that a picture of the field within which the drug is an economic product begins to consolidate, with collaborations with the Botanic Garden, the Agriculture Department, and so on. Arnold's arguments on botany in India are relevant here, as a field where the presence of indigeneity in the form of plants and plant collectors has been most visible.

We also see, in the deliberations of the Committee, that the control over drug trials is advised to be retained by the larger institutions, effectively keeping out the 'Hospital Assistants in charge of dispensaries' – in effect, native practitioners trained in Western medicine – who are 'in many cases hardly qualified to judge of the actions of the drugs supplied' (p. 79) from the exercise. This is after the distribution of trial drugs has already occurred, and it is unclear whether some of these drugs are then withdrawn from the dispensaries at Gauhati, Nowgong, Tezpur, and other places where they had been distributed for trial earlier, in October 1898.

The debate between using economic and scientific criteria continues. As the introductory note to the provisional list of indigenous drugs says – 'An endeavour has been made to select indigenous drugs which are reputed to be equivalent in therapeutic action to drugs official in the British Pharmacopoeia and also as far as possible to select those of very general occurrence in the drug shops of India'

(Report, Appendix XIV, p. 178). At the same time, it is reiterated that for a very large number of indigenous drugs, the claim to therapeutic efficiency is unsupported by chemical investigations or physiological actions – an indication of the sciences of biochemistry and physiology being given arbiter status over and above practitioner experience, with these experts being also proposed to be brought on board the local committees, and a source of the familiar caution in declaring these drugs therapeutically valuable. This is in contrast to the stress on the practitioner as the centre of the system that we have seen in the Ayurvedic preceptor accounts, and it is here that we see the separation from and dismissal of 'native practitioners', as also their separation from the category of indigenous drugs, emerging in this interface between the institution and the 'messy outside'. As the Committee notes, 'in these days of standardisation of drugs it would be [a] distinctly retrograde step to recommend the use of a preparation of linseed oil and Narcotine of indefinite strength, mixed with the inert impurities of crude opium' (Report, p. 56). Given that standardization is in place, the Committee then is able to consider the supply of standard samples not only to Indian Medical Schools but also to 'a selected number of Colleges in Europe … where voluntary co-operation with the Indigenous Drugs Committee might be anticipated' (pp. 56–7) – a co-operation, perhaps, that is likely to elevate colonial medicine to metropolitan status, an aspiration that Chakrabarti has noted in his discussion of colonial science. Conversations also continue at this time on aspects of packaging, labelling, and appearance – further markers of credibility and validity via standardization. As far as supplies go, discussions around the responsibility of supplying these drugs to various hospitals or to storekeepers/medical depots, lead to exploring the possibility of asking provinces other than Bengal to supply these. The only conversation that seems to have relied on practitioners is of the part of the plant and the method of administration.

It is during the deliberations of the 11th meeting of the Committee on 20 March 1899 that a Report from the Pharmacopoeia Committee of 1894 on the proposed Indian and Colonial addenda to the British Pharmacopoeia is discussed. This is the first suggestion that there was a parallel committee with the same or similar mandate as that of the Central Indigenous Drugs Committee. Here begins a protracted battle on authority to pronounce therapeutic value and addenda to the British Pharmacopoeia, with each Committee offering their own provisional lists, with the Indigenous Drugs Committee dismissing some drugs in the Addendum that are not in its own lists on the grounds of poor widespread availability, or the wisdom of listing lesser and locally known species when existing populous remedies were already in place. Through all of this is also evident the conflict between the Madras and Bengal presidencies is also evident, with the Pharmacopoeia Committee having taken more from the knowledge of the South and the Indigenous Drugs Committee from Bengal and Bombay, while actively dismissing remedies from the South on specious grounds like 'it would be well to exclude [a] drug of purely South Indian origin and habitat' (Crawford, 17 August 1899, p. 329). The squill comes up for debate again here, with *Crinum asiaticum*, proposed by the Pharmacopoeia Committee as a substitute, being dismissed as an inferior and adulterant drug compared to the Indian squill, which is allied to the European squill. The long and short of this debate becomes clear as the mandates and processes of each are made clearer. The Pharmacopoeia Committee, it is said, was 'not called upon to report on the indigenous drugs of this country that might be recommended as substitutes for the drugs imported from Europe' (Report, p. 67) and therefore should not have accepted without wider consultation the 'Madras list' of drugs on the basis of *reputation* rather than *merit*. While it is beyond the scope of my exploration to explore these hierarchies across knowledges of southern and northern parts of the subcontinent, it is important to flag this unevenness as a possible vantage point from which to read the struggle to establish a single canon for indigenous medicine in India.

In further deliberations, the Committee is at pains to demonstrate how the most successful and therapeutically effective drugs like *Podophyllum emodi*, purportedly 'the first indigenous drug investigated by the Committee, and supported by papers published in the Edinburgh Medical Journal and Chemical Society of 1898, should be one wholly unknown to the natives of India' (Report, p. 74). These are deliberations of the same time as the battle lines with the Pharmacopoeia Committee have been drawn, and it is impossible to miss the thrust – that anything deemed indigenous that can be declared and brought to public attention and use has not happened through native agency but through the untiring efforts of Englishmen practitioners and researchers. This is another significant pointer at the emerging character of institutional (Western) medicine.

It is also useful to be attentive to who seems to be the driving force in the Committee, namely the Reporter on Economic Products, George Watt, who is also Honorary Secretary to the Committee. Whether it be arbitrations on parts of the plant that have the most active drug principle, or communications with researchers in England or with eminent specialists there, Dr Watt prevails. He is also able to direct the conversation away from the nationalist interpretation of the indigenous, away from almost every suggestion made by Dr Dey, who up until then has been seen along with Watt as having written the most influential papers on indigenous drugs, and towards the economic sense, instead, in accepting or rejecting a drug into the list or for investigation, focussing on where the supplies were available, how they could be recognized accurately, how they were to be preserved, and the pricing and agencies for distribution. Watt discusses the value of issuing standard samples of the drugs under investigation to foreign institutions like Medical Schools of the United States and the Glasgow University that have asked for these, saying that they could participate in the 'very complicated problem of the chemical, therapeutical and physiological investigation of the drugs of India' [98], indicating meanwhile the many dealings that are already in place between himself and gentlemen like Edward Morrell Holmes, the curator of the Museum of the Royal Pharmaceutical Society of Great Britain. He is also instrumental in attaching, with the identification of every new indigenous drug for investigation and possible addition to the lists, the idea that these are 'quite unknown to the Natives of this country but ... nevertheless should be included' (Report, p. 76). This translates into a resolution by the Committee that 'in future the limitation to enquiries to be prosecuted should be fixed by the term "Indigenous" ... [as] ... already ... accepted by the Government of India in ... October 1896' (Report, p. 77). As such, the proposals for an Indian drug emporium at Calcutta, or medicinal plant farms as suggested by Dey, or pharmaceutical preparations for medical stores, all get followed or rejected to differing degrees, with the enthusiasm for the inclusion of indigenous drugs in the Pharmacopoeia dissipating into territoriality, caution in the face of 'sophistication and adulteration' (Report, p. 109) of these drugs, and a recalibration of the idea of the 'indigenous'.

Patronage?

This is also the time when conversations around involving *Kobirajes* in testing indigenous drugs in hospitals, with beds set aside for these, begin to come up, and we may see links with Committee members' attempts at bringing their views into Committee decisions. Babu Bolye Chunder Sen makes this request, on 5th December 1895, to Surgeon-Lieutenant-Col J.F.P. McConnell of the Indigenous Drugs Committee, on the grounds that existing works in English on indigenous drugs are built not on experience but mere translations from Sanskrit, and that there are Kobirajes[17] like Sham Kishore Sen willing to undertake this labour, hoping for some recognition in return. We may see the familiar system of patronage being invoked here. We also see, in the Committee's reports, a list of indigenous drugs by Amulya Charan Bose, which he offers as a practitioner's experience (Report, Appendix IX, p. 148). Surgeon-Lieutenant-Col Warden suggests a 'permanent scheme for collecting information regarding and ascertaining the therapeutic values of indigenous drugs', noting with some frustration the continuing issuance of pharmacopoeias from Waring's 1868; he suggests that a useful step would be to

> ask Government to select certain schools of medicine where native students are taught, and to equip these ... with indigenous drugs ... to the exclusion of all imported vegetable ones ... [o]ne great reason for pushing the use ... [being] that the cost of medicines will be considerably reduced.
>
> (Warden, p. 150)

We see that Warden's proposals for finding cheap remedies differ from those of Watt, as evident from minutes and resolutions of the Committee. The resolution of 8th May 1896 that proposed both Local Committees and the supply of samples of indigenous drugs to selected hospitals also states the value of 'a better system of supply of indigenous products' that is likely to result from such a plan. Wherever the local committees provide lists, the local and popular names are both listed. As Watt says, in his note recommending Local Committees to be formed to support the work of the Central Committee, are the many indigenous drugs being spoken of

> sufficiently cheap to compensate for any loss in remedial value as compared with imported drugs? ... important task of directing the attention of the village practitioners to a selection of the indigenous drugs of greatest merit ... when viewed in the light of the teeming millions ... and the limited funds at the disposal of the Government ... the labours of this Committee might

fairly well be directed to making a selection, and by giving the weight of its superior knowledge, urge the few of undoubted merit to a more extended use.

(Dr. Watt's Note, Report, pp. 141–2)

For this selection to be blameless, he suggests that 'we call to our aid Native and European practitioners of high repute and pharmaceutical chemists, ... local committees be appointed ... and collect information' on these questions. To that extent, he agrees on the gaps in the literature on indigenous drugs, the information hitherto available being limited to the centres of Bombay, Madras, and Calcutta.

Regulate, standardize

It might be useful, at this point, to recall briefly some of the debates around professionalization and practitioner presence in a medical market in available scholarship. Mukharji (2009) discusses different analyses of the medical market as a 'topos to understand and describe preprofessional medicine' (p. 14), as an influence 'in shaping the identity and content of "indigenous" medicines' (ibid), and the links between the medical market and state medicine. He also suggests the need to historicize the practitioner identity. Pratik Chakrabarti has written of 'bazaars' in India as a site of 'the formation of a non-Western medical marketplace' (2007, p. 197), influencing the practice and texts of European medicine in India as well as back home in the late 17th and 18th centuries. I suggest, in light of the arguments I have been making, that the period at the cusp of the 19th to 20th centuries is also the site of emerging regulation of 'indigenous medicines' – in terms of their packaging, description, and inclusion in pharmacopoeias, availability and testing of these, and teaching medical students of their clinical value as 'substitutes'. It is this impulse that we find translating and consolidating in the contemporary in the form in which dominant Ayurvedic medicines appear – packaged as tablets rather than hand-made *golis*, with dosage and content information in standard allopathic formats. While this might appear as a linear and complete history of standardization, I am more interested in the preparations that do not make it to these standardized formularies, and the practitioners who fail to move from markets to professions, remaining attached to the *bazaar* as a marker of their professional inadequacy and corruption, linked to, in the case of *dais*, their 'inferior caste' status. This of course applies only to the engagements happening at the borders of the Western medical institution; for those outside the regulatory frameworks of profession, commerce, and governance, practice continues to this day. The archive of the somewhat exhausting details of the Indigenous Drugs Committee and its workings could be seen to tell this story.

Indigenous knowledge, native gentlemen, and colonial science

There is another impulse at work here, that of the value of colonial science. There are marginal discussions on collectors and their communities – like *Kurumbers* for Kino in Malabar, their ability to recognize medicinal plants, and their experience in collecting (Parker, 21 February 1896). These are what were listed as minor products, beginning to be recognized as a source of revenue, and here the question of notified tribes also comes up, with the legislation around these communities. Observations on these communities, available in the Committee papers, are mostly recognitions by storekeepers who are responsible for sourcing. As per the communication by Major Crawford, member of the 1894 committee and of the local branch, to the President of the Indigenous Committee, carrying extensive explanations for the contexts in which the Madras list of drugs was given to the Pharmacopoeia Committee, there is mention and appreciation of the work of 'lower classes, natives, gardeners, peasants, etc., [among whom] there is a very accurate knowledge of many ... drugs which have a vernacular nomenclature' (Crawford, 26 October 1899, Report, Appendix XXXVII.F, p. 332). Between these researchers at the Imperial Institute in London and the Central Committee, there is competition on authority to declare authenticity and merits of the drug in question, and this might also be examined through the interpretative lens of colonial science. Despite exhortations from Professor Attfield, editor of the new British Pharmacopoeia and of the proposed Indian and Colonial Addendum, that '[t]he Indian and Colonial officials here encourage direct communications with the Medical Council' (Attfield, 29 August 29 1899, cited in Report, p. 333, Appendix XXXVII. F.), this conflict, and the confusion over mandates and their interpretation, continues. It might be useful here to understand the role of the colonial administrators in determining which of these officers are finally representative and given authority to represent and take forward policies, and therefore, bear the flag of colonial science vis-a-vis the metropole. The second Madras Committee gets declared as 'entirely without any status' in this context in May 1900 (Hewett, 19 May 1900, p. 495).

The involvement or not of native practitioners in the work of commenting on and determining the indigenous drug, has been on since at least 1893, when a suggestion is made in the Bombay Pharmacologist that 'native gentlemen' be considered for pharmacological research work after suitable training, and for the post of Professor of Pharmacology. This is quickly put to rest, however, referring to the tropical climate that Arnold speaks of, unless these men be called Pharmacologists and not professors, that this be done to 'encourage native talent and work' [114] and with the understanding that such pharmacology will be inferior and at a disadvantage in the Indian climate, and therefore such experiments would be more accurately conducted in Europe. The proposal, therefore, is not granted. The provincial committees are dissolved in 1900, citing unresponsiveness, impersonal constitution, and wide dispersal, and a new system suggested, involving particular officers of select hospitals, medical storekeepers and chemical examiners, to name and determine drugs to be included. Meanwhile, the practice of sourcing of drugs named in some of the Addenda and provisional lists continues and shows the presence of collectors, or *malis* (gardeners), in their identification, collection, and even therapeutic evaluations. Parallely, the Assistant Surgeons and Hospital Assistants, native Indians, have also begun, by the end of 1899, to make suggestions for substitute drugs of indigenous origin, and in many of the reports of these experiments, the Hindustani names reappear.

After this debate is closed, unsatisfactorily but firmly, in 1900, inasmuch as the work of the Indigenous Drugs Committee is concerned, it emerges again, in among others the reports of Dr. M.R. Ry. Rao Bahadur M.C. Koman Avargal of the Indian Medical Service, on his investigation into indigenous drugs. Dr. Koman, placed on special duty in July 1918 for a period of four months, following debates in the Legislative Council calling for an investigation into Ayurvedic and Unani drugs and other indigenous drugs of India, specifically undertakes a study of the properties of the drugs considered important by *vaidyans* and *hakims*. The report is submitted in December of the same year, where Dr. Koman eventually comes to the opinion, seconded by Major General G. Giffard, Surgeon-General to the Government of Madras, who reports that as per Dr. Koman, 'the hospitals and dispensaries under Government and local boards are doing far better work for the public than the Ayurvedic dispensaries' (Giffard, 11 February 1921, p. 2), citing the multidisciplinary character of the hospitals in being able to respond to surgical and obstetric cases as also to the conditions of ear, nose, throat, etc. In sum, Dr. Koman cites some drugs as useful but mostly suggests the need for more investigation before 'they can be universally recommended' (ibid); a repeat of the cant of the Indigenous Drugs Committee, with the difference that a native medical officer conducts the investigation in the heart of Ayurvedic medicine and puts out the report. Koman also refers not only to the work of Dey, UC Dutt, and Mohideen Sheriff but also Charaka and Sushruta in translation, and several Ayurvedic compilations in Malayalam, a language of the region within what is today the Kerala state. This investigation and the consequent dismissal of any claims to efficacy by Ayurvedic drugs in general, observing that 'the science of Hindu medicine is still sunk in a state of empirical obscurity' (p. 3), assumes significance in juxtaposition to contemporary contexts where the Southern regions, and in particular Kerala, are understood today as the cradle of globally promoted Ayurveda as a tradition and as a Pharmacopoeia – a completely opposite scenario. The other, paradoxical perhaps, significance is of the naming of *systems of medicine* – here Ayurveda and Unani – as structures within which to investigate these drugs, thus simultaneously according history and codification while invoking the non-scientificity of these fields. Berger has discussed, in some detail, the taking up of the cause of Ayurveda by a different group than practitioners in the second decade of the 20th century, and the fascinating turns this takes in the career of the field. I am interested also in exploring further the return of the civilizational into this discourse, and through this, the production and consolidation of what I call the canonical indigenous. I trace this history through an exploration of two spaces – the legislative assembly debates around the teaching of indigenous medicine, particularly to native doctors, and the classificatory exercises around tribal communities that are home to many of the groups titled as collectors in the botanists' and practitioners' accounts of these drugs in this and the earlier period. Such a turn will, I propose, shed some light both on the murky and dangerous outside that continues to feature in colonial accounts of the indigenous and the interface between the institution and the indigenous that we have already been discussing. In doing so, the murky outside of the colonial also becomes that of the nationalist, canonical indigenous.

Of the diseases that are considered benefitted by these drugs, if at all, it is uterine, some intestinal, those of malnutrition, and febrile illnesses that feature in Koman's report. Given the larger contexts then and now of 'women's diseases' finding a hearing among the marginal disciplines, these comments – 'this drug is reputed in Ayurveda to be a specific in all uterine affections especially in menorrhagia' (Appendix II, p. 10), for example – are to be kept in mind, and I will attempt to explore this idea more in the *gharoa chikitsa* that I explore in Chapter 5.

One of the modes of investigation adopted by Dr. Koman involved visiting Ayurvedic dispensaries and practitioners of Ayurveda and Unani, which he reports on with comments varying from the antiquated nature of diagnostic equipment to an unwillingness to share therapeutic procedures. One of the experiences that Dr. Koman reports with incredulity – that of the refusal by a Unani *hakim* to divulge the composition and method of preparation of his remedy on the plea that this would take away his livelihood – is instructive. This is the 'murky outside' that I spoke of above, much the same as the *dai* that is described in the Ayurvedic translations or in the Dufferin Fund reports that I will discuss in the next chapter. Variously described as quacks in colonial and nationalist accounts, as folk practitioners or therapeutic subalterns in critical scholarship, these shadowy, 'irrational' figures continue to drop in and out of the institutionalization that is emerging in the therapeutic domain. They are seen as coming in the way of good science, resulting in the exasperation that the good doctor experiences; given the secretiveness of the indigenous practitioners, the good doctor has to grope in the dark for possible uses of these drugs, and to fit patients to medicines instead of the other way around. As such, the search for meritorious drugs must be conducted in a climate where these must be rescued from the practitioners themselves.

Tamil and Sanskrit names are included in the notes on each drug in Koman's report, another subtle change from earlier. Each drug note has a comment on speed of action, mostly 'slow'. Almost despite this scepticism, it would seem, Koman notes the need for 'time, labour, skill, patience and money in their preparation in accordance with Hindu Pharmacy, if they are to serve the purposes' (p. 10) – a grudging respect for the labour, skill, and time that somehow also reinstates the civilizational aspect of the knowledges in question here, while taking the official evaluative line. As is evident from the tabulated lists that follow these drug notes, several of the drugs are also stated as locally or 'bazaar-made', without adulteration – a term which was a powerful metaphor for anything *bazaar* in the discussions on the Indigenous Drugs Committee. The cure and relief rates together are also said to be clearly higher than failure rates. There is also space given, in the report, to claims by Malabar *vaidyans* in curing many diseases considered incurable by other practitioners, and therefore focus on their treatment methods as a possible source of success. There is detailing here on douching either on the scalp or other parts 'for which the services of an experienced and skilful *vaidyan* is required and certain apparatuses are necessary' (Appendix No. 9, p. 65), as also on massage, etc., and this is where we see the beginnings also of a different kind of focus, on methods rather than preparations, and the specificity associated with these, that in more contemporary times become the exotic imagery associated with Ayurveda, and by extension, Hindu India. A new orientalism is now at work, it would seem. I will explore this in more detail in the last chapter, along with the 'way of life' argument that is visible in these spaces today.

Koman is very aware of the report of the Indigenous Drug Committee, the Indian Pharmacopoeia, and other reports that have explored the same terrain, and as he draws a picture of the field from his engagement with practitioners and texts, he finds that '[t]he Tamil medical works were … originally written in high Tamil (Yelacanam) which is … peculiarly energetic and richly cultivated … [and] said to be less shackled with the mythological doctrines of the original Ayurveda, to contain a great number of formulae and to show a minute attention to the discussion of morbid symptoms' (p. 3), while he continues to comment on the exaggerations and focus on evil spirits that pervade these texts too. Another development in this round of examination of indigenous drugs is the critical although perfunctory examination of texts by Koman, where he expresses embarrassment at the focus on humours in the time of advanced physiology; and yet, the tone is less derisive, more acknowledging of the existence of a *different* system, albeit an inadequate one, and a grudging admiration of it, with a constant reference to the 'ingenuity and skill … by the ancient Sanskrit writers in their methods of classification and descriptions of the causation and symptoms of disease' (p. 4). The problem, then, is presented as these systems not standing the test of 'rational science of the present day' (ibid). In light of the historical validity, if not resilience, of these texts and the ancient practitioners, it is the present-day *vaidyans* and *hakims* who are seen to be the problem, not being erudite enough, or rational enough, and making do only on experience and mystification of their profession. In his final report, while noting some of this, and more details on modes of preparation, composition, and administration of the drugs across the western, eastern, and southern regions, Koman concludes that 'there is very little if anything for us to learn from the methods of treatment followed by the *vaidyans* and *hakims'* (p. 5), the useful drugs – for fevers, digestive complaints, leprosy, tubercular disease, and diabetes – themselves being too slow. And yet, he ends by suggesting that he has heard that 'in the lectures on Materia Medica at the Madras Medical College, the practice of including some of the important Indian drugs has of later been dropped. I would suggest the inclusion in that course of the indigenous drugs noted in Appendix No. 8, as it would serve as a guide to those students who are inclined to widen their knowledge on the subject' (p. 5). Most of Koman's observations on the outdatedness of Ayurveda, the irrationality of the explanations, and the efficacy of drugs vis-a-vis their cost, are taken on board in the final government order of 11 February 1921, while his suggestion on the teaching of some indigenous drugs in medical colleges does not find mention. Koman finally makes suggestions for extended trials of some drugs – a recommendation that finds place in the order. While Koman's suggestion itself may be read, literally, as a recommendation for the token presence of Ayurveda within the medical curriculum, the overall tone of the report would suggest that this is also a response to the prevailing political climate of the time, where particularly Ayurveda has begun to become part of the nationalist discourse. We will look at some of the legislative assembly debates to examine this more carefully. The location of evaluators like

Koman is also relevant here. As Indians within the IMS in the 1920s, Koman and others may possibly experience the same divided self that Nandy speaks of in his psychobiographies of Bose and Ramanujam; his ambivalence towards a complete dismissal of indigenous practice, and his leaving of a window open to this practice, as his appraisal of these practices as readable into a system, all provide support towards such a reading.

A messy indigenous public sphere

It is useful to consider the role of the many journals that reached and produced a vernacular reading public in the middle to late 19th century in the United Provinces, Bengal and the Delhi region. While some of these were presented as medical journals, several spoke of a desired public code, a perspective on ways of being modern, and were perhaps directed not uniquely to practitioners but the communities they were embedded in. Alavi locates, in this aspiration, medical literature that not only spoke of a system of treatment and healing, but its cultural milieu, and its potential as reference for individual practice. Among the many journals titled *Tibbi Ayeena* (Mirror of Health) being published in the late 19th century, 'in line with the title of the genre of polite literature on conduct and etiquette published for princes in Mughal India' (2008, p. 238), Alavi points to the common space created here for both those trained in Western and Unani medicine, bringing material from both realms into one text. *Akhlaaq* – 'moral self-improvement' (p. 238) – remained a cornerstone of these texts. This perspective enacts a movement from an earlier moment, in the 1820s, when British surgeon-practitioner-teachers at the Calcutta Madrasa were translating Western medical texts into Arabic and printing Unani texts in the same to replace manuscript versions, in a stated attempt to break the stranglehold of a few families on the knowledge, as Alavi details. By the time of the *Tibbi Ayeena* edited by the curator of the Agra Medical School, and the *Oudh Akhbar* – a widely circulated Urdu newspaper released in Lucknow from the Nawal Kishore Press and largely catering to the elite – the discourse had moved towards advocating for class segregation, an acceptance of caste discrimination, a trenchant criticism of unlearned indigenous practice, and a sharp critique of racial discrimination in the dispensaries, with a conspicuous lack of indictment of Western medicine itself. Munshi Newal Kishore is said to have been supported by the colonial administration post-1857 with an invitation to start a press in Lucknow, and *Oudh Akhbar* demonstrates the nature of his collaboration with them as well as with the local elite, attempting to build public opinion in favour of Western medicine and an institutionalization of Unani. Here begins an exercise of de-subalternization and centring of expert power, with powerful *hakimi* families being brought back into public favour as original curators of Unani, 'Urdu-reading self-taught and self-styled hakims who had proliferated in the nineteenth century' (p. 299) being derided as quacks, and colleges like the Takmil-ut-Tibb at Lucknow being set up through philanthropic efforts by established *hakimi* families like the Azizi family, with the tacit support of the colonial administration. These colleges present a new formalization of what counted as authentic Unani, with courses in

Western medicine being included in the syllabi, 'as a way of embellishing Unani's own robust scientific tradition' (p. 245), while claiming antiquity for itself, much like Ayurveda did. Training in midwifery was also offered at the college 'to 'literate' women ... the aim [being] ... to train 'properly such women who are at present involved in *daigiri*' (p. 298).

With the formalization of Unani education along the lines of Western medical education, Alavi says, '[t]hose whose learning skills did not correspond to this textual regimen were no more seen as hakims' (p. 299). This included the self-taught hakims, the '*jarrahs*' or barber surgeons, and of course the '*jahil dais*' indicted by Hakim Abd al Aziz (Alavi p. 299), who invited practitioners to train at the Unani college instead. The *Oudh Akhbar* played a significant role in this discourse, with the powerful hakims, in authoring views on health in its columns, taking on the role of 'public intellectual' (p. 243), demanding professionalization of Unani through 'tighter state regulation of Unani's public face: practitioners, pharmacists, and clinics' (p. 244). 'Ordinary people' were also included in the developing discourse, with complaints from individuals who were being convinced by self-styled *hakims* to disavow Western medicine; the moral was to educate *hakims* more effectively so that Unani could flourish. We see, then, the emergence of the Muslim public intellectual as an advocate for standardized Unani practice, re-establishing a rarefied textual realm for Unani, although not a handed down but a codified version, learnt at colleges run by the families who had earlier had historical control over the profession, and who also called for state benevolence and support towards this shift. *Qaum* (community) is consolidated here, as also partly connections with Graeco-European knowledge histories, and with Islam.

Arnold observes this strategy of pushing out of 'folk practices' as part of the process of centring Ayurveda too as the 'culturally appropriate alternative', as I have mentioned in Chapter 2. Some impulses towards standardization we have seen in the commentaries by native nationalist doctors above; another route to indigenous therapeutics constituted through a vernacular reading public has been discussed by Arnold (2004), and Girija (2017). Girija (2017) speaks of the emergence and practices of print media that invited, via medical magazines like *Dhanwantari* in the early 20th century in Kerala in the south of India, a diverse range of practitioners of *vaidyam* to share, for the public good, their oral wisdom and the manner in which this translated into the absorption, subsumption, and partial extrusion of these in the formation of a singular canon, with those extruded being labelled quacks, while the parts written in being re-written as esoteric, classical, inaccessible outside of the expert domain. An *Aryavaidyam*, Girija shows, is born out of a large and unstable collection of practices of *naattuvaidyam*, through this and related acts of appropriation. 'When esoteric is used to represent a classical tradition, its meaning is equivalent to scholastic, which cannot be accessed by layman with his common sense. When esoteric is associated with marginalised practices, then the meaning is equated with secrecy, quackery etc' (p. 15), she notes.

Berger, in tracing the dynamic story of Ayurveda in modernity, speaks of the emergence of a standardized language of Hindi, written in Devanagari script, in the United Provinces, and the links of this emergence to the consolidation of a national identity in the late colonial period. Print culture in the early 19th century had a significant role to play in the genesis of this 'imagined community', as historians and scholars of cultural studies have observed. Mukharji traces the role of journals like *Bhishak Darpan, Chikitsa Sammilani,* and *Swasthya* in creating both a vernacular reading public and a community of indigenous consumers of Ayurveda in Bengal from the 1870s (2009, p. 93). As in the case of *Oudh Akhbar,* these journals were part of medical literature and provided a ground to discuss both Western medicine – in fact to access advanced research in the field – and the indigenous, alongside discussions of institutional functioning, syllabi and examination papers. Mukharji suggests that 'this helped to consolidate a professional identity for the Bengali *daktars*' (p. 95). *Chikitsa Sammilani* seemed to engage with indigenous medicine more explicitly, with separate sections for *daktari* and *kaviraji,* a commitment to 'improve' as well as learn from Ayurveda as 'the "national" medicine' (p. 96), while being the ground for Bengali *daktars* to establish connections of their therapeutics with cultural context, and thereby their local embeddedness. This is somewhat in alignment with what *hakims* in northern and central India were saying about Unani being the medicine of the *mulk*. Again, like the *Oudh Akhbar,* the readership included not only medical practitioners but other elite professionals, landed gentry, and a middle-class populace of less privileged folk. Mukharji goes on to qualify this further, indicating a readership that was 'overwhelmingly Hindu' (p. 99), and a concomitant near-total absence of 'Unani *tibb* or *hakimi* medicine' (ibid) in these journals.[18]

Alavi (2008), Berger (2013), Mukharji (2009), Bhadra (2005), Sharma (2009), and others have discussed the forms, commerce, meanings, and significance of advertisements in producing an indigenous reading public. As Alavi puts it, the newspaper 'did not just create a new concept of the author; it also created a new concept of the public' (2008, p. 278), and to that end, 'advertising was the new technique that both cemented the vernacular public as well as used it as a viable commercial market for the sale of drugs, medical texts, and medical services' (p. 279). Munshi Newal Kishore, as editor and publisher of *Oudh Akhbar,* played an important role here too, promoting Western as well as certain indigenous medicines that were being advertised, making the advertisements into 'advertorials' (p. 280), putting the weight and reputation of the newspaper behind these. Newal Kishore also provided a column titled '*Zaroori Itilaa Awaam Ko*' '(Important Message/ News/Information to the Public) that often accompanied advertisements in the Oudh Akhbar' (p. 281) where he mediated dialogue between doctors and the Indian public; there were also warnings against 'spurious drugs' (p. 282). The newspaper also provided a path from the pharmaceutical agent or the doctor to the patient consumer, with agents for pharmaceutical companies or doctors often located within newspaper offices. The *hakims* too advertised their services, texts, and *nusqhas,* via advertisements in these newspapers, thus developing a different path to potential patronage than earlier, as did pharmacies and pharmaceutical companies. In addition, the Urdu press also hosted commentaries that spoke of 'new themes like the significance of chemistry in pharmacies' (p. 287), and supported translations of both Unani and English medical literature into local languages. Following Alavi, we might conclude that the *Oudh Akhbar* thus became a site for the growth of an indigenous public sphere where therapeutic models, elite concerns around the nation, commercial interests, and relationships with the colonial government intersected, with the active mediation of the editor/ publisher. Mukharji elaborates on the role of the advertisement, or *bigyapan*, in the Bengali public sphere in the mid to late 19th century, suggesting the produc-tion of a space where a 'non-specific surface identity for different medicines and medical books' (2009, p. 102) – of *kaviraji, hakimi,* or *daktari* – could be hosted. Mukharji also goes on to discuss an exoticism, located in the names of various drugs and their stated origin – from regions as diverse as China, Japan, Tasmania, and Greece, rather than simply the 'West', that seemed to inform *daktari* medicine. It is this messy co-presence of reference nomenclatures rather than therapeutic sys-tems that I suggest as the soil for an indigenous therapeutic public sphere. Berger too focusses on medical advertising in the 20th century as a space where both formal and informal knowledge of the body, expressed through advertisements around 'diseases of men' as well as 'healthy babies' (pp. 100, 102), came together in the 'education of desire, ... the deployment of nationalism, ... to the cementa-tion of cultural values within the middle class' (p. 100). While this set of ideas has found purchase in other scholarship too, Berger's exploration of the 'consumption of indigeneity' (2013, p. 99) via medical advertising, considered alongside Alavi's and Mukharji's exploration of a period just prior, suggests a loose consolidation of indigenous desire, perhaps, into a more recognizably nationalist form in the late colonial period.

The intersection between intellectual, political, and therapeutic debates informed other pharmaceutical and publishing practices too. Shinjini Das presents a rich account of homoeopathy and a vernacular reading public from the mid-19th century onwards, looking at the family, the market, and the vernacular, opening up the grounds of an indigenous therapeutic community outside of a seeming contest between Unani and Ayurveda in the Bengal context. Das speaks of the 'paradoxical production and dissemination of homoeopathy by large sections of the intelligent-sia as an unorthodox European science, peculiarly suited to Indian culture, tradition and constitution' (2019, p. 7), and following on her sharp analysis of the processes by which this comes about, we see somewhat more of the possible character of this indigenous therapeutic public sphere. Homoeopathy too, in Das' exploration, participates in the extrusion of the 'spurious', while often being indicted on the same grounds, emerging as the safe and accessible go-to for the domestic sphere. *Gharoa chikitsa,* that we will detail in Chapter 5, leans heavily on this paradigm and, in that sense, absorbs this layer of the indigenous therapeutic space.

It is in these multiple enactments, as also the indigenous intellectual masculine as the 'natural' inhabitant of the public sphere that I alluded to at the end of Chapter 2, that we see the emergence of the indigenous therapeutic public sphere in this time. The performance of Hindi nationalism in the early decades of the 20th cen-tury via clothing, purity of speech, and ideology as the grounds for 'grouping over and above kinship or community ties' (Berger, 2013, p. 79), and the use this is put to in medical writing, would be the logical culmination of this process.

Keeping in place: native practitioners, indigenous populations, indigenous practitioners

Vernacular medical education

A government order of 15 August 1916, containing a letter from P.W. Monie, Secretary to Government, to be forwarded to the Surgeon General of the Govt of Bombay, and to principals and superintendents of various medical colleges and hospitals in the country, asks for opinions on whether, 'assuming for the purpose of argument that suitable text-books in the four vernaculars and suitable teachers could be obtained, boys who had been educated in the vernaculars only would be educated sufficiently to profit by courses of instruction in the vernaculars in science and medicine' [Monie, 15 August 1916, in Medical Matters, p. 14]. In the accompaniment to this Government Order, there is reference to 'a secondary school [that] was opened in connection with the Medical College, Calcutta, for the instruction of native doctors for the ... Service' in 1839. The document also notes that 'native doctors' have anyway been taught often in 'Hindoostanee or Bengalee languages [although in] Madras and Bombay the candidates ... are required ... to give evidence of a sufficient knowledge of ... English'. It is useful, as we explore the interface between the institution and the outside, and as we unpack the outside in order to understand the emergence of the preferred indigenous, to look at the legislative assembly debates behind this order. In the proceedings of the Imperial Legislative Council of 9th March of the same year, Dr. M.N. Banerjee had moved a resolution to consider 'the advisability of establishing institutions for the purpose of giving medical students a special course of training conducted in the vernaculars so as to qualify them for ordinary medical practice in rural areas' (Banerjee, 9 March 1916, Proceedings, p. 5). As the many responses to the resolution show, and as Arnold has traced (1993), these are all activities that occupy the space of a felt need to expand the IMS, at a time when Indians have already been allowed entry, but numbers are perceived as not enough. Since an increase in numbers as demanded by a populace that is under British rule is possible only through a greater intake of natives, is such a number containable in a separate cadre, one that can be allocated to the rural (read poor) populace and safely away from the English in India? The Hon'ble Sir Pardey Lukis' suggested clause in the Imperial Council discussions, that these practitioners be limited to the rural areas, and that the institutions be kept separate, would seem to suggest so. It is acknowledged, during the course of the debate, that the question of vernacular medical education emerges alongside the 'evolution of the service of dressers (in Madras), hospital assistants (in Bombay), and native doctors (in Bengal), subsequently designated hospital assistants in all three Presidencies, and latterly known as sub-assistant surgeons' (Wheeler, 22 June 1916, Accompaniment to the G/O), all of the Subordinate Medical Service.[19] Arnold has written on this cadre of practitioners in some detail, indicating the hierarchies, and particularly the debates around inclusion of native Indians in the service (1993). The idea of introducing medical training in the vernacular is also discussed when native women are to be included for training under *purdah*; it is also mentioned in the debates around this resolution that vernacular education has worked perfectly with women students. 'Bengalee classes' had opened up in 1852, with about 15 such schools functioning across India by the time of the resolution. It is towards standardizing and regulating this system that the resolution aims, given that, as Banerjee admits during his tabling of the resolution, there are already 'a number of capable men who, though outside the Register, have been useful as country practitioners and as medical assistants in the service of Government and of the various industries, such as tea, jute, mining and shipping' (Banerjee, 15 August 1916).

The proposal itself, while a logical extension of the earlier entry of native Indians into the service, is an opening of borders of institutionalized biomedicine to the native language and its embeddedness in local cultures. Such an exercise may carry the danger of consolidating the identity of the 'native' body that is already inside the system. The 'native' is always to be suspected of having divided loyalties but can be kept in check nonetheless by separating him from his root culture and language. In the 1920s, when self-governance has already been partially instituted in India, this need to keep the 'native expert' divided, having a fragmented sense of self, is that much higher, and this is the affect that we sense lurking in the rooms, whether of the Assembly or Wellesley Place earlier where the Indigenous Drugs Committee met. Ashis Nandy's psychobiography of native scientists (1980) remains a useful reference point in this regard.

The debate in the assembly goes into the history of an earlier effort in 1826 to 'train and maintain a cheap class of medical practitioners of inferior attainments ... [with a] Madrassa for training Indian doctors, but as it proved unsatisfactory, it had to be given up six years later' (Thomas, 7 August 1917). We also see discussions of a shift, from the various exercises of determining the standard of the English qualification examination for hospital assistants, ever since the absorption of the 'Bengal class of native doctors' into the civil hospital assistant category in 1878, to recommendations in 1893 to raise the standard of English examinations, and where it might be possible to do this. Finally, in 1901, the government, 'with the object of improving the quality of the [civil medical] service, ... decided that an absolute prohibition should be enforced against the employment of students familiar only with the vernacular' (Wheeler, 15 August 1916). The United Provinces and Punjab took similar steps in 1905–6, with the students in Agra and Lahore apparently resisting the prospect of vernacular education on the grounds of 'their status and methods of instruction' not being satisfactory, while 'lecturers protested that they found teaching in the vernacular difficult, confusing and generally unsatisfactory'. At the time of the Council resolution in 1916, it was noted that highly trained medical men were unwilling to work in rural areas on account of the poor income; and the medical aid available in these areas was unsatisfactory. The vernacular schools had all adopted training in English, the Sealdah school in particular was turning out practitioners who had encyclopedic knowledge but no skills, reducing the available numbers of men for 'ordinary practice'. There might be, as Banerjee says, 'the *Kabirajes*, *Hakims* and practitioners of other methods. But times are changed and the majority of the population are for the western method of treatment, being impressed with its efficiency' (Banerjee, 15 August 1916). These modern methods must therefore be brought to the service of the general public, and it is in this

background that the suggestion of evolving a middle class of 'humble village practitioner' much along the lines of the Englishman general physician, with practical
knowledge, who could 'at least treat the simpler cases and would be an improvement on the quack' (Wheeler, 22 June 1916, Accompaniment to the G/O), gains
ground. Such a suggestion of a middle cadre had come up in 1891 in the Bengal
government but was dismissed on the grounds that these practitioners would 'raise
their fees and devote themselves to a more wealthy class'. We will see the same
logic being used in the case of the trained *dai*, with a similar set of considerations
around who could qualify to do the work, in the next chapter. During the course
of the Council debate, Sir Pardey Lukis suggests that these vernacular schools
be entirely separate from existing institutions, that these vernacularly trained village practitioners be allowed to practice only in rural areas, and that some form of
supervision be instituted to maintain standards.

Madan Mohan Malaviya and the clamour for or against the indigenous 'system'

Mukharji has written in detail about the class of 'native doctors' in Bengal, more
specifically about the figure of the *daktar* as a socially significant identity, a figure that perhaps sits at the cusp of Western medicine and Indian society. There
are, Mukharji suggests, references to south Asian physicians as far back as 1676
(Mukharji, 2009, p. 2), and to hospital assistants in Bombay in the 1700s, with
most of these early practitioners being either Eurasians or Brahmins (ibid, p. 3).
The Native Medical Institution is established in 1822, with classes being held at
the Calcutta madrasa and the Sanskrit College at Calcutta; this exercise actively
produces the category of native doctors trained in Western medicine. The more
privileged castes among these mostly achieved Sub-Assistant Surgeon status,
were considered more respectable and of a good 'family background', and were
posted at dispensaries (pp. 3, 4). We find the native doctor of Bengal being referred
to multiple times in the debate around vernacular medical education, and it is in
terms of an intervention in the fashioning of this class that Pandit Madan Mohan
Malaviya makes his two significant points in response to Dr. Banerjee's resolution.
One, for the restriction on place of practice to be removed for this proposed group
of practitioners, and two, the 'great need, the insistent need, for the Government to
recognise, even at this day, the justice of providing means for imparting instruction in the indigenous systems of medicine' (Resolution re Vernacular Medical
Training, p. 10, *The Hon'ble Pandit Madan Mohan Malaviya*, 9 March 1916). He
makes this intervention while expressing deep admiration for Western medical science and its role in the 'amelioration of human suffering' (ibid), but indicates the
role of indigenous systems in serving the vast population, the numbers they attract,
and therefore the need for the government to 'help and encourage these systems'
(ibid). An immediate furore follows in the assembly, as evident from the Vice
President's attempt to bring the house to order, and Pandit Malaviya is asked to
stay strictly within the scope of the resolution.

Opposition to the resolution, voiced primarily in worries over maintaining standards, may also be read in the context of the anxieties around the 'native within'.

Whether it is Sir Pardey Lukis who proposes a clause prohibiting these auxiliary practitioners from practising in urban areas, or Vijiaraghavachariar's insistence on no auxiliaries, no mediators, on account of this being the route to bogus practitioners, the impulse of keeping the institution exclusive and its borders opaque, is clear. Indeed, if mediation or translation be required, Vijiaraghavachariar (active leader in the Indian National Congress and later the Hindu Mahasabha, an organization founded by Pandit Malaviya) would prefer that it happen with Unani and Ayurveda, so that students would know where to look for further knowledge. As such, the preference for bringing these systems under direct supervision, is much higher than the impulse to grant more power to native practitioners to translate Western medical knowledge into communities, or to grant entry into knowledge communities for natives at reduced labour cost. The trope used, of course, is of standard, or merit.

Individual medical colleges respond to the proposal differently. Grant Medical College had accepted such a proposal first in 1861; the proposal underwent discussion in the form of a possible separation of Europeans and Indians within the service on the grounds of 'country, colour or caste, between Europeans and Indians ... [that only] referred to the division of the service in which they were to be employed' (Grant Medical College). This was followed in 1877 by a proposal to shift the teaching to local centres at Poona and Ahmedabad, and make English the medium of instruction. Finally, the proposal is accepted by several medical school superintendents and administrators, some asking for postponement. There are also, however, a barrage of apprehensive responses, as also alternative suggestions to improve the healthcare system through state subsidization of the remote dispensaries and clinics where equipped practitioners are not able to make a good enough living. Apprehensions also centre around the impossibility of translating

> scientific works properly from English into the vernacular, ... the science of medicine changes ... rapidly ... translation ... will be out of date in a very short time ... and ... the spread of the English language as a means of unifying the peoples of India should be helped.
>
> (Sale, 19 October 1916)

Even where support is available, the role of such practitioners is seen primarily as supplementary, or for maintenance of hygiene, as dressers, for instance. Also, the restriction of practice to villages by such trainees as suggested by Sir Lukis comes up again and again for rejection in the light of both the difficulty of such regulation and the poor income that would then discourage such practitioners at all.

One set of apprehensions centres around the IMS itself being tied to the Army, without what Simeox, the Collector of Ahmedabad, calls an 'organized medical profession' (Simcox A.R.A., 18 September 1916), and there are appeals for opening of a special course in the vernacular for training medical students.

Some responses are far firmer in defending the 'native Vaidyas', stating that 'it is important not to confound native Vaidyas with quacks. Unfortunately native medicine is looked upon with suspicion born of ignorance' (Memo, response to GO of 15 August, 16 October 1916); this observation goes on to give details of dispensaries and pharmacies like the Zandu Pharmacy and the Ayurvedic Aushadhalaya of Dr. Popat Prabhuram in urban areas like Bombay that are both popular and useful. The separation from quacks might be possible, 'without danger to the public and without bringing the western science of medicine into disrepute', by perhaps using compounders, says one response – 'The Gwalior State has adopted a scheme of sending out experienced compounders to work in villages' (Henderson, 12 October 1916), as also keeping them under supervision, since otherwise they were found to be operating as medical practitioners. It is also suggested in some of the responses, that if 'established *vaids* and *hakims* choose to avail themselves of such a course they should be welcomed' (Superintendent, Byramjee Jeejeebhoy Medical School, Poona, 19 October 1916). The government, at this time, seems to think that the indigenous practitioners have a strong hold on the people, even of the 'better classes'. How do we reconcile these views? One of the directions seems to be to offer vernacular-trained practitioners as competition to the Unani and Ayurvedic practitioners. Poona is suggested as an experimental centre for the same. Lt. Col. P.P. Kilkelly, superintendent, BJ Medical School, Ahmedabad, for example, joins the chorus of severe reactions to the proposal, talking about there being no dearth of English-speaking applicants for medical training, that the 'Sub-Assistant Surgeon are the back bone of the profession in India, … and every endeavour should be made to raise rather than lower their standard of education', and that a larger number of nurses would instead be preferable to training in the vernacular (Kilkelly, 23 September 1916). Kilkelly also further alleges that the scheme 'is in reality an attempt to spread Ayurvedic treatment [as] clearly shown by the remarks of the Hon'ble Pandit Madan Mohan Malawia before he was called to order by the Vice-President' (ibid). The Personal Assistant to the Surgeon-General also receives a rather sceptical response from the Principal of Grant Medical College, stating that while education in 'their own languages' will no doubt benefit 'Indian boys', the 'practicability of such a system in India at present' is much in doubt (Principal, Grant Medical College, 27 October 1916). Among other reasons, it is noted that up-do-date textbooks are available only in English.

Those approving of the resolution all suggest supervision through these schools and courses being attached to big hospitals. To recapitulate, then, we see three categories of response – support with supervision, complete rejection on account of damage to public health and to Western medicine, and support with suggestions to include indigenous medicinal systems, or that 'the Vaids and Hakims should also be encouraged' (Desai, 14 October 1916). Finally, a year down the line, on 7 August 1917, Thomas Esq, Secretary to the Government of Bombay, writes to the Secretary to the Government of India, Home Department, Simla, stating that the Bombay Government is entirely opposed to the proposal. Meanwhile, '[b]etween 1913 and 1922 Indian recruits outnumbered European … prompting post-war government anxiety over the future of the service' (Arnold, 1993, pp. 60–61), and these anxieties may well have played a role in the closure of this proposal.

Institutionalizing indigenous systems

Both favourable and unfavourable responses to Dr. M.N. Banerjee's resolution acknowledge the undeniable presence of Ayurveda and Unani in the institutional discourse of the time. Some of the responses to the proposal for short medical courses in the vernacular also bring up the question of the utility of indigenous medicines and institutions for training in indigenous systems as a way of addressing the gap in numbers and affordability of healthcare. One Dr. R.B. Naik of Dharwar, in response to a question from the Collector of the district, takes this line, speaking of 'our ancient and useful systems of medicines'. He refers to the kindness of Viceroy Lord Hardinge who 'laid the foundation stone of an indigenous medical institution in ... Delhi'. He also expresses gratitude towards a resolution in the Imperial Legislative Council by Sir Asad Ali Khan to 'investigate the possibility of placing the ancient and indigenous systems of medicine on a scientific basis and increasing their usefulness', further going on to attribute to Sir Pardey Lukis the idea that 'what appear to be inventions now in the west, were discovered hundreds of years ago by the eastern medical science, that 90 per cent of the Indians have faith in the indigenous systems, and that therefore it is desirable to improve upon them' (Naik, 19 October 1916). We have already seen Pandit Malaviya's plea to increase curricular attention to indigenous systems of medicine. Banerjee's resolution is thus placed alongside this attention to indigenous systems sought from the government, citing existing administrative support for the same. On the other hand, other medical practitioners refer to medicine being only 'a part of the method of Western treatment', other parts being ideas about 'food and diet, light and ventilation, heat and cold, changing of clothes, giving bath and even the system of giving medicine' (Kulkarni, 3 October 1916). Dr Kulkarni, a private medical practitioner, hints at the civilizational difference that I have been speaking of earlier, that is experienced at the heart of difference between medical systems, while naming Western systems as superior in overcoming prejudice – 'The English education brings about a regular revolution in the ideas of an Indian, e.g. in regard to the pollution of touch of men of inferior classes as also in regard to drinking water mixed with medicine by men of inferior classes etc. ...', and '[t]o train a man in the Western Medical Science and Surgery without giving him the necessary English education is to construct a tank without water-springs'.

It is in this time that we also see the suggestions to support, or supervise, Ayurvedic or Unani dispensaries. The Commissioner of Sind is particularly poignant in his response (Commissioner in Sind, 21 November 1916), speaking about the rapidly dying practice of the *hakims* in the face of Western medicine and consequent loss of patronage from the wealthy even in villages. Such a scheme as proposed by Dr. Banerjee is seen as a possible route for the *hakims* to revive their livelihood. And, rather than the rebuke earned by Malaviya in the Imperial Assembly, the Commissioner of Sind indicates that the

Indian politicians who are patriotically anxious to preserve the Unani and Ayurvedic systems from extinction should be given an assurance that practitioners of this new and, so to speak, composite school will not come under the ban of the Medical Council. It is very important to secure the harmonious co-operation of Western and Eastern Science.

One of the responses to and mobilizations against colonial regulatory attempts, loss of patronage, and perhaps a feared loss of presence in the therapeutic domain was the formation of associations of practitioners. The Akhil Bharatvarshiya Ayurved Mahasammelan (ABAM) was formed in 1907, and focussed on textuality, accurate translations, and ancientness as tropes of authenticity (Berger, 2013, pp. 60–62). While the idea of associationalism followed the models of professionalization, however, the ABAM would seem, following Berger's analysis, to take an esoteric rather than a voluntarist approach, primarily focussed on the affect of 'being left out', and thus we see that it does not feature significantly in the political nationalist public sphere. Other movements towards professionalization, like the Takmil-ut-Tibb established by Hakim Aziz for, in his words "'*mulki* and *fanni* khidmat" (service of the nation and the profession)' (Alavi, 2008, p. 312), seem to follow a closer link with family, community and practitioner networks via the *nuskhas* and *darrs*, as well as claims to nation. A possible connection or collaboration across Unani and Ayurveda via these associations does not seem to have taken off successfully, however, although there are suggestions in the first decade of the 20th century, when communal tensions were already reflected in the therapeutic and political discourse, for a combination of the Unani and Ayurveda systems, a suggestion 'the Azizi family fiercely resisted' (Alavi p. 311). This resistance also found a formal consolidation in the Anjuman-i-Tibia – an association for *hakims* who supported a pure Unani – that opposed Ajmal Khan's All India Vedic and Unani conference in 1911. At any rate, these associations do not seem to have garnered much attention from colonial government, except for the Takmil-ut-Tibb college at Lucknow. This college, established in 1902, was an example of medical philanthropy that Arnold speaks of that became popular among urban elite in several parts of the subcontinent, resulting in the endowment of medical colleges in Bombay and other regions, for example. In the case of the Takmil-ut-Tibb, it was held forth as a dedication to the Crown, referring to the coronation of Edward VII as the occasion for its inaugural – a possible message to the colonial government that the *hakimi* families believed in the need to regulate and standardize indigenous medical education and practice, and finding common cause to eliminate 'illiterate hakims' and spurious practice.

Pushing back: regulation and prohibition of Indigenous dispensaries

In the year before the deliberations around creating a class of native practitioners trained in the vernacular, a flurry of communications between the Governments of Bombay and the Centre are to be seen, around the proposed closing of the Poona Ayurvedic Dispensary that was reported in *The Hindu* of 13 August 1915, and cited in a letter from the Home Department to the Government of Bombay, asking for a report on the same (Government of India, 2 September 1915). The instructions for closure or alternatively to put it under the charge of a registered medical practitioner, had apparently come from the Collector following the provisions of section 11 of the Bombay Registration Act of 1912 – one of the steps towards regulation of medical practice in India. *The Hindu* goes on to talk of the history, repute, and work of the Poona Ayurvedic Dispensary, that has 'been approved as a suitable agency for giving medical relief to the numerous classes of the citizens who are habituated to the native systems of medicine'; and application of the Act which was 'admittedly intended to apply to only medical institutions conducted on ... Western principles'. Following the outrage in public and administrative circles, the secretary to government of Bombay decides to 'amend section 11 of the Act by reserving to himself the power to allow in special cases unregistered persons to hold the appointments specified ... and has permitted the Poona City Municipality to continue the maintenance of the institution' (Rieu, J.L., 7 October 1915). The order bringing this into force is enacted on 8 January 1916.

Arnold has written on the contest between Hindu and Western science, using this particular debate and the resistance to the Act as example, in the context of the revival of indigenous medicine in India (1993). A close look at the language of the conflict suggests, rather than a successfully repressive regime, however, an administration under siege, dealing with much more complexity with regard to the indigenous than it was prepared for. Prior to this, the dispensaries or *shifakhanas* had been, since the first decade of the 1800s (Alavi, 2008, p. 159), sites for the dispensing of medicine to the local populace of towns, the site of dialogue between British doctors and Indian *vaids* and *hakims*, the contribution of this dialogue to the commerce in indigenous medicines, as training centres since the 1850s for native trainees in the vernacular, and conduits for the dissemination of vaccination during epidemics. Local elites and aristocracy were major benefactors of these dispensaries. It is the 1830s, also the period of institutionalizing of training – which is systematized with the Bengal Medical Regulations of 1851 – that Alavi marks as the communal profiling of Unani and Ayurveda in these dispensaries, with the colonial administration using what they saw as the segregation of clientele of Unani and Ayurveda on caste, class and religious lines, in order to press the advantage for colonial medicine. Meanwhile, *hakims* like Inayat Hussain expressed the Unani philosophy of health as embedded in locale – 'not just climate and environment but also the political and social context' (Alavi p. 193) – as a critique of Western medicine, while offering research reports on diseases. Needless to say, this evoked strong reactions from the administration who expected him only to report on 'impediments to the spread of European medicine' (Alavi p. 194). It is in this developing climate, then, that we see the later clampdown on dispensaries.

Amidst this confusion of pushback, tolerance, and administrative struggle, there is also talk of surveillance on grants to Ayurvedic or Unani teaching institutions (1918). Already, in 1868, there were efforts to disseminate the learnings on indigenous drugs among practitioners across the provinces. About 2000 copies of the *Pharmacopoeia of India* had been considered at the time for distribution to different provinces for further dissemination to 'Native and European military hospital library ... and likewise ... to each Native dispensary within British territory' (Memorandum, 6 August 1868). A further suggestion is made, 'that copies be presented to such dispensaries in Native States as may be known to exist ... an act of recognition like that suggested would, besides bringing the work into notice, have an encouraging effect' (ibid). Such an empathetic position shifts hugely by the decade of 1910–20, as we see in the Medical Registration Act and the pressure to regulate and standardize small dispensaries as well as large institutions.

The practitioner who isn't: the depressed classes, the criminal tribes, and the dai

At various points during this history from the late 1800s to the 1920s, the question of quacks comes up. These are men seen to be either selling impure drugs in the *bazaar*, or claiming therapeutic knowledge they don't have. Prior to this, however, when Kanai Lall Dey puts out his indigenous drugs list both in 1870 and 1896, he talks about the men of 'professional castes' who have been known to collect medicinal plants for processing; these are also men of the 'lower' castes. Arnold has usefully discussed the skill attributed to the native practitioner, as also the role of native collector granted to some of these men in the colonial botany that emerges in India in the 19th century. It is useful to put this discourse around the skilled but non-knowledgeable native practitioner alongside some of the active measures towards classification and upliftment, and thereby governance, of tribal communities in the first half of the 20th century. While these two sets of conversations do not seem to intersect in any visible way, and are in fact the domain of different departments of government altogether (the general and home departments), the attempt to regulate these communities is worth exploring to see if there is overlap in their knowledges and the ones under scrutiny under the category 'indigenous'.

The point of maintaining registers of 'every male adult ... of some castes and sub-sections of castes, eg – Harranshikaris, Chorkaikadis, etc' was the assumption that these 'tribes are criminal' and should be controlled by a combination of surveillance and reform (General Department, 1916, p. 2). While the exercise of colonial categorization and surveillance of what are named criminal or nomadic tribes, on grounds of gender expression or public performance, is well known and critiqued (Philip, 2017; Hinchy, 2017, 2019), it is useful to see this alongside the exercise of educational and health reform of the 'depressed classes and backward tribes'. This latter exercise, developed following an earlier template of upliftment of certain communities through 'Mohammedan education', follows representations from Indian journals, and charts the difference of such an exercise for these groups who are a 'vast congeries of very various types, possessed of no solidarity of opinion, and containing the merest sprinkling of well-to-do individuals' (General Department, 1916, p. 1). The press note released on the issue, while making this distinction, goes on to talk about the prevailing status of primary education for these groups, the focus on scholarships, the rise in numbers of students, the prejudice among ordinary Hindus, and reflections on possible futures for these groups. On 16 March 1916, a resolution regarding amelioration of the depressed classes is brought by Mr Dadabhoy. While the language of the resolution is acutely reflective of racism and race privilege, what we are concerned with here is the directions the amelioration strategy took. Education as a source of empowerment is common to all the steps taken, and the categorization of these marginalized groups and the evaluation of their status as knowledge makers is an echo of earlier documents and texts. Sohrawardy speaks in his *Prosuti Mongol* text of 1925, for instance, of the extremely unhygienic *dhatri* (midwife) of the *dom, houri, chamar* and other 'lower castes', at whose doorstep the high maternal mortality rates can more or less be placed. The *Doms* of Benares are referred to in the Depressed Classes resolution as well, as 'hitherto [having] been condemned to menial or even predatory habits' (Dadabhoy, 16 March 1916). There is, in Dadabhoy's speech and the dynamics of the members in legislative assembly, both an indictment of privileged-caste Hindu society for this condition, and pressure on the central government to push for educational reform, in order to make sure the provincial governments follow through. The trope of unsanitariness and consequent danger to civilized society that is embedded in Sohrawardy's text as also almost all other texts of the time and earlier, however, are shared within this resolution and indeed in the entire discourse of the 'depressed classes', alongside tropes of illegality, criminality, and backwardness. Nowhere is there any reference to the ways in which these communities, particularly the 'hill tribes', are also those that have a great deal of skill and indigenous knowledge in medicinal plants and remedies. The same holds for *Bhils*, named in this resolution as also in Kanai Lall Dey's list as 'professional castes who deal in these substances' (medicinal plants). These very skills have been mobilized by colonial botanists, but there is no acknowledgement of this in the management of population exercise. Even when the work of the Forest Department is referred to, we hear that the 'hill tribesmen, who are otherwise apt to be addicted to crime ... finding themselves with regular employment and looked after by intelligent officers, soon learn to do useful work' – a reference to achievable docility, not to community knowledge, initiative, or skill. While social reform is called for in this document, it is left to society, and educational, industrial, and political change proposed as the role of government. To a proposal for a committee to look into the needs of such groups, there is opposition from several members of the council, and a resistance to official acknowledgement of marginalization and discrimination that such a Committee would mean. As one of the members, Mr Madhusudan Das notes, 'when it is a contest between a desire to improve and between old customs and traditions – customs based in most cases on religion – then we must look forward to the work of evolution; a revolution should be avoided' (ibid). With these communities – regular constituents of the murky outside – being now produced and bounded through categorization and via this framework of upliftment, moreover with elite Hindu society participating in this exercise, the knowledge communities they constitute find no place in the discussion. As Sir Reginald Craddock notes, he finds in this position even 'two Hon'ble Members, with whom I often have to disagree, as the staunchest supporters of Government' in this regard (p. 18 of the Resolution Proceedings) – referring to Surendra Nath Banerjee and Pandit Madan Mohan Malaviya – who we have earlier seen speak so passionately of the need to preserve indigenous medicine and knowledge. Given the colonial administrative positions on non-interference with native social and religious customs, the marking of the problem of the depressed classes as a social and religious problem rather than a political one, thus absolving government, is significant. This is what the mover of the resolution, Mr Dadabhoy, accurately describes as 'a policy of benevolent indifference', with no regard for the disempowerment inherent in the refusal to acknowledge knowledge skills. The *Bhil* plant collector, or the *chamar dai*, then, do not qualify as practitioners, and one more step in the construction of the canonical indigenous – a product of the Hindu society that all the members of the legislature are speaking of and from – is further consolidated. Following the withdrawal of the resolution in the Assembly, efforts to consolidate the categories of 'depressed classes' into 'untouchables', aboriginal and hill tribes, and criminal and wandering tribes, continue, with numbers of each population listed, more or less on a war footing.

It is much later, at the time of the Simon Commission in 1927–8, that we see a 'Memorial on behalf of all Marathi-speaking Untouchables of the Bombay Presidency' submitted to the Indian Statutory Commission by Dnyandev Dhruvanath Gholap, President of the Satara district of the Mahar Seva Sangha on 20 May 1928. Here the community makes a specific representation, not holding privileged-caste Hindus responsible for their plight, stating rather that 'we have to make no complaint against them … [t]hey are our co-religionists'. Rather, this sub-mission holds up their own poverty as the source of suffering. They therefore ask for specific industry that may relate to their traditional occupation of rope-making, for opportunities in government service, for residential schools, for making 'a gift of government waste lands' for cultivation. In asking for other support, they spe-cifically ask for medical and sanitary services, 'facilities for medical education … in all provinces of India', and particularly ask that 'unqualified practice whether by Vaids, Hakims or magicians should be mercilessly suppressed' (Waidande et al., 1928). Thus, while making a fairly nuanced case for rural support services, the trope of modernity and science are reinforced.

It is thus in the coming together of vernacularziation, an emerging canonical indigenous, and the extrusion of specific groups via the terms of validity for this idea of the indigenous, that the non-legitimate practitioner is born.

Conclusion

At multiple points in the debates around training in the vernacular for village prac-tice, responses talk about the greater need for midwives to be thus trained. Both sets of conversations are happening in 1916, by which time the Dufferin fund, Victoria Memorial Scholarship, and other schemes have been in effect for long, and have in fact become the subject of retrospective evaluation and recasting. These are also histories that have been well documented. I will, in the next chapter, try to open up some of these histories, trying to relate them to the emergence of the canonical indigenous in India.

Notes

1 Including what would be, in the modern world, recognized as consent, reproductive health, and so on, under the sections '*garbhadharan ki ayogya stree*' [the woman unfit

for conception/pregnancy], and '*streegamanvidhi*' [the manner in which to have sexual relations with a woman] p. 573. These are presented as prescriptive clauses, with the addressee being solely male.

2 Conditions of conception are reflected upon as having an impact on the childbirth process – an interesting parallel because these also suggest a different classification of stages of pregnancy than the modern obstetrical – we might call it a more porous or overdetermined staging.

3 Madhavakara, who Nagendranath names as the author to whom the second set of organizations of Charaka and Susruta is attributed, after Vagbhatta, is also suggested, casually, as possibly 'that Madhava who is known by other appellations, viz. Sayana and Bharatirtha Swami, the great commentator of the Vedas' (vii). This is posed as an open question by Nagendranath, and thereby, a closer link to the core Hindu texts suggested, as well as an excuse for the exclusivity of the practice and knowledge to the higher castes.

4 We do know that this is the time of the Dufferin Fund, Victoria Memorial Scholarship Fund, and other forms of training of *dais* coming up in the context of concern being expressed on questions of maternal mortality among Indian women. The discourse around the precarity of maternal health, therefore, particularly puerperal fever in the context of the 'unhygienic indigenous dai', is well in place. We will, in Chapter 4, come back to this context.

5 'Orthodox Hindus, who have a prejudice against ship-borne salt' (xxxii).

6 Treatment of women's ailments as per homoeopathy.

7 Facts of pregnancy.

8 Care during pregnancy.

9 About pregnancy.

10 Pertaining to childbirth and the welfare of the infant.

11 Health and Baby Show.

12 The pointer to vitality, popularly and in colonial administrative parlance, associated with 'martial' communities in western India are hard to miss here.

13 Translating as 'Women are wont to say such-and-such, but Bhagvan Atreya prescribes differently' (p. 546).

14 Some of the terms are retained in the text in what I have been calling common-use language, including the particular 'corruptions' of English terms easily recognizable within communities. Castel (castor oil) and tarpin (turpentine oil) are examples.

15 Treatment of female diseases.

16 The spelling as listed.

17 The spelling used in the Report.

18 While communalization, particularly in the period of dyarchy, has been one of the lenses through which this has been read in most scholarship, it might be useful to think of segregation as a received trope that fashioned most of the therapeutic discourse in the subcontinent during this period. The period of the late 19th century, in the context of competition for a reduced patronage for indigenous medicine, the self-fashioning of Ayurveda as a separate entity would likely have definitely found anchor in the increasingly polarized political debates building up to dyarchy, but this may yet not qualify as the communalism of independent India.

19 A Commission was appointed in 1866 to consider measures to improve the Subordinate Medical Services.

References

Books and articles

Alavi, S. (2008). *Islam and healing: Loss and recovery of an Indo-Muslim medical tradition, 1600–1900*. London: Palgrave Macmillan.

Alcoff, L., & Dalmiya, V. (1993). Are old wives' tales justified? In L. Alcoff & E. Potter (Eds.), *Feminist epistemologies* (pp. 217–244). New York and London: Routledge.

Arnold, D. (1993). *Colonizing the body: State medicine and epidemic disease in nineteenth-century India*. Berkeley and Los Angeles: University of California Press.

Arnold, D. (2004). *Science, technology and medicine in colonial India* (The New Cambridge History of India, Vol. 5). Cambridge: Cambridge University Press.

Arnold, D. (2006). *The tropics and the traveling gaze: India, landscape, and science, 1800–1856*. Seattle and London: University of Washington Press.

Bala, P. (Ed.). (2009). *Biomedicine as a contested site: Some revelations in imperial contexts*. Lanham, Boulder, New York, Toronto and Plymouth: Lexington Books.

Bala, P. (Ed.). (2012). *Contesting colonial authority: Medicine and indigenous responses in nineteenth- and twentieth-century India*. Lanham, Boulder, New York, Toronto and Plymouth: Lexington Books.

Bala, P. (Ed.). (2019). *Learning from empire: Medicine, knowledge and transfers under portuguese rule*. Cambridge Scholars Publishing.

Berger, R. (2013). *Ayurveda made modern: Political histories of indigenous medicine in Northern India, 1900–1955*. New York: Palgrave Macmillan.

Bhadra, G. (2005). *From an imperial product to a national drink: The culture of tea consumption in modern India*. Tea Board India, Department of Commerce, Kolkata.

Botre, S., & Haynes, D. E. (2017). Sexual knowledge, sexual anxieties: Middle-class males in western India and the correspondence in Samaj Swasthya, 1927–53. *Modern Asian Studies, 51*(4), 991–1034.

Chakrabarti, P. (2007). Medical marketplaces beyond the West: Bazaar medicine, trade and the English establishment in Eighteenth-century India. In M. S. R. Jenner & P. Wallis (Eds.), *Medicine and the market in England and its colonies, c. 1450–c. 1850*. London: Palgrave Macmillan.

Chakravarti U. (1989). Whatever happened to the Vedic Dasi? Orientalism, nationalism and a script for the past. In K. Sangari & S. Vaid (Eds.), *Recasting women: Essays in colonial history* (pp. 27–87). New Brunswick, NJ: Rutgers University Press.

Chatterjee, P. (2019). Women and nation revisited. In P. Ray (Ed.), *Women speak nation* (pp. 19–28). India: Routledge.

Chattopadhyaya, D. (1992). *Lokayata: A study in ancient Indian materialism* (7th ed.). New Delhi: People's Publishing House.

Das, S. (2019). *Vernacular medicine in colonial India: Family, market and homoeopathy*. Cambridge, New York, Victoria, New Delhi and Singapore: Cambridge University Press.

Devji, F. F. (2018). Gender and the politics of space: The movement for women's reform in, 1857–1900. In Z. Hasan (Ed.), *Forging Identities: Gender, communities and the state in India* (pp. 22–37). London and New York: Routledge.

Ghosh, A. (2006). *Power in print: Popular publishing and the politics of language and culture in a colonial society, 1778–1905*. New Delhi: Oxford University Press.

Girija, K. P. (2017). Interface with media and institutions: The reordering of indigenous medical practitioners in twentieth-century Kerala. *History and Sociology of South Asia, 11*(1), 1–18.

Guha, A. (2018). *Colonial modernities: Midwifery in Bengal, c. 1860–1947*. London and New York: Routledge.

Gupta, C. (2005). Procreation and pleasure: Writings of a woman Ayurvedic practitioner in colonial North India. *Studies in History, 21*(1), 17–44.

Hinchy, J. (2017). Obscenity, moral contagion and masculinity: Hijras in public space in colonial North India. In *Contestations over gender in Asia* (pp. 111–132). Oxon and New York: Routledge.

Hinchy, J. (2019). *Governing gender and sexuality in colonial India: The Hijra, c. 1850–1900*. Cambridge: Cambridge University Press.

Langford, J. (2002). *Fluent bodies: Ayurvedic remedies for postcolonial imbalance*. Durham and London: Duke University Press.

Mukharji, P. B. (2008). Pharmacology, 'indigenous knowledge', nationalism: A few words from the epitaph of subaltern science (195-212). In B. Pati & M. Harrison (Eds.), *The social history of health and medicine in colonial India* (pp. 1–14). London and New York: Routledge.

Mukharji, P. B. (2009). *Nationalizing the body: The medical market, print and Daktari medicine*. London and New York: Anthem Press.

Mukharji, P. B. (2016). *Doctoring traditions: Ayurveda, small technologies, and braided sciences*. Chicago: University of Chicago Press

Mukherjee, S. (2001). *Disciplining the body? Health care for women and children in early twentieth century Bengal*. In D. Kumar (ed.), *Disease and medicine in India: A historical overview* (pp.198–214). New Delhi: Tulika Books.

Nandy, A. (1980). *Alternative sciences: Creativity and authenticity in two Indian scientists*. Mumbai: Allied Publishers.

Nandy, A. (Ed.). (1989). *Science, violence and hegemony: A requiem for modernity*. New Delhi: Oxford University Press.

Philip, K. (2017). English mud: Towards a critical cultural studies of colonial science. In A. Balsalmo (Ed.), *Cultural studies 12 (3).* (pp. 300–331). London: Routledge.

Prakash, G. (1994). Subaltern studies as postcolonial criticism. *The American Historical Review, 99*(5), 1475–1490.

Sharma, M. (2009). Creating a consumer: Exploring medical advertisements in colonial India. In B. Pati & M. Harrison (Eds.), *The social history of health and medicine in colonial India*. London and New York: Routledge.

Sivaramakrishnan, K. (2006). *Old potions, new bottles: Recasting indigenous medicine in colonial Punjab (1850–1945)* (New Perspectives in South Asian History, number 12). Hyderabad: Orient Longman.

Thapar, R. (2002). *Early India: From the origins to AD 1300*. Berkeley: University of California Press.

Visvanathan, S. (2003). Progress and violence. In A. Lightman D. Sarewitz, & C. Desser (Eds.), *Living with the genie: Essays on technology and the quest for human mastery* (pp. 157–180). Washington: Island Press.

Watt, G. (1890). *A dictionary of the economic products of India*. Volume III. Dacrydium to Gordonia. Calcutta: Government Press.

Archival sources

From British Library, UK -

Devanagari/Hindi texts -

Author unknown. (1892). *Garbharaksha-athahidayatnama-daiyanali.* A Supplementary Catalogue of Hindi Books in the Library of the British Museum acquired during the years 1893–1912. By J. F. Blumhardt. Open Access Asian & African Studies Reading Room ORC HIN PBS 2 (VT 1241).

Author unknown. (1900). *Aushadhikriya.* A Supplementary Catalogue of Hindi Books In the Library of the British Museum acquired during the years 1893–1912. By J. F. Blumhardt. Open Access Asian & African Studies Reading Room ORC HIN PBS 2 (14043.c. 45 (2). UIN:BLL01002223054).

Bajpai, P. R. (1891, January). Susruta Samhita bhashanuvaad. [A treatise on medicine, translated from the Sanskrit, Lucknow]. In *A supplementary catalogue of Hindi books in the library of the British Museum acquired during the years 1893–1912*. By J. F. Blumhardt. Open Access Asian & African Studies Reading Room ORC HIN PBS 2 (14156.c.4. UIN: BLL01002223054).

Gopal, P. (1874). *A catalogue of drugs indigenous to the Bombay presidency, arranged according to "drury's useful plants of India".* Byculla, Bombay: Education Society's Press. (Asia, Pacific & Africa T 35502, UIN: BLL01007260132).
Heeralal Mulazim Manve. (1867). *Vaidyaksaar: jisko Janab Machhu Khan sahib ke mananusar unke granth vaidak mein se sangrah kar arthat vaidak ka saar le ... Hindi bhasha mein banaya.* Agra. (No. 16 of 1076).

Bangla texts –

Compilation. (1924). *Homeopathic mate Streerog Chikitsa: Garensi, Jwar, Minton probhriti bibidho homeopathik utkrishto grantho hoyte sankalit (dwitiyo sanskaran, sanshodhito o paribardhito).* Calcutta: Batokrishno Pal & Company. (Ben B 3701).
Mukhyopadhyay, B. (1926). *Prasuti o Paricharja.* Calcutta: Batokrishno Pal & Company. (Ben D 478).
Sen, J. (1929). *Prasuti Tattva* (Ben B 5005).
Sohrawardy, M. H. (1925). *Prasuti o Sishu Mongol.* Calcutta: Wellington Square Art Press. (Ben B 4382).

English texts -

Dey, K. L. (1867). *The Indigenous drugs of India; or, Short descriptive notices of the medicine, both vegetable and mineral, in common use among the natives of India.* Calcutta: Thacker, Spink, and Co. (Asia, Pacific & Africa T 35541. General Reference Collection 7509.ccc.14. UIN: BLL01001924756)
Dey, K. L. Assisted by William Mair. (1896). *The Indigenous drugs of India: Short descriptive notices of the principal medicinal products met with in British India* (2nd ed., Revised and entirely Re-written). Calcutta: Thacker, Spink, and Co. London: W. Thacker and Co. (Shelfmark(s): General Reference Collection 07509.h.1. Asia, Pacific & Africa T 12628. UIN: BLL01001924757).
Koman, M. C. (Madras, 1921). *Reports [3] on the investigation into indigenous drugs.* India Office Records and Private Papers. (IOR/V/27/850/41).
Sen Gupta, N. (1901. 1907). *The Ayurvedic system of medicine, or, An exposition, in English, of Hindu medicine as occurring in Charaka, Sucruta, Bágbhata, and other authoritative works, ancient and modern, in Sanskrit / by Kaviraj Nagendra Nath Sen Gupta.* Calcutta: K.R. Chatterjee [etc.]. (Asia, Pacific & Africa T 35442, UIN: BLL01007260216).
Waidande, M., et al. (1928). In Gholap, D. D. E-Bom-416: Memorial on behalf of all Marathi speaking Untouchables of the Bombay Presidency, submitted to the Commission by Dnyandev Dhruvanath Gholap, President of the Satara District Mahar Seva Sangha. (20 May 1928). India Office Records and Private Papers. (IOR/Q/13/1/5, item 33).
Waring, E. J. (1868). Pharmacopoeia of India prepared under the authority of her Majesty's Secretary of State for India in Council. India Office. W. H. Allen and Co: London.

From Internet Archive online –

Sen, N. (Compiled). (1960). *Vaidyak shiksha, arthat charak, sushrut, vagbhat, ... Ayurvedic shastra ke yavatiya janne laayak vishayon ki sanchit pustak* (1st ed.). Kalkatta. Retrieved from the Internet Archive https://ia804608.us.archive.org/23/items/uuYQ_vaidyak-shiksha-by-nagendranath-sen-nagendra-printing-works-calcutta/Vaidyak%20Shiksha%20by%20Nagendranath%20Sen%20-%20Nagendra%20Printing%20Works%20Calcutta.pdf

From Maharashtra State Archives, Mumbai, India –

Central Indigenous Drugs Committee. (1896–1901). *Report of the central indigenous drugs committee.* (N10883).

Central Indigenous Drugs Committee. (1896–1901). *Report of the central indigenous drugs committee, Appendix I to Para I of the report, resolution of the Govt of India appointing the committee.* (N10883).

Commissioner in Sind. (1916, November 21). To The Secretary to Government, General Department. In Accompaniments to the letter to the Government of India, Home Department (Medical), no. 5499, dated the 7 August 1917. No. T.-32. (No. 1452, Box 162, S-M 161–2).

Crawford, Major F. J. M.D., IMS, Honorary Secretary, Indigenous Drugs Committee, Madras. (1899, August 17). To – George Watt, Esq, M.B., C.M., C.I.E., etc, Reporter on Economic Products to the Government of India and Honorary Secretary, Central Indigenous Drugs Committee. In *Report of the Central Indigenous Drugs Committee.* Appendix XXXVII. F. to paras 97.98 and 114 (3) of the Report. No. 17, Madras Medical College.

Crawford, Major F. J. M.D., IMS. (No. 2226, 1899, October 26). To The President, Madras Branch, Indigenous Drugs Committee, Medical College, Madras. In *Report of the Central Indigenous Drugs Committee.* Appendix XXXVII. F.

Desai. (1916, October 16). Memo: The G.O. no. 5530 dated 15 August 1916 is returned herewith – with compliments with the following views and suggestions which occur thereon. (No. 1452, Box 162, S M 93–99). Na[n]diad.

Finance Department, Calcutta. (1918, January 14). Letter to the Honorable P. R. Cadell, Chief Secretary to the Govt. of Bombay. Maharashtra State Archives, Bombay (General Department, No. 37, Box no. 2, S-M 1).

Government of Bombay. (1916, March 9). Extract from the Proceedings of the Indian Legislative Council assembled under the provisions of the Government of India Act, 1915 (5&6 Geo. V, Ch. 61). Resolution re Vernacular Medical Training (S-M 17–28). In Medical Matters (No. 1452, Box 162).

Government of Bombay, General Department. (1916, August 15 Order no. 5530). *Medical Matters: Regarding the advisability of establishing institutions for the purpose of giving medical students a special course of training conducted in the vernaculars.* (No. 1452, Box 162).

Government of Bombay, General Department, Order no. 178 (1916, January 8). Letter from the Government of India, Home Department (Medical), No. 926, dated the 2 September, 1915. In Dispensaries: Regarding the closing of the Poona Municipal Ayurvedic Dispensary, and the amendment of the Act. (General Department, No. 1326, Box 159).

Henderson, C. G. (1916, October 12). Camp Surat, Assistant Collector. No. G.E.N. 50 of 1916.To Collector, Your M.E.D. 185 of 14-9-1916. (No. 1452, Box 162, S-M 107–8).

Hewett, J.P., Esq., C.S.I., C.I.E., Secretary to the Government of India, Home Department. (No. 930, Simla, 1900, May 19). To George Watt, Esq., M.B., C.M., C.I.E., Reporter on Economic Products to the Government of India, and Honorary Secretary, Central Indigenous Drugs Committee. In *Report of the Central Indigenous Drugs Committee.* Appendix LVI.

Kilkelly, P.P. (1916, September 23). Letter To the Personal assistant to the Surgeon-General with the Government of Bombay. No. 931 of 1916. (No. 1452, Box 162, S-M121).

Kulkarni, Private Medical Practitioner (1916, October 3). To The Collector of Dharwar. [in response to letter no. 3255 dated 15 September 1916, on opinion regarding advisability of establishing institutions for the purpose of giving students a special medical course of training in the vernaculars (No. 1452, Box 162, S-M 79–85).

Naik, R. B. (1916, October 19). To The Collector, Dharwar. No. 388 of 1916. [Regarding views regarding the advisability of establishing institutions for the purpose of giving training in the vernacular to medical students]. (No. 1452, Box 162, S-M 69–77).

Parker, Lieutenant-Colonel J. IMS Medical Storekeeper to Government, Bombay Command, to the Reporter on Economic Products to the Government of India – No. 1364 -G. (21 February 1896, extract from). In *Report of the Central Indigenous Drugs Committee, Appendix XXV. B.*

Press note. Ca 1916. Education of Depressed Classes and Backward Tribes. In Depressed Classes. Improvement of the moral, material and educational condition of the. (General Department, 1916, No. 785, Box No. 144).

Principal, Grant Medical College. (ca 1916). Resubmitted after issue of orders with reference to para 1 of the Secretary's note dated the 11 July 1916. (No. 1452, Box 162, S-M31-36).

Principal, Grant Medical College. (1916, September 27). To The Personal Assistant to the Surgeon General with the Government of Bombay, Poona. (No. 1452, Box 162, S M 113).

Resolution re Amelioration of the Depressed Classes. (1916, Thursday, March 16). In Extract from the Proceedings of the Indian Legislative Council assembled under the provisions of the Government of India Act, 1915 (5&6 Geo. V, Ch. 61). Council Chamber, Imperial Secretariat, Delhi.

Rieu, J. L. (1915, October 7). Letter to The Secretary to the Government of India, Home Department (Medical). (General Department, No. 1326, Box 159).

Sale, E. L. Esquire, B. A. I. C. S., Collector of Belgaum (1916, October 19). To The Commissioner, Southern Division. Course of medical training in the vernaculars (No. 1452, Box 162, S M 53–55).

Simcox, A. R. A. Esquire, I. C. S., Collector of Ahmedabad (September 18, 1916). To The Commissioner, Northern Division. (No. 1452, Box 162, S M 87–89).

Superintendent, Byramjee Jeejeebhoy Medical School, Poona. (1916, October 19). M119. Note on vernacular medical training (vide Govt order, General Department, no. 5530, 15 August 1916). (No. 1452, Box 162, S-M 117–119).

Thomas, G. A. Secretary to the Government of Bombay. (1917, August 7, Bombay Castle). Letter to The Secretary to the Government of India, Home department (Medical). (General Department, No. 1452, Box 162, S-M 159).

Warden, C. J. H. Surgeon-Lieutenant-Colonel, M.D. *A Permanent Scheme for collecting Information and ascertaining the Therapeutic Values of Indigenous Drugs.* In *Report of the Central Indigenous Drugs Committee. Appendix X.*

Watson, J. F. (1868, August 6). Memorandum, K. 641/497. (General Department, No. 37, Box no. 2, M-S 92).

Wheeler, H. Secretary to the Government of Bombay. (1916, August 15). Letter to the Secretary to the Government of Bombay, General Department. In Accompaniment to the Government Order, General Department, no. 5530. (S-M17-20, No. 1452, Box 162).

4 Revisiting the clinical encounter II

The emergence of the dai in the management of populations

Introduction

My formulations in this chapter are the following. One, as I attempt to open up what I have called, in the previous chapter, the murky outside, I suggest that the *dai*, as available or absent in canonical or popular medical texts, administrative accounts, nationalist discourse, or proto-feminist literature in the 19th and early 20th centuries, is not presented as an indigenous knowledge practitioner or as a participant in the dialogue or conflict between institutionalized western medicine and what might be deemed the indigenous.[1] This is one of the differences I would mark from British or European midwifery, which have been regularly visited by feminist scholars as exemplars of an alternative model of knowledge than the propositional scientific (Dalmiya & Alcoff, 1993).

Two, the hyperbolic and vitriolic rejection of the *dai* in early missionary and later colonial administrative documents, justified on the grounds of her failure to be learned, trainable, or responsible, is, I propose, more accurately read as a caste rejection, one that extends into attempts at reform and training in the 19th century. This is an impulse that also travels into post-independence policy documents.

Three, the analogy of the *dai as a traditional birth attendant*, a concrete and fairly pan-Indian agent of childbirth, rather than being a more porous figure, having different roles and stakes, and diverse responses even in childbirth scenarios, in fact, being more than one individual, is actually *produced within the discourse of the colonial* – and by this I mean the exhortations of missionaries, Englishwomen physicians who are seeking the setting up of *zenana* hospitals, the push towards the institutionalization of Western medicine, and the focus on women's reproductive health and education by elite middle-class, privileged caste reformers and nationalists, maintaining caste lines and the status quo, thus creating an implicit collusion of the scientist and the casteist in the late 19th to early 20th centuries.

What, then, is the feminist epistemological question that might be asked of this category/figure/space? How do the discourses of knowledge (including non-codified ritual and bodily knowledge), skill, care, and stigma intersect, and what might be the connections with the idea of the 'indigenous'? These are the questions I hope to ask in this chapter.

DOI: 10.4324/9780367824051-4

Missionaries, Englishwomen physicians, and the naming of the *dai*

Concern over the health of women in India was a recurring theme in multiple non-administrative sectors, including missionary work, since at least the 1860s. Modern missionary work is said to have begun in the 1790s (Fitzgerald, 2005); the London Missionary Society established a mission in the United Provinces in the 1820s (Semple, 2008, p. 562). Semple has talked extensively about the hierarchies prevailing in mission work, among wives and daughters of missionaries, single British women who were introduced into missionary work from the 1870s, local Anglo-Indian women, and native Biblewomen, in terms of pay, expert status, those doing *zenana* visits and those in teaching work. I have discussed, in Chapter 2, the meanings of these for a historiography of colonial science that has paid no attention to women as actors. Here, I focus more on the incitements available in the records of these missionary societies, on the 'women of India and what can be done for them' – a constantly repeated concern. Before that, however, I offer a few notes on the gendered structure of mission work.

Rosemary Fitzgerald, Rhonda Semple, and others have written about the history of women in mission work, particularly in India and China, from the early to late 19th and early 20th centuries. 'Women's work with women' was the framework in which women missionaries were drawn in; while the first to get involved were the wives and daughters of the male missionaries, this was followed by single professional women in the 1870s. Fitzgerald discusses the nature of gendering and segregation that projected the women of Christian missionary families as models of domestic and familial life, thus allowing for what she calls a 'domestic evangelism' (2005, p. 67). Fitzgerald reads a shift of missionary work into the 'social as well as the spiritual' (p. 65) in the later years of the 19th century. Evangelical work, the domain of ordained men in the missionary societies, took second place to more secular 'civilizing' activities in the work of these women (Brouwer 2019, pp. 11–12). Within the missions themselves and at the London Missionary Society (LMS), conflicts over focus on evangelical or secular work were common, as also were conflicts over the role and scope of work for 'native brethren' and Biblewomen, for example (Semple, 2003, pp. 71–114). It is in this context that we must see the comments of medical women attached to missions on the health and conditions of women in India. The mission women – professionals and others – were also often individual negotiators on what could constitute important work or demanded more funds, and this is the other relevant context here. By the time professional single women enter, and the first female medical missions are initiated in the 1860s and 1870s, mission attention has shifted to the 'zenana', or what is seen as the 'inner social life of India' (Elmslie, a medical missionary in Kashmir, quoted in Fitzgerald, 2005, p. 69). *Zenana* women, seen as guardians of 'indigenous culture' (Fitzgerald, 2005, p. 70) by missions as well as administrators, or of the spiritual domain by nationalists (Chatterjee, 1989, 2019), were also seen as victims of 'the barbarous practices of native midwifery' (Williamson, quoted in Fitzgerald, 2005, p. 70), and the latter seen as the justification, as also the way, to enter into these inner recesses. Needless to say, this segregation of domains was articulated by all parties more in northern Indian contexts than elsewhere. The results sought of this 'good work' were social transformation, modelled on the Western Christian world, with the medical work 'act[ing] as an "entering wedge"' (p. 65).

It is useful to mark some of the language of the mission literature. One tract, titled *The Women of India, and what can be done for them*, comes out in 1888 and is part of a series of papers on Indian reform that range from commentaries on character and debt to sanitary reform, caste, and religious reform (Christian Vernacular Education Society, 1888). One of the primary laments of this particular paper is the condition of women in India who, it says, are denied 'their full share of the air and light of Nature's free gift' (Dorabji E. Gimi, quoted on p. 96), on account of being disallowed from public spaces. While this, and its contestation by elite nationalists, is an old debate that I will address more fully in the next chapter, the implications of this taboo for women's health are what we are concerned with here. The absence of air and light is something that 'Hindu practitioners' also refer to in the early years of the 20th century, and there as here, it is seen as a source of debility and proneness to maternal morbidity or mortality, both before and during childbirth. As has been discussed in the scholarship around gender segregation, the paper also refers to the observations of 'a Native writer in the *Indian Magazine*', on how, owing to 'the delicacy, to communicate even to their male relatives the character and symptoms of their complaints, native ladies either directly consult or, through their maid-servants, obtain whatever help they can get from village midwives and quacks of their own sex, and the result generally is very serious' (p. 102). And,

> in the lying-in chamber ... *Vaids* and *Hakims* do not study the character of puerperal diseases, nor as a rule undertake to attend to them, and the whole duty of puerperal management devolves on our midwives, who, as a body, are utterly incompetent. They belong to the lowest grade of society, and are never trained in their work. When widowed and old, women of the lowest caste, such as *Domes*, *Chamars*, and *Podes*, &c., first seek employment as attendants on women in confinements, and after a time set themselves up as midwives. There is thus no help for Indian women at the most critical period of their lives, except what may be obtained from these so-called *Dhaies*.
>
> (ibid, p. 102)

Before we go into the work of medical women in India, it might be useful to underline a suggestion that this paper makes and that establishes itself more fully in the nationalist discourse about a decade later. The wife, whose health and well-being are under consideration here, is of the educated upper-caste nationalist and is in danger from the 'lowest caste' women. These dangerous women are non-familial, outside of the structures of endogamous marriage and family as we know it, being older, widowed, or single women. Alongside the other aspects of reform, these women, then, are those from whom distance must increase, for the nation to acquire greater health. All these exhortations to a better life for the wife are attributed to one Raja Sir Madhava Row, to whom the paper is dedicated, and whose pronouncements on the self-inflicted evils of the 'Hindu community' make him a prime reference for the paper.

It is with this set of dangerous women that the Countess of Dufferin Fund and others must contend as they attempt to provide 'competent female medical attendance' (p. 32) to the suffering Indian woman-as-wife.

Sanitary reform, professionalization, and the management of populations

Sanitary reform as the removal of the offensive

As part of the reform papers of the Christian Vernacular Education Society, there is also one on sanitary reform (Murdoch, 1888), relating to the need for such reform, the definitions of health, the common causes of morbidity including cholera, smallpox, and other infectious diseases, and the mortality and morbidity rates in the population. Referring to public health talks and accounts from 1885 (Sir Joseph Cunningham, 'Public Health in India'), the paper also highlights the practice of registration of births and deaths. The paper goes on to describe and decry the 'supposed causes of sickness' (p. 3) of cholera and smallpox, in particular, believed to be caused respectively by Kali, *Mari-amman*, or the goddess *Sitala*. The paper goes on to list the 'true causes of sickness' in the 'properties of bodies', and eventually pronounces that 'Filth is the mother of sickness ... the true *Mari-amman*, Mother of Death' (ibid, p. 5), and that 'health is largely secured by' good water, pure air, suitable food, and cleanliness. The paper refers to the histories of plague and other epidemics in England and Europe, making a reference almost in passing to the 'discovery of vaccination' after which smallpox deaths in England dramatically reduced, going on to make a comparison between the 'sanitary condition of India at present ... [and] that of England in the seventeenth century' (p. 7), and therefore the 'need of sanitary knowledge', so that '[s]anitary regulations [which] are regarded by the masses as mere freaks of their rulers ... [or] as a kind of zulum (oppression)' (ibid, p. 9), may be better observed. The paper goes on to detail these regulations and knowledge, and to relate the value of these particularly in the context of inadequate numbers of doctors and *dais*. The point of this discussion for our purposes is to indicate the language of sanitation and hygiene as it appears in para-institutional spaces in the last decades of the 19th century and the link made in these to maternal welfare.

Frank Snowden (2019) presents a detailed account of the histories of sanitary reform in France and England in the 1830s and 1840s, on the premise of what he calls the 'sanitary idea' (p. 185). Snowden states that the idea that filth bred disease was first born in Paris, where scientists sought to find a measurable correlation between the smell of effluents in Paris and the prevalence of disease. This idea, travelling to England, translated, in the work of the influential Edwin Chadwick and his colleague Thomas Southwood Smith, into the 'filth theory of disease' (p. 189), broadly meaning that microenvironments in urban localities were the cause of disease, that disease caused poverty rather than the other way around as other medical opinions of the time would suggest, that these were aggravated by alcoholism and were therefore individual responsibility, and that filth must be removed through centralized state initiatives. This led, in 1848, to a Public Health Act. Chadwick had also been instrumental, prior to this, in introducing poor law reform through the Poor Law of 1834, promoting the notorious idea that welfare would breed laziness, and therefore proposing to make welfare itself so painful that all but the 'deserving poor' would be pushed to work, no matter how exploitative. Put together, these interventions in poverty and disease provided a mode of social control, responding to indigent distress by proposing that longer lifespans, that would purportedly be brought in by good health promoted by cleanliness, would introduce more productivity and responsibility as the population – the male population – aged and matured (Snowden, 2019, pp. 184–203). Snowden goes on to indicate the Christian ethic of behaviour also underlying this line of thinking, as well as the denial of just working conditions, daily wage, or working hours, having anything to do with health or disease. This civilizing mission for England's poor could not but have had echoes in the colonial government's moral and humanitarian impulse, with the trope of racial inferiority offering a ready placeholder for poverty, and the tying of sanitary science with caste discriminatory vocabularies of 'filth', non-cognitive work, and indolence. The 'indigenous' or '*bazaar dai*' as a category could logically be born in this scenario.

We may recall here the work of Mary Douglas on the hyphenated questions of power and danger. Turning Douglas' anthropological impulse towards colonizer societies allows us to locate the 'ignorant', 'filthy' *bazaar dai* via the framework of 'social inarticulateness' (1984 [66], p. 103) that Douglas offers, for 'marginal … people who are somehow left out in the patterning of society, who are placeless' (p. 96). Douglas speaks of different forms of power – that accorded to authority figures, that exercised by the system when there is dissent or defiance, and that attributed to the 'formless', the ones whose 'status is indefinable' (ibid); in what she calls a secular and not ritual context, this is someone 'credited with unreliability, unteachability, and all the wrong social attitudes' (p. 98). This powerful trope to understand the 'witch' in Western societies might well have been a placeholder for the *dai* in colonizer accounts; the hyperbolic and almost identical language through which this figure is referred definitely invites such an interpretation.

Another element of the discourse on public health in the colony is that of who constituted the 'public'. Partho Datta traces some of the positions on public health and the notion of the 'public' in this frame through the work of Sudipto Kaviraj's articulation of a 'protopolitical public in colonial India' that was 'highly restricted and regulated' (Datta, 2009, p. 17). Datta sees the urban planning efforts toward 'road building, slum clearance and regulation of markets' (ibid), as well as the setting up of hospitals, as public health initiatives to contain and prevent epidemics in the late 18th century. The hospitals, Datta avers, were also segregated to respond to a differentiated public, with the destitute being picked up for the Police Hospital in Calcutta, and other hospitals catering exclusively to the European or native residential populace. Datta goes on to discuss Ranald Martin's 1837 *Notes on the Medical Topography of Calcutta*, published at a time when the germ theory was displacing environments as a cause of disease in Europe, but medical topographies persisted in the colony, tied as they could be to commentaries on native racial inferiority and the consequent need to govern and regulate. At any rate, the idea of a differentiated and differently important public, accompanied by miasmic theories that persisted in the colony, promoted a vision of ghettoized and segregated urban planning.

The idea of the 'public' relates to ideas of patronage as well. Almost all histories of medicine in the colony have recognized the role of epidemics in the framing of public policy (Harrison, 2009; Arnold, 1993; Berger, 2013), and I would extend this to suggest that epidemics and their management had a major influence on emerging therapeutic regimes of the time. Alavi, for instance, has written of the contest over 'welfare management' between local rulers and the Company in the early 19th century, with vaccination against smallpox becoming a collaborative exercise between these actors; the Peshwa at Poona offering his 'consort as the "subject" of vaccination' (Alavi, 2008 p. 104), thus not only bringing the local populace to heel but also retaining power over and patronage of newer therapeutic practices, while the contest between local Brahmin variolators and medical vaccination remained, with medical officers of the Company like J.Z. Holwell endorsing the variolators' rationale and practice. This complicates both the idea of a common 'public' and the idea of a straightforward contest between indigenous and biomedical practice, or a suppression of one by the other. We see, however, that the management of epidemics and ideas of welfare management flowing from the experience offer another site of segregation of the public – in this case between indigenous practitioners and royal families who withdrew patronage from them, as also between the local commoner population that could be offered for experimentation, and the king himself. It is in these contexts of understanding of a native public that we examine some of the texts on sanitary reform coming out of this time.

A revised edition of *The Elements of Sanitary Science*, a handbook meant for medical and sanitary officers and 'addressed primarily to the educated classes' in India, appeared in 1903 from the government press in Madras. It had been prepared by Captain J.W. Cornwall of the IMS, who was also the municipality Health Officer, vaccination inspector, sanitary commissioner, and professor of hygiene and practical bacteriology at the Madras Medical College. We see, then, that close on the heels of the sanitary movement in England, and around the time when the germ theory of disease was exploding on the biomedical horizon, an organization of disciplines, institutions, and professions was developing in the colonial context as well. I have discussed, in Chapter 2, the question of whether colonial science followed the metropole or whether this was a more overdetermined development. This particular handbook claims to articulate hygiene 'almost entirely from an Indian point of view' (McNally & Cornwall, 1903, p. iii). It takes, however, almost entirely Chadwick's point of view with respect to poverty and disease instead, stressing a causative correlation between bad sanitary conditions and poverty, the vast majority of deaths being preventable, ignorance and apathy being the root causes of these deaths, these being linked to poverty, the value of removal of filth for reducing poverty and disease, and citing the successful example of England to justify such intervention. Such intervention, moreover, must be done by 'the governing, educated, and wealthy classes of a community' (p. 4), since the poor have been devitalized by disease. In a clear tie with productivity concerns and those of building/retaining military strength, the public health measures, supported by statistical accumulation of data, become the concern of the State, for 'a healthy long-lived community has enormous advantages ... as it possesses a larger proportion of working adults' (p. 5). Snowden's analysis of 19th-century English sanitary reform is uncannily applicable to this 1903 document.

What of the 'Indian point of view' does this document offer? While an Indian perspective is hardly visible, problems considered unique to Indian society are brought up. In the chapter on removal of waste, for example, water carriage as a means to remove human waste from habitations is preferred, because 'when it is in operation the populace is less at the mercy of that very intractable community who are variously entitled *bhangis, halalkhors, toties,* and *mehters,* and who can be influenced by nothing but the rod, which it is not legal to apply' (p. 110). The disadvantaged, thus, occupy the place of *ungovernability,* much like the *dai,* and need to lose even their exploitative occupation if the populace is to be saved. We may see the links to the practitioner who isn't, that I refer to in Chapter 3, in these descriptions of ungovernability.

Like several of the colonial evaluations of Indian conditions, commentary on race is front and centre of this discourse. In justifying what is presented as a positive intervention into the lives of the poor and diseased, unsanitary conditions are said to affect the health not only of the debilitated but also the 'strong, whom they debilitate, and in this way, they tend to produce a depraved race; ... for each one who dies, a considerable number recover with more or less damaged constitutions ... therefore [causing] ... degeneration of the race' (McNally & Cornwall, 1903, p. 7). The chapterization of the handbook reads like a foundation for the field of preventive and social medicine that enters medical curricula in India in the 1950s, providing statistical tools to identify variations from norms of health as well as illness, and to incorporate the effects of the environment – geographical, climatic, racial – on these deviations. In the critiques of modern medicine, preventive medicine may be seen as helping shore up the universalizing impulse of modern western medicine through the same tools. Sometimes this branch of biomedicine has been used as a vantage point to describe what is 'wrong' with society, as also what is 'lacking' in modern medicine i.e. the social disparities that determine access, attention, and so on, and therefore the gaps in public health policy that need to be addressed. While the tracing of the continuities between colonial sanitary policy and preventive and social medicine in later periods is beyond the scope of this discussion, we do see that public health administration had begun in India with the appointment of a Sanitary Commission in 1869 (Thakur, Pandit, & Subramanian, 2001). Here, aspects of hygiene – protocols on sourcing drinking water, and the ideas of a balanced diet, and nutrition, for instance, take shape, apart from centralized state infrastructure for sanitary reform. The City of Madras Municipal Act 1884, amended in '84 and '92, the Madras District Municipalities Act 1884, and the Indian Penal Code 1860, are some of the laws and state actions put into place in this time, in the interest of corralling and managing populations.

Sanitary reform in this time, however, is not only about laws on urban behaviour and their enforcement via punitive measures but also about the regulation of such behaviours, practices, and occupations. A list of 'offensive trades', including tanning, paddy boiling, oil boiling, indigo dyeing, and bone boiling, often the occupation of rural migrants and particular 'lower' and middle castes, occupied the time and attention of the municipality of a rapidly expanding Madras city in this time. Links between these forms of criminalization and the ghettoization of urban space have been made, and we may make further links with caste segregation and ghettoization as a foundational component of urbanization. The idea of spatial segregation and governance has been explored, for example, in scholarship around urban planning, particularly in the context of Madras, with the segregation of Black and White towns, the coastal location, and their role and place in European commerce (Balachandran, 2008; Lewandowski, 1975; Neild, 1979); I cite the example of occupations to also flag a linkage with caste-based occupations that get classified as criminal in the 1870s, thus denying certain forms of livelihood as well. For my purposes, the language of sanitary reform, as it contributes to the foundational principles of preventive and social medicine, and thereby to the modern therapeutic regime, via caste exclusions, is relevant here.

The chapters on hygiene and custom in the reform paper also stress women's roles and responsibilities in educating children on good social habits. Regarding marriage and motherhood, the *Manusmriti*, among other texts, is invoked to discourage early marriage, stating that the texts of Manu advocate marriage for a woman when 'she is fit for it', and interpreting this to mean that before her physiological development is complete, she cannot be considered fit for marriage and maternity (McNally & Cornwall, 1903, p. 161); therefore, such improvident marriages will result, again, in the degradation of the race. Childbirth practices are, of course, a natural target of critique.

Sanitary policy and maternal health in Bombay and Calcutta

Biswamoy Pati and Mark Harrison, in writing about the history of public health in colonial India, remind us that sanitary reform in Indian colonial contexts evolved along British lines much earlier than in newer colonies like Africa, with 'disease-specific campaigns … absorbed into other areas of public work' while therapeutic interventions came later (Harrison & Pati, 2009, p. 4). The East India Company, too, managed a tenuous entry into this role of welfare management via the dispensaries set up in the same period. This collaborative tension and co-patronage continued between local rulers and the Company, as also between native physicians and the work of management of epidemics in the early 19th century, as discussed above. Mridula Ramanna makes a link between sanitary reform and maternal health, writing about sanitary reform in colonial Bombay with reference to two periods – 1845 to 1895, and 1896 to the 1930s. Ramanna marks the start of the sanitary policy in Bombay Presidency in the 1860s, with the Health Department being created in 1865 (2012, p. 39), and discusses the fraught debates around the need for sanitary reform and how it should be instituted, whether by top-down or dialogic means.

This included conflicts around the availability of safe drinking water, the imposition of taxes for sanitation and infrastructure, the closing of burial and cremation grounds, and salary cuts for those employed in scavenging. This structure-setting exercise seemed to have dissipated into a series of departmental wrangles until the 1888 Act rendered the municipal corporation the 'supreme governing body of the city' (Ramanna, 2002, p. 115). Ramanna also focuses on the cusp of the 20th century as the start of '[s]emi-official initiatives to provide maternal health care ... in 1901 with a scheme to provide free milk to the poor' (2012, p. 117), for instance, and the combination of nationalist reform positions, philanthropy, and individual vision that got the process started, with membership-based bodies like the Bombay Sanitary Association (BSA) formed in 1904 that advised the health department. Ramanna focuses on the attention that maternal health receives in this scenario; despite the practice of recording infant and maternal deaths in the Bombay Presidency in the late 19th and early 20th centuries, causes attributed included conjectures on poor maternal health, early marriage, unhygienic conditions, and overcrowding, among others. Ramanna observes that one medical paper presented at the Bombay Medical Congress laid the blame at the door of mismanagement by the *dai* and poor childrearing practices. The municipality of Bombay at this time is being encouraged to set up 'lying-in hospitals for the poor with free medical attendance, the education of Indian midwives and licensing of women who attended confinements, legislation ... to prevent unlicensed women ... and municipal milk depots to be started' (ibid, p. 117). Efforts like the Lady Willingdon scheme established by the BSA in 1914 for maternal care and training of 'Indian midwives' ensured, apparently, in the words of Sir Mangaldas Mehta, Medical Officer, Wadia Hospital, that 'dais had been wiped out of the city' (ibid, p. 119). Of course, a newspaper, *Sanchitra Vinod*, also notes in this time, Ramanna says, that 'the midwife was insignificant in Hindu society' (ibid), with most women in Bombay being poor and unable to afford paid childbirth care – one of the few sharp alternative positions in maternal care discourse on the seemingly ubiquitous hold of this all-powerful figure.

Ambalika Guha, writing about the role of the Calcutta Municipal Corporation from the 1910s, speaks of maternal and infant welfare efforts instituted by the corporation, particularly in the context of and popularity of baby shows being organized from the 1920s onwards. With the appointment of a permanent health officer in 1886, the organization of public health under this officer in 1899, and the Calcutta Municipal Act of 1923, followed by the appointment of nationalist men like Chittaranjan Das and Dr Sundari Mohan Das at its helm, Guha notes the active role of the corporation in maternal care, particularly for the urban poor, taking both care and supervision outside of hospital settings, as also making 'slums and lower-middle-class enclaves ... new sites of obstetric research' (Guha, 2017, p. 127). Some of this research was conducted under the auspices of the All-India Institute of Hygiene and Public Health. Positions on which women trained to some degree or another were appointed for supervision ranged from 'female sanitary inspectors' to 'health visitors' to finally 'corporation midwives' in 1915, leading to the setting up of corporation maternity homes by the 1920s and 1930s across Calcutta. Guha suggests that these maternity homes, set up outside of the Dufferin Fund, seemed to take the approach of catering to women of 'all classes' (p. 138), while the earlier colonial provisions in this regard were confined to formal sector sites like the textile mill workers in Bombay or the jute mill workers in Calcutta. I will return to this later in the chapter.

Ramanna's and Guha's work, while tracing the emergence of indigenous maternal welfare as a state subject, also helps us see the growth and spread of the institutional healthcare apparatus in itself, with the alignment of medical professionals with the discourse on public health. The first decades of the 20th century, particularly the period 1916–18, saw multiple institutional regulatory measures emerging parallelly. These measures included debated decisions over training in indigenous systems of medicine for medical trainees, decisions over whether native medical students should receive medical training in the vernacular, whether a separate class of students trained in medicine in the vernacular was acceptable, whether indigenous systems of medicine were to receive funds, and whether their dispensaries were to be shut down as per the Bombay Medical Act. Additionally, it is in the 1920s, says Ramanna, that 'the discourse of childbirth and health took place against a changed political background. Motherhood and fertility were no longer regarded as predominantly moral issues but as social problems linked with … living conditions. … Infant and maternal health were the most important of all these concerns' (Ramanna, 2012, p. 131). It is in these shared contexts, then, that the data on maternal and infant mortality and the blame on the *dai*, already diagnosed as an unsanitary, lower-caste, unskilled, and rigid agent, assume significance.

The shift and reform within the institution here in the form of maternity benefits, creches, leave, etc., are the route sanitary reform takes, in addition to *dai* training. Health Visitors are able to visit homes where there have been births, to encourage conversations on child welfare. Organizations like Bombay Presidency Women's Council, and later the National Council of Women in India, all participated in pushing for these reforms, as per Ramanna. These were the labour policy reforms taking shape in a context where women formed a sizable chunk of mill workers in Bombay.

By the late 1920s, medical training for women in India had begun to reflect both the early sanitary movement and the later germ theory of disease. It is stated, however, that regular medical training is not enough for women to do or supervise health work unless 'medical women for specialised maternity and child welfare work' (Eighth Annual Report of the Chelmsford League, 1928, p. 124) are trained. The Lady Reading Health School in Delhi had, by this time, specialist lecturers in tropical diseases, psychology, and economy. In Bombay and Bengal provinces, the health workers and health visitors passing out from the health schools were seen as needing to respond to industrial textile and jute mill worker concerns around maternal mortality and morbidity. Factory owners bore the expense in some districts. In many provinces, including Bengal and Madras, it was the 'mofussil' and rural areas that are seen as the primary target of this work, acting as a mediator and negotiator of medical intervention. In some sense, communities of maternal and infant health awareness were being built through this work, creating spaces to carry modern therapeutic vocabulary within communities – of disease and hygiene, for instance. As the list of activities of the Madras Presidency Maternity and Child Welfare Association speaks of in regard to centres for child care:

> Children under four years old have hot baths, children over four and under eleven years old have cold baths. After the bathing, the children's hair is combed and cleaned, and any minor ailments ... attended to. Codliver oil is given to children suffering from rickets ... The children are all fed at the centres ... Mothers ... [b]efore and after maternity ... are given 'ragi conjee' when necessary ... between 2 and 5 o'clock, each nurse visits the houses in her locality, giving advice to expectant mothers on health and ... trying to persuade them to have a properly trained midwife or go to a hospital for their confinement ... Each nurse has ... a maternity register.
>
> (Eighth Annual Report of the Chelmsford League, 1928,
> p. 112)

'Mothercraft', in other words, was born. There are also references to social work as an apt descriptor for this work, although social work as a discipline had yet to enter educational curricula in India. The health workers themselves, however, were kept in touch with, much in the nature of alumni networks, with newsletters, reunions, and so on. The health visitors were often recruited into vaccination drives for children.

How does sanitary reform thinking within the institution impact the 'murky out-side' that we have been speaking of? What is the place of the *dai* in this scenario? Does she, once defined and named, get appropriated into the system as part of the reform agenda? It is this possibility in particular that I explore in the remaining part of this chapter.

Forbes has commented in some detail on the regulations around the *dai* in the late 19th to early 20th centuries, and her analysis shares some commonalities with Ramanna's insights on the Bombay presidency. Forbes suggests that the formal sec-tor, 'factories, mines and plantations – were impacted by new international standards that required the provision of some health care' (2005, p. 91). She talks about how 'medically qualified inspectresses' were proposed for factories so that they 'could then supervise trained midwives ... [who] could [also] be used to report on' (p. 92) women who took maternity leave but worked elsewhere in the time – some of the possible early accounts of labour surveillance. Plantation owners were also encouraged to offer trained midwifery services but asked to hold back maternity bonuses if these services were not used. Alongside this, by 'the 1930s, the three all-India women's organizations were determined to abolish *dhais* and replace them with midwives trained in Western techniques' (p. 94). And the 'National Council of Women in India ... [while] involved in schemes to encourage maternity benefits for women ... called for additional schemes to train nurses and midwives and thought that both should be registered ... [and] asked the government to ... make special appeals to get "refined girls" to enter the profes-sion' (p. 94). While it is anybody's guess who this 'refined girl' might be, this attempt at control might be better understood as an attempt at regulation rather than exclusion, particularly when seen in the context of emerging healthcare systems. What we see in this process of regulation is the emergence of a category of trained midwife, to which the *dai* must aspire but will never reach, given her already declared untrainability – a good rationale given the astoundingly poor success of the training programmes. It is in the trained midwives now emerging and being employed by district hospitals that we see this new category at the bottom of the scale, that later dovetails somewhat with the trained nurse, that will eventually continue into post-independence health workers who eventually are re-invented as link workers. I will explore the historical journey of this category post-independence in more detail in Chapter 6.

Regulation of women's therapeutic work

Professionalization and English medical women in the colony

By the later years of the Dufferin Fund, the annual reports began discussing training in sub-disciplines such as pathology and pharmacology, apart from the clinical and patient-interfacing fields of surgery and medicine. The tone of these reports indicates two things. One, the prospect of greater cadre-building and professional opportunities for women, particularly after the establishment of the Women's Medical Service (WMS) in 1914. The principal of the Women's Medical School in Agra, for instance, reported in 1923 that 'during the short time the Pathology laboratory has been open two students have shown marked aptitude for the work, and expressed a wish to go on with it after qualifying' (tenth annual report of the Women's Medical Service for India, p. 23). What opportunities, however, do these suggest for a women's colonial science? What connections with the sanitary movement and the later germ theory of disease? Arnold has referred to the first decade of the 20th century as the period when, in recognition of the limited participation of English scientists in medical research on tropical diseases, several governmental institutions were established to conduct medical research – including the Central Research Institute at Kasauli in Punjab in 1906, Pasteur institutes for rabies research, the Haffkine Institute in Bombay, and the King Institute of Preventive Medicine in Madras around 1900. The Calcutta School of Tropical Medicine opened in 1921 to study tropical diseases (Arnold, 2004). Apart from the organization of these spaces as already elite and separate from sanitary reform agendas, requiring '"mental and physical qualifications" that were apparently not to be found in "races bred in a tropical climate"' (Arnold, 2004, p. 146), the presence of even Englishwomen physicians and researchers in these spaces is not apparent. Instead, the push among British medical women seems to have been towards clinical and institutional space in the colony.

Dufferin Fund

The formal retrospective report of 50 years of the Dufferin Fund (Balfour & Scott, 1935), looking back at the period 1885–1935, begins with the by-now mythologized account of the letter-in-the-locket in 1881 from the 'Maharani of Punna' to another Queen – Victoria – through Dr Elizabeth Bielby, who had been working as a missionary in India and was to now receive medical training in England; the letter 'appealed for help for the women in India' (p. 3). Elizabeth Hoggan, in her 1882 account of the same, re-reads this appeal 'rendered into Western and constitutional language, ... [as] a demand on Government for a new public service, and for a recognition of the right of Indian women to have their so-called prejudices ... respected and not outraged' (Hoggan, 1882, pp. 1–2). In fact, Hoggan speaks in the face of the misogyny of English medical men like Sir Joseph Fayrer, professor of surgery at Medical College, Calcutta, as also in the light of support and appeals from Indian statesmen like Sir Salar Jung, to point to the abysmal access to medical services faced by Indian women, and to indicate that the reason for this was 'the absence of skilled medical women' (ibid, p. 6). Hoggan goes on to speak of the need to support trained English medical women, who are otherwise 'left to fight their own unaided way to success' (p. 8), in the service of this needy constituency. It is the right time, she avers, to 'consider the expediency of introducing English medicine to the women in the only way in which, admittedly, it can be done, through medical women' (p. 10); the only reason not to do so would be prejudice against women entering the profession. In the face of the thin argument that Englishwomen physicians would not be safe in rural practice, she wonders why this argument has not been considered for nurses or midwives going into the country – whether the fact that they are poor women makes them less deserving of protection. Hoggan's particular argument – a demand for respect for both English and Indian women – does not get traction, however, and the Dufferin report goes on to describe the strictness of purdah among the women of the 'Hindu as well as of the Mahommedan community' (Balfour &Scott, 1935, p. 3), the refusal of Indian women to be allowed visits by male doctors, the '[i]gnorance, carelessness, and unsanitary practices' (p. 4) of the indigenous hereditary *dai*, that are responsible for the poor health of women in India. The report acknowledges 'other beginnings' like 'the first class of women students, headed by Mrs. Scharlieb, [who] had commenced work in Madras, and the 1882 "Women of India Fund" which led to the opening in 1886 of the Cama Hospital' (p. 4). The Dufferin Fund, formally titled *The National Association for Supplying Female Medical Aid to the Women of India*, is presented, however, as the first organized effort in this direction. Beginning with conversations between Lady Dufferin and those she perceived as stakeholders – 'Indians and Europeans, missionaries and officials ... wives of Governors and Lieutenant Governors' (p. 5), Lady Dufferin puts together a prospectus, laying down the 'proposed constitution and principles' (ibid) of the work, and the Association is formally registered in 1888. It declares the following objectives:

(1) Medical tuition, including the teaching and training in India of women as doctors, hospital assistants, nurses and midwives; (2) Medical relief, including the establishment under female superintendence of dispensaries and cottage hospitals for the treatment of women and children; the opening of female wards under female superintendence in existing hospitals and dispensaries; the provision of female medical officers and attendants for existing female wards; ... the founding of hospitals for women where special funds

or endowments are forthcoming. (3) The supply of trained female nurses and midwives for women and children in hospitals and private houses.

(ibid)

While the Fund was to be administered by a Central Committee with Lady Dufferin as the President, all administrators, from the Queen down to the Lieutenant Governors of the various Provinces, are patrons and life councillors. It is under the aegis of this Fund, in 1888, that Lady Dufferin proposes training, compulsory registration, and licensing of *dais*. I have indicated, in the section on sanitary reforms earlier in the chapter, the manner in which regulation of *dai* work operated in labour contexts in the mills in Bombay, as also plantations and other factories, in the first decades of the 20th century. It becomes clearer, as we examine the operations of the Fund, both the status of this impulse vis-a-vis the Fund's other objectives and its operationalization. Overall, it would seem that, given the 'women's work for women' frame, and the need to 'save' the Indian woman, creating a full cadre of women at all levels of reproductive work in particular, and reaching out to *zenana* women to spread awareness about hygiene and modern healthcare, is one route the Fund took. We see, however, that not only westernization, but also professionalization and *regulation of therapeutic work by women* was one of the key impulses in the Fund. With rich scholarship available on all these aspects save perhaps the last, this is where I will focus now.

Regulation of therapeutic work by women

While the 'women for women' framework developed in early missionary work, different actors and categories of work appeared within the framework across the period until the 1930s at least, until a tentative institutional structure emerged. The underpaid and less appreciated Englishwoman physician, the Women's Medical Service (WMS) professional, the Indian lady doctor, the Dufferin *dai*, the indigenous *dai*, the *dai*-cum-nurse, the nurse, and the trained nurse all appear in this structure. The framework already included, in the early to mid-19th century, maternity and child welfare, and funding moved from parastatal to philanthropic to a public-private model during this time. Bodies that determine and control these actors are the Dufferin Fund and its allied institutions – the Victoria Memorial Scholarships fund, the Lady Reading Women of India Fund, and the Lady Chelmsford All-India League for Maternity and Child Welfare. By the time of the setting up of the Women's Medical Service in 1914, the Government of India's contribution was well ahead of the expenditure.

As laid out in its objectives, the Dufferin Fund raised money for salaries and scholarships for medical women for graduate and post-graduate studies, building grants for the Lady Dufferin Hospital, and several Dufferin hospitals across the country. It was administered through a Central Committee and several provincial committees, with a United Kingdom Committee that offered scholarships to medical women at the London School of Medicine and passage to India for them. While the retrospective report is ambivalent about great progress having been made, it talks about the institution of 'definite rules for pay, promotion and leave' (Balfour & Scott, 1935, p. 9) across grades and the structure of a regular service, in the United Provinces, where the Fund's provincial work seems to have flourished the most. Apart from women's medical schools in Agra and a Nursing School at Cama Hospital, Bombay, women's hospitals were opened in Shikarpur, Hyderabad, Karachi, Surat, Rangoon, Nagpur, Jubbulpore, Amraoti, Akola, Shegaon, Yeotmal, Sibi, Quetta, Fort Sandeman, Gaya, and Bhagalpur, and several Indian states, under the aegis of the Fund. Some of these hospitals and medical schools were taken over by the state in the early 20th century. The report refers obliquely to the missionary service where medical assistants could easily be obtained from their 'schools and orphanages' (p. 10) and therefore is better provided for, while the medical women of the Dufferin hospitals had to go to much trouble to find and train staff. The report also talks of the suspicion and doubt that the Fund faced from a populace that was encountering new therapeutic practices – surgery, for instance, although a lot of this work continued to be non-surgical well into the 1920s, as women preferred 'to die rather than be operated on' (National Association for Supplying Medical Aid by Women to the Women of India, 1928, p. 24). The salaries of medical women also continued to be low, dependent as they were on local uncertain grants or funds. Government aid began to the Fund in 1914, with the setting up of the Women's Medical Service, designed by Sir Charles Pardey Lukis, Director-General of the Indian Medical Service, and Sir James Roberts, Honorary Secretary, in consultation with Sir Harcourt Butler of the Central Committee and Lady Hardinge, then president of the Fund. In 1913, Sir Lukis, who later sharply intervenes in the question of vernacular medical education as we have seen in Chapter 3, has spoken of the medical needs of India at the London School of Medicine for Women. He begins with the seemingly progressive perspective that the medical woman in India must not limit her work to reproductive health but may do 'pioneer work by disseminating knowledge of the laws of health and the value of preventive measures', given that 'we shall never make any real headway in promoting the knowledge of domestic and personal hygiene until we have convinced the women of India as to its necessity and they have thrown their powerful influence into the scale', since '[h]ere the medical man is powerless – the purdah bars the way, and it is to the medical woman that we must look for educational propaganda inside the zenana' (Lukis, Oct. 1, 1913). This rationale for the introduction of British medical women into Indian service has been written about in other scholarship (Burton, 1996; Sehrawat, 2013); we may add the contexts of the severe criticisms by then accumulating against the Dufferin Fund and the status of women professionals therein, the increase in professionalization and regulation of Western medical practice in the colony, as also the increasing presence of the state in the sector, as contexts for the encouragement to Englishwomen physicians at this time. Following the concerted campaigns by the Association of Medical Women of India (AMWI) from its establishment in 1907, and with the establishment of the WMS, came pay increases, and complete professional control over the hospitals the medical women were at, in contrast to earlier interference and humiliation at the hands of senior male colleagues, as Forbes, Ramanna, and others have recounted. Margaret Balfour, in 1921, is given the title of Chief Medical Officer of the WMS, followed by Dr Agnes Scott in 1924. A

Women's Medical Training Reserve is organized in 1925, employing women graduating in medicine from India, with a track to enter the WMS after further training in England if they are found suitable. Lukis also announces, alongside the setting up of the WMS, the setting up of a medical college to exclusively train women – The Lady Hardinge College – and the need to train 'native' women too into the profession. This is perhaps the beginning of the entry of Indian women into the service and onto the Central Committee, later a Council. While medical education for women in India was available by the late 19th century, positions for women post their graduation however continued to be dismal.

The later years of the Fund see the Victoria Memorial Scholarship Fund for training indigenous *dais* in 1903, but also the setting up of the Lady Hardinge Women's Medical College in Delhi in 1916 and the Association for the provision of Lady Health Visitors and Maternity Supervisors in 1918. The creation of these largely supervisory posts ties in with efforts to educate the public – talks and lectures in girls' schools are part of their mandate. These last are the professionals Forbes, Ramanna, and Guha refer to, in relation to women working in factories or on plantations. Also, in 1923, the Women of India Fund was set up to, among other things, provide scholarships for the training of Indian nurses, and in 1928, a sum was procured by Lady Irwin for research by medical women into maternal and infant mortality.

As discussed earlier in the context of sanitary reforms, labour conditions in factories were not seen as causally related to maternal or infant mortality in the late 19th early 20th centuries. Employers contributing to the setting up of crèches or medical centres near factories, however, could manage the imperial administrative agenda of benevolent attention to maternal health in a piecemeal fashion, bringing 'childbearing practices of such mothers within public scrutiny', as Guha notes (2017, p. 139). Women's organizations, particularly in Bombay, that lamented on the need to find the 'right girls' for training in midwifery also contribute to the discourse of training, supervision, and regulatory recognition/legitimation of therapeutic work by women, with the implicit casteism behind the search for the 'right girls'.

The institution enters the zenana

These positions are similar and yet somewhat at variance with the 'women's work for women' frame of the mission societies in the late 19th century. While medical women continue to be seen as the entry into the *zenana*, and as doing the work of secular civilizing and reform, as well as being a professional replacement for unskilled medical missionaries, the focus seems to be much more on the woman inhabitant of the *zenana* than the woman polluting it, i.e., the *dai*. By this point, professionalization has become the goal for women, whether it be in medicine or nursing; *dai* training programmes have failed quite comprehensively, and the institution has become more visible, if not more effective, in regulating childbirth within hospitals for the *zenana* woman. By the time of the Women's Medical Service, it is reported that there is a steady increase in the 'number of purdanashin ladies' attending the Dufferin hospitals (National Association for Supplying Female Medical Aid to the Women of India, 1913, p. 7). Apart from the upper-class women that this category signifies, working-class women like mill workers in the Bombay presidency are also being brought into the frame, and in the focus on increasing hospital deliveries as well as public health measures, the *dai* as problem, already established, is no longer the absolute adversary.

The *zenana* hospitals, however, are also failing at this time in breaching the boundary of the *zenana* that, from missionary times, had posed a challenge. The privileged-caste upper-class woman continues to remain within the home, drawing upon Englishwomen or Indian women physicians for their childbirth needs and comprehensively avoiding hospitalization, in fact, being pulled out of hospital settings even after reaching them (Forbes, 2005). Administrators attempt a response, trying to retain an exclusive environment that might attract privileged-caste women. In fact, as Forbes notes, 'In Gaya, officials took the drastic measure of ruling that only women who could "produce a certificate from one of the Indian members of the Committee, stating the applicants are *Pardanashins*" would be admitted to Lady Elgin Zanana Hospital' (Forbes, 2005, p. 135). This push to retain *zenana* hospitals for privileged women continued well after this period, with the AMWI actively critiquing the Dufferin hospitals for not maintaining sufficient *purdah* restrictions, indeed alleging that allowing the entry of marginalized-caste women as patients was an obstacle to privileged women's access, and thus the cause of poor admission rates of privileged women. As evident in writing by medical women at this time, there is acknowledgement that women's hospitals should be both 'attractive but also easily accessible' (Campbell, 1918, p. 122), via good leading roads, availability of transportation and communication, although the facility is not advised to be free, so that 'a feeling of self-respect is thereby engendered, and even well-to-do caste people now think it is no indignity to have their ladies come to us for delivery' (ibid). Needless to say, the poorer women who were accessing hospitals were not the focus of these efforts, either by the colonial administration, women's organizations lobbying for medical care for women, or Indian nationalist men.

Samiksha Sehrawat, in her rich study of the contexts of colonial medical care in northern India (2013), traces the relationship between the Dufferin Fund imperatives and state funding, the 'women for women' model, and the overall poor focus on healthcare expenditure in favour of greater investment in economically advantageous projects. While this relationship is not the focus of this chapter, Sehrawat's study helps shed some light on the complicated mobilization of a heterogeneous public of native women into the regime of institutionalization. We will return to this idea in Chapter 5.

Indian women and the Indian woman doctor

These contexts might be relevant to the entry of Indian women into the service. Bombay University and the Grant Medical College received, in 1883, letters from the working committee for the Medical Women for India Fund of Bombay, asking that medical degrees be conferred on women and that Government diplomas of apothecary or hospital assistant be given to women as well as men, along with five scholarships for women students. Under the chairmanship of Sir George Kittredge, the committee included Mr Sorabjee S. Bengallee, among others. While the first exercise of the committee was to recruit Englishwomen physicians from England, it put into motion several initiatives that paved the way for native women to be allowed entry into medical training, as well as to provide medical aid to poor women and a hospital for women and children. We also see in the workings of this Fund, an impulse to work with financial support from the wealthy Parsi and other communities of the city rather than seek government assistance, thus introducing what the committee called the 'first non-official non-sectarian female medical relief into India' (Kittredge, 1889, p. 30). This was a time when London hospitals were still closed to women surgeons, and Dr Edith Pechey, an experienced physician, agreed to be the first to accept the post of Senior Medical Officer at the Jaffer Sulliman Dispensary, and later the Cama hospital, in Bombay, in 1884 and 1886, respectively, to cater exclusively to women; Dr Charlotte Ellaby comes in later in this position. In the work of the committee that lasted until 1889, when these hospitals were given over to government management, there is a reclaiming of the history of Bombay for its community members – be they Parsi, or Muslim. Whether this may also be read as a national or nationalist science, is a question.

Medical colleges opened their doors to Indian women in staggered ways. Medical education in the vernacular for women was one; but the regular medical colleges were also admitting a few women with higher qualifications in the 1880s. There is much scholarship on the fractious debates around 'letting women in', and then 'letting Indian women in' to formal or semi-formal training (Forbes, 1999, 2005; Ramanna, 2012). The Bombay University granted the request for medical degrees to matriculated women, the Grant Medical College offered certificates to non-matriculates, and '[t]welve female students (5 Parsees and 7 Europeans or Eurasians) commenced attendance at the Grant Medical College in January 1884' (Kittredge, 1889, Medical Women for India Fund, First Annual Report, p. 4). What we do see with the coming in of Indian women doctors graduating from medical colleges in India in the late 1800s and early 1900s is a significant presence of these women as indigenous reform agents, as Ramanna has pointed out (2008). Not only do these practitioners take strong positions on reproductive health and rights to contraception, they are also well represented in women's and social reform organizations like the All India Women's Conference, the Arya Mahila Samaj, the Red Cross, and so on. Also significant, they were elected to state legislatures and involved in state work on welfare for women. On the issue of *dais*, they seem to have been more inclined towards training rather than replacement (Ramanna, 2008, p. 78).

The WMS, taken under the control of the Dufferin Fund, underwent a revision of rules in 1923, with preference for candidates in the service of the Fund, with later consideration 'to the claims of candidates who have qualified in local institutions and of those who are natives of India' (National Association for Supplying Medical Aid by Women in India, 1923, p. 44). Which women were to be let in, therefore – European, Anglo-Indian, or 'natives' – was a matter of undeclared surveillance in the service. The racialization of the service manifested in a number of ways – positions, numbers – with the Anglo-Indian practitioner standing in for the European in so many words when necessary. By the late 1920s, annual reports of the Fund state that 50% of the service are Indian.

Looking at the composition of the initial pool of 'native' trainees offers an interesting account of the demographic and their constituency. In the Bombay presidency, this ranged from privileged-caste and wealthy women to privileged-caste women of reform and/or nationalist families, some with links to mission work. In Bengal, too, privileged-caste women as well as women of Brahmo families entered training, and with the stated demand for female medical practitioners who could be paid considerably less than their male counterparts for district work, several young widows who wished to work and thus escape family (Ramanna, 2008; Forbes, 1999) entered the service. These women, the 'lady doctors' (Sen, 2012, p. 59), engaged with *dais*, *kabirajes*, and *hakims* in the district hospitals they were placed in or allowed to run (Forbes, ibid). Many of these hospitals did not see the typical *zenana* woman that the colonial administration sought; rather, the indigent and working-class woman was more likely, and it was thought that failure to observe strict caste segregation was the cause, as mentioned earlier. This Indian lady doctor, however, was beginning to be called in to attend to the *pardanashin* or upper-class woman in her home as well. What position they took in these homes vis-a-vis the *dai* does not seem to be recorded, and it is a matter of speculation whether they may have favoured the canonical indigenous systems finding favour with the nationalist elite by then – a space the *dai* definitely did not occupy. What seems to be the case from memoirs like those of Haimabati Sen (Forbes, ibid) is the uncritical stance taken toward caste purity or *parda* by some of these professional women, but this is not substantiated.

From the evidence of these women being visible in women's and reform organizations as well as in legislatures, and the voting patterns of some prominent women doctors like Muthulakshmi Reddy on matters of abortion and contraception in women's conferences in the 1930s, it would seem that abstinence was the virtue and method preferred to 'birth control' for family planning, and the rationale for birth control – a phrase sparingly used as Ramanna suggests – is the need to preserve the strength of the race (Ramanna, 2008). What other manifestations this would have for the life of the *zenana* or privileged-caste women, and the women doctors' relationship with this constituency, is a question I will come back to in the next chapter.

Gender segregation or institutionalization?

A phenomenon that has not received much attention in the scholarship around midwifery or *dai* traditions in Indian contexts is the place of male physicians in the field. The known argument is of *zenana* women not willing to be examined or treated by men in childbirth or other health conditions. Ambalika Guha's insightful study of midwifery being included in formal western medical curricula in Bengal, and the role of male physicians as specialists, authors of textbooks, and popular treatises, offers a more differentiated picture of the period between the 1840s and

1947 (Guha, 2017). Guha writes of the 1840s as the period when midwifery is incorporated into the medical curriculum of Calcutta University – a step largely facilitated and sustained through the agency of male physicians, several of whom also wrote advice pieces on the rationale of a scientific turn in midwifery in the vernacular medical periodicals of the time. I have, in the previous chapter, alluded to Mukharji's discussion of the place of the Bengali *daktar* in indigenous discourse, and the provincialization and vernacularization this *daktari* signified. Guha deploys this argument to point to the '"medical" view of childbirth [that] was discursively constructed in the pages of vernacular medical journals' (p. 112) and thus disseminated to the reading public, including the semi-formal literate public. Following this, we might say that epistemic authority in this discourse was held by the male expert and popularizer, a pattern common enough in the histories of science in India, and one that Guha logically reads as tied in with the nationalist discourse on racial strength relying on healthy motherhood. We have seen Sohrawardy and others wax eloquent on this in their speeches and writings. Guha tells us about the technologization of childbirth in India at the time too, with respect to the debates around the forceps that needed to be refigured for the smaller pelvis of the Bengali woman, for instance – resulting in the devising of a 'remodelled "Bengal forceps"' by Kedarnath Das in 1913 (ibid, p. 116).[2] This interpretation is closer to the critical analysis of the institutionalization, technologization, and masculinization of childbirth that feminists have offered of western societies (Martin, 2001; Findlay, 1993; Stone, 2009). While we might ask whether the inclusion of midwifery in medical curricula in Bengal could be read outside of the derivative nature of medical curricula and discourse in the West (as I discuss in Chapter 2), I find Guha's argument incisive for other reasons when considering the category of the indigenous as it forms in this period. At the very least, we learn that there are more stakeholders and a more complicated terrain than that of the colonial administration and the onus it seems to put on medical women – English and Indian – to take care of the *zenana*. Taken further, this shows us the emergence of a networked community of carers linked to the institution that actually participate in the institutionalization of childbirth. Two, the appearance of agency for Indian medical women in childbirth practice must be read against the institutional and knowledge hierarchies that we see fairly starkly spelt out in the memoirs of Haimabati Sen, for instance, as she speaks of the humiliation, harassment, and dismissal that she faces at the hands of male supervisors. Three, the place accorded to the woman hospital assistant, the trained *dai*, and the lady health visitor, with, as Guha says, the 'corporation midwives at the bottom and the medical professionals on top' (p. 121), is more symptomatic of childbirth beginning to become the subject of regulatory governance mechanisms, and 'not so much … a gendered demarcation of the sphere of action' (ibid). I will, in the last chapter, attempt to follow this through as I look at the contemporary link worker scenario in the Indian healthcare assemblage.

We will see, later in this chapter in the section on papers by medical women, the many proposals by Englishwomen physicians towards the improvement of maternal health services, which also give supervisory powers to the medical women themselves. It is unclear how many of these find fruition in the work of the Dufferin and

Victoria Memorial Fund. The annual report of 1912 of the Dufferin Fund has on its agenda the formation of the Women's Medical Service in India, which finally took off in 1914. An important aspect of this formation is the amendment to Rule 20 of the Memorandum of Association of the Fund that now indicates that the women employed by it will 'ordinarily be expected to act in co-operation with, and where necessary in subordination to, the Medical Officers of Government' (National Association for Supplying Female Medical Aid to the Women of India, 1913, p. 2). It was the clause 'in subordination to' that continued to be the bone of contention inasmuch as women's professional autonomy vis-à-vis regulation was concerned, although 'where necessary' purports to offer reasonable autonomy. As Miss Vaughan submits, '[m]edical women ... have asked that the objectionable clause "in subordination to the medical officers of Government" should be removed' (p. 22). This was not accepted, however, and marks a significant moment in the context of complaints by medical women that their autonomy was being curbed by men in the service. This plays out as both a race and gender question, with, for example, the lady doctor of Rampore not being allowed to be independent of 'an Indian State Surgeon', and she having left in consequence (p. 19). With the institutionalization of the women's medical service becoming real, then, is also to be seen an acknowledgement, however reluctant, of their professional skills and authority, although the appointments themselves were not permanent or necessarily at adequate remuneration owing to the 'charitable and more or less struggling Association which endeavours to provide as full medical relief as possible' (ibid, p. 3).

The argument for the need to segregate the *zenana* woman manifests in medical training as well. The Bishop of Lucknow is said to have written a letter 'telling his Indian Christian congregations that he wished particularly that girls should not enter the Dufferin service, that they should not go into medical work at all, where they were employed in the same places with Indian men without any proper protection' (National Association for Supplying Female Medical Aid to the Women of India, 1913, p. 19). While this position may not have been sustained, it highlights the anxieties that accompanied the entry of Indian women into the profession. The amendment, and the felt need to not be professionally subordinated to medical men, particularly Indians, may also be read in this light. The eventual course of the amendment continues to reflect the gender struggle over professional authority, as well as sexual anxieties over racial intermixing.

Not just gender

The institutionalization of childbirth at this time and later is also layered through with an accompanying institutionalization of caste hierarchies. As we read of the design and structuring of hospital buildings, for instance, the separation of wards and rooms occupied by 'caste' and marginalized-caste patients is evident, as is also the construction of latrines separately for the 'menial staff' and patients (39th annual report, p. 20). There is also scattered mention of 'Hindu wards' in reports from local hospitals, for example, the Lady Elgin Zenana Hospital, Gaya (National Association for Supplying Medical Aid by Women to the Women of India, 1928, p. 36).

We see, then, in the attention to maternal health in labour-intensive industries, state-sponsored sanitary reform, education, and appointment of Indian women as hospital assistants, a vast layering and dispersal of institutionalization around women's roles in healthcare. Standards of education for these women were considerably lowered, and some of the experiences of the women hospital assistants, as well as the rhetoric around women's work for women, suggest that women's health, including reproductive health, continued to be largely the black hole that allowed corrective measures to be arbitrary and ad hoc, rather than affirmative. Most of this discussion stays within the domain of civilizational 'need', and is also, as Forbes notes, directed at international audiences. Civilizational shortcomings have become, by now locatable in the figure of the *dai*, the lower-caste untrained woman, who can now be cordoned off and controlled, partly by replacement, partly by processing through the institution. I therefore now focus on the institutional discourse around *dai* training. While this is a space that is quite saturated with research, my attempt is to look back at it with two views – one, to trace the repetitive/imitative quality of the discourse around the *dai* as the trope of the *failed indigenous*, and, two, the positioning of this figure as abjectly included in the emerging therapeutic landscape and language in the late 19th and early 20th centuries in India. Before the involvement of the state and institutionalization in these explicit ways, the need to contest 'primitive midwifery' had been announced by the missionaries, and this contestation was established as the voluntary 'good work' of civilizing – the task of almost every good European. We go back, therefore, to the concerns and questions of *dai* training, as they emerge from the missionary time to the mid-19th century, and the Dufferin and other philanthropic funds that take up this seemingly humongous task.

The institutional and the affective discourse around the dai

Anthropologists investigating contemporary childbirth practices in India have talked about how midwife occupations began to be called by the ubiquitous term *dai* in the colonial period. They also indicate the progressive loss of livelihood and knowledge status that these women have faced historically and point to the oppressed-caste status that their marginalization is associated with (Van Hollen, 2003; Forbes, 1999; Chawla, 1994; Sadgopal, 2009; Pinto, 2008; Jeffery, Jeffery, & Lyon, 2002). Cecilia van Hollen speaks of the putting together of a variety of 'traditional midwives under the term "*dai*"' (2003, p. 40) across regions and communities. Van Hollen goes on to explore a diverse set of etymologies and semantics around midwifery in India as a means of exploding the homogeneity imposed by the universalist usage of the term 'dai'. Sarah Pinto, in talking about the multiple roles of women in birth work, splits the term in another way, as an umbrella used to describe a variety of hierarchically related roles (2008). Mira Sadgopal, writing on the *dai* traditions, the history of *dai* training, the question of plurality and epistemological dialogue among medical systems, and policy implications, is concerned primarily with the need to locate and legitimize *dais* in present-day maternal health services. She traces the shifts in state-sponsored maternal healthcare services where, with the undue focus on family planning, primary healthcare took a back seat, *dais* were either treated as stop-gaps or community volunteers, and since 2000, taken out of training programmes altogether. We may note the non-unitary notion of who the *dai* is in Sadgopal and Pinto's texts; as also the focus on different kinds of non-biomedical practices, and the non-medicalization of pregnancy. Janet Chawla takes a different approach, talking about the 'ritual facilitation methods of the midwife [that] can be appropriately designated as "shamanic"' (Chawla, 1994, p. 81). This she poses against what she terms the 'Brahmanic effort to desacralise those aspects of the female and the feminine which were not able to be appropriated and controlled' (p. 80). She argues that 'both the demonic feminine and the purity and pollution concerns can be seen as resulting from a tension between the beliefs and ritual practices of basically localized worshipping groups and the emerging brahmanic priestly caste' (p. 80). As against biomedical parameters of knowledge, she posits 'a "community of women" who assembles at the time of birth [c...]haracterized by different beliefs and ritual performances than those of the dominant religious groupings', and claims that 'the dai can legitimately be viewed as a "transpersonal specialist" and "experiential guide"' (p. 81) to childbirth. Chawla points to the 'absence of references to traditional midwifery in the historical and sacred' to indicate gender and caste bias that devalued these women and their work. Chawla sees this view of the *dai* as a ritual practitioner as both a 'woman-centered and caste-sensitive' interpretation (ibid, p. 83), primarily therefore asking for an evaluation of the *dai's* work in this regard rather than through a biomedical lens.

Chawla's argument is useful inasmuch as it suggests an epistemic difference, and a resistant subjectivity located within that, although Chawla takes pains to trace the *dai's* as a woman-centred practice. As I go into this already explored terrain, I ask a different set of questions, as laid down in the introduction to this chapter. These include the grounds on which this figure is constituted, what the terms are on which she is included in the therapeutic, and what claims to knowledge communities she is denied. I will, in the last chapter, explore more fully the question of epistemic difference. I am interested in exploring how these grounds became important to establish for one the incapacity to self-govern, the physical removal of the Dalit woman from the privileged-caste household, the collusion between nationalist elites and the colonial administration on this, and the emergence of the 'true' indigenous as the therapeutic concomitant to her forcible removal from within the privileged household.

The one obstacle to maternal welfare

[T]he more medical women practised in India, the more did they find themselves faced, in maternity work, with a problem which appeared almost insoluble. That problem was (and still to a large extent is!) the indigenous midwife, or *dai*. For ages the *dai* had been the genius presiding over childbirth and her sway was undisputed ... [she] admitted to no gaps in her knowledge ... [t]he profession of midwife in India is hereditary.

(Balfour & Young, 1929, p. 126)

This report, titled *The Work of Medical Women in India*, one of many, while beginning to reflect on the various *dai* training schemes in the 20th century, following an earlier period of greater ambivalence, lays the grounds thus. The value of the report is in its affect more than its information – the focus on what kind of woman is required to attempt the training of these untrainables, for instance – not an Indian sub-assistant surgeon but possibly an Englishwoman carrying missionary legacies, women of education and character and personality. Interestingly, this is accompanied by another description of the indigenous *dai* – as an 'illiterate, downtrodden menial' who must be handled with patience – a classical provision for the secular aspect of the civilizing mission where the object of improvement is infantilized, and her resistance read as obstinacy. There is, however, reference to accounts like those of one Miss Bose, which takes into account the experience of the *dais* and thus considers them better trainees than other midwives. This is, however, by far the minority opinion, and gets buried beneath the rhetoric of untrainability.

A significant repair mechanism suggested is to put more effort into antenatal care, in order to detect 'abnormal conditions in time' (ibid, p. 139). This is expected to better equip the pregnant body for the trials ahead, and, accompanied by strict instructions to the *dai* to attend only normal cases following the 'principles of surgical cleanliness and diagnosis by external examination only' (ibid), is expected to improve maternal mortality rates.

As we have seen in the discussion on professionalization, the attention to and organization of multiple layers of health work around women, and the opening up of these layers to women accessing education and/or seeking employment in India, is one of the outcomes of Dufferin Fund work. While this creates professions for women entering education in India as well as for Englishwomen physicians who found work here while marginalized back home, and also begins to make space for these professions outside of missionary institutions, the one group of women it struggles to deal with are what are referred to as the *bazaar* or indigenous *dais* in the papers by medical women. These are the only non-familial women already engaged in therapeutic work in communities and in the *zenana* space that the Dufferin Fund is trying to enter; these women, therefore, are the direct adversaries in any 'women for women' frame that may be created. I have indicated, in the sanitary reform section, how, with the coming of the category of trained midwife, as well as that of medical inspectresses and health visitors, this adversary becomes less threatening. Here, in the minute workings and attitudes of the Fund, we will see how this adversary also gets boxed in, described one-dimensionally, in fact, produced as an individual figure – what Forbes has called 'the transformation of the *dhai* into the evil witch of progressive India' (2005, p. 81). To understand this further, I examine in more detail some of the papers by medical women in the period.

Papers by medical women

Several papers by medical women are part of the Victoria Memorial Scholarship Fund reports. These papers focus both on conditions of childbirth in the country in the experience of these medical women, and discuss means of improving these. In one of the reports discussing 15 years of the work of the Fund, there are four causes listed for unfavourable conditions of childbirth in India – and the first is 'The Dai: unskilled midwifery' (1918, Chapter III, Appendix V, p. 69).

> Any scheme of improving the conditions of child-birth in India must differ in some points according to the part of India to which the scheme is to apply … The great problem, in fact the crux … is the part played by the Hereditary or Indigenous Dai; if by legislation we could exterminate the whole race of these women the problem would have a comparatively easy solution but we cannot; their hold on the people … is too strong.
>
> (Wylie, p. 90).

The accounts go on to talk of the 'dai or untrained native midwife [who] *inherits* her office and her skill (or lack of it!) from a relation who has been a dai before her' (p. 69). As seen in the Dufferin reports, the earlier missionary and journalist accounts, and the many accounts by medical men in the first three decades of the 20th century, the description of the *dai* being a member of the 'lowest class' on account of her work being considered unclean, is laid out. The papers carry personal accounts of most of the medical women in this regard. One account speaks of having encountered 'cord-cutters' from the 'very lowest of the seven castes' of the 'Hindu sweeper-class', for instance, 'in the sacred city of Benares' (ibid). Apart from her unclean visage and apparel, the account also speaks of the manner in which she feels compelled to '"do something" for the patient', since she is being paid; and therefore often interfering in the labour process where she needn't have. It is unclear from these accounts whether these are single instances, whether they indicate a shift in *dai* practices in the context of increasing curbs and loss of livelihood; across the papers, the description is almost identical.

What, however, is the place this *dai* goes that she must not? In every one of these descriptions, it is vaginal examination with no knowledge of 'dirt and sepsis … [with a] dirty hand, which perhaps has just been cow-dunging a floor or attending a case of puerperal fever' (p. 70) that results in puerperal fever and death, or chronic '*sterility* and of *painful adhesions*, for the rest of the patient's life' (p. 70, italics in the original). The surroundings – the much-described ill-ventilated and unlit *aturghar* or *sutika griha* (lying-in room) – in both rich and poor homes – are also listed as contributing to mortality. I have discussed, in Chapter 3, the scathing mention of these conditions by male physicians in the first decades of the 20th century; there is not much difference in the descriptions there and here, except for more dedicated attention to the authority and consequent failure of the *dai* to protect the mother, and a few references to the vulnerability of her occupation and the possible value in exploring her practices. Damning patterns in these practices are spoken of:

> The dai traditions though interesting from any point of view are most difficult to combat – they vary in different parts of the country, but the following are fairly constantly present. It is considered unwise to give *any nourishment to a*

> *woman in labour*, and so one finds women dying almost of exhaustion ... [i]
> f the *labour is long delayed* ... [a]n egg may be beaten up and smeared over
> the vaginal walls to lubricate the passage, or plugs of "*medicine*" placed in
> the vagina ... [composed] of earth alone (hence the cases of *tetanus*) ... date
> seeds are placed in the mouth of the uterus to dilate it.
>
> (ibid, p. 70, italics in the original).

Further graphic descriptions are available of her attempts, in cases of a small pelvis resulting in difficult labour, to 'extract the child *by main force* ... with the
resulting *large vesico-vaginal fistulae* so common in Indian women' (ibid, p. 71,
italics in the original). The incredulous description of this therapeutic agent who
'seems quite unable to recognise any limitations to her art!' (ibid) grows. Add to
this the irrational and unreasonable, irresponsible attitudes attributed to her, who is
'*jealous of her reputation* and even if a Doctor-Miss-Sahib is within reach delays
summoning her aid till ... the patient is *in extremis*' (ibid, italics in the original).
Also, after the birth, the child is not allowed to breastfeed for the first 3 days, being
fed instead 'a mixture of spices, with ... something of the nature of lucky coin or
charm (usually old and dirty), or some incantations ... cooked with them' (ibid).
While some of these practices, including not giving the mother milk, or allowing
them to wash, are perceived as caste-based, these are also laid at the door of the
dai. The cutting of the cord is another event that is described in horror as unclean,
highlighting the use of 'a rusty nail, an unspeakably dirty and blunt household
knife', and the application of earth leading to 'septic cords ... and the incidence of
tetanus' (ibid). The *dai* is also accused of treating gynaecological conditions like
leucorrhoea and sterility, of performing female circumcision in Sind, each of these
associated with lasting damage – '*pelvic cellulitis* ... is the *usual result*' (ibid, italics in the original).

   We are invited to see, then, a powerful and arrogant individual who is holding
on to her practices, to her authority hitherto unquestioned, unwilling to cede to
better informed and safe therapeutic work. Or, we see a caricature of an individual, apparently *the same* across at least the northern regions of the country, whose
capacities for bodily damage are so great that they defy description, and training
whom is meaningless – '[e]ven if a dai attends a hospital and learns the rudiments
of midwifery, *the forces against her applying them are very great*' (ibid, italics
in the original) – on account of the resistance of a *mother-in-law* or some ancient
dame [who] superintends the confinement ... [and] *insists on* ... observance [of old
traditions]' (ibid). She also enjoys community patronage, so that '[e]ven where a
woman doctor is supposed to be in charge of a case, it is not unusual to find a *dai
is also being consulted*, and in the intervals of the doctor's visits, applying her own
methods of treatment, the evil effects of which are usually later attributed to the
western methods of the unfortunate medical woman!' (ibid). This powerful figure
is, then, not only harmful in her practices, but also responsible directly for defama-
tion of western medical practice, and *therefore cannot be ignored*. We see, then, an
almost illogical turn towards training:

The dai, therefore, is an important factor and one which cannot be over-looked in any scheme for improving the condition of childbirth in India. In the future we may hope to see midwifery in the hands of trained nurses, (and every effort should be made *to increase* the number of such women), *but till the patient herself ceases to desire* and employ a dai it is necessary to acknowledge the existence of the dai class, and to limit their power of doing harm by – (1) attempting to lessen their ignorance (2) improving the conditions of their work.

(p. 71–2, italics in the original)

Till such time as 'the patient herself ceases to desire and employ a dai'. We have seen the *zenana* woman as the ultimate victim of tradition from missionary accounts onwards. This reproductive familial being, the young woman of the couple unit, has been for Biblewomen the target of proselytization and then of secular 'good work'; she will become the upholder of the spiritual domain of nationalism soon enough. Till this *zenana* woman acquires some measure of agency, however, the *dai* must be managed.

The word becomes the woman

Who is the *dai*? Forbes has spoken of the 'construction of the dhai into the evil witch of progressive India' (2005, p. 81). Other than the cord-cutter of Benares, who has a specific task, however, the term is used in papers by medical women to describe a vast array of harmful practices that are neither tied to anything indigenous (although the untrained *dai* is termed the indigenous or *bazaar dai*), nor is it clear whether there are different practitioners among these who attend to different ailments or complaints. Popular translations of Ayurveda and discussions of popular remedies, or *gharoa chikitsa* texts, at this time, prescribe precautions and pre-emptive steps for the *dai*, mostly referring to hygiene and character. The popular medical text by the Indian male doctor sometimes uses terms like *dhatri* and *dai* for different and hierarchical roles in birth work, but the language used indicates the derivative and poorly evidenced nature of the argument. Otherwise, for all intents and purposes, it would seem that the shadowy figure of the *dai* is always already inside the *aturghar*, performs all these malfeasances, and is not to be seen otherwise. She is not tied to the indigenous male practitioner; in fact, there are references in popular writing to the failure of *vaids* and *hakims* to bother with women's ailments. There is no writing or biographical material available outside the anecdotal evidence presented in these papers. In some sense, then, this figure exists in an epistemic vacuum; there are no bridges or contests whatsoever between her and the textual canon of the indigenous, for instance. All descriptions are of practice, practice understood as hereditary, and non-authorial. Do women's reproductive health concerns then actually occupy such a black hole in the indigenous textual canon? Is that the source of the *dai's* seeming absolute authority?

Prasuti tantra and the missing practitioner

A very brief examination of commentaries on the Ayurvedic canon might be useful here. These commentaries speak of *Prasuti tantra* (doctrines of childbirth) through a detailed reading of the standard texts attributed to the Ayurvedic corpus, the *Caraka Samhita* and the *Susruta Samhita*. The subject of *Prasuti-tantra* is not fully available in one *sthana* or chapter; rather, it is scattered throughout whole books, sometimes along with other subjects. Of the eight branches (*ashtanga*) of Ayurveda, *kaumara-bhrtya* – the subject concerned with the *bharana* (bearing) of *kumara* (child) – contains topics related to *prasuti-tantra*. There are entire sections of the Susruta Samhita devoted to the delineation of *Stree rogam* (illnesses of women) and to the care of the woman in pregnancy and during and after childbirth – *Prasuti tantra*. It would be pertinent to say that in Ayurveda, there are some roots that may be linked with the Sramana tradition that showed influences of Buddhism and Jainism, later taken up by Vedic traditions – promoting an abstract, other-worldly intellectual-philosophical outlook. These regard the body as something to be vigilant about – in this view, phenomenal existence, or *loka tattva*, is considered to be not only unimportant but evil. These are in direct contestation with *kayasadhana*, a combination of *dehatattva* (bodily constitution) and *dehasvabhava* (bodily behaviour), which work with an emphasis on nature and balance within the body – definite influences of Tantrik traditions. The subject of *Prasuti tantra* comes under *kaumara-bhrtya*, one of the eight branches of Ayurveda. For this particular speciality Caraka seems to have used the term *kaumara-brtyaka*, Susruta *kaumara-bhrtya* or *kaumara-tantra*, Kasyapa *kaumara-bhrtya*, and both Vagbhata and Harita *bala-cikitsa*. Concepts like the *putresti yajna* in monarchies that laid a certain weight on the son as heir to the throne, *rtukala* as perhaps the optimum period for fertilization, *garbha, dauhrda* as perhaps the clinical features of pregnant women, *udavarta* and *kikkisa, panca mahabhutas* as perhaps descending into the embryo, *rajasika/tamasika* as features of the foetus, are to be found. Out of the *Susruta Samhita* concepts like the *stri-sukra, artava, raja, garbha-srava, garbha-pata, garbha-vrddhi, garbha-kyasa, garbha-sanga, makkalla-sula, rakta-vidradhi* (references to physiological and ritual aspects, and ailments of pregnancy and childbirth) are used. The details of the anatomy and the physiology of the female body, of menstruation, and of the descent of the embryo as described in *sarira-sthana* would also come up for discussion; the notion of the nine *grahas* and the treatment of *skanda, apasmara, sakuni, rewati, putana, andha, mandika, sitaputana, naigamesa* would also be dealt with. Out of the *Astanga-Samgraha, Astanga-Hrdaya, Harita-Samhita, Madhava-Nidana, Sarngadhara-Samhita, Bhawaprakasa, Yogaratnakara* and the specific source book of *kaumara-bhrtya* – the *Kasyapa-Samhita* – the concepts of the *yoni samvarna, rasausadhis, jataharini, varana-bandha, avis* (as perhaps labour pain), notion of the possible vitiation of breast milk by *grahas, stana vajra, ulbaka* as perhaps the diseases of the newborn, and the treatment of the umbilical wound, *yoni-bhramsa, sutika rogas,* and *jarayu-dosa* may be found. Nowhere in any of these discussions is the practitioner visible. Although that is the case in the entire text, we have seen how, in the mid to late 19th century, translations and commentaries present the male practitioner at the centre of the system. In this case, however, there is no such voice.

Practice and knowledge

I have discussed, in Chapter 2, Dalmiya's articulation of the challenge to epistemological models available in European midwifery. A consideration of writing by British midwives from the 15th century onwards shows an authorial political voice that resists the takeover of their livelihood and knowledge by male obstetricians during the 17th and 18th centuries. Given the active nature of this history, extending also into the fraught debates around labour anaesthesia versus natural childbirth that took the British public by storm in the 19th century, or the serious criticisms by British midwives of experimental instrument use by unlicensed male practitioners, it is curious that no whiff of similar debates, or at least an alternative empathetic view of midwifery as experiential knowledge, is to be found among these papers.[3] Instead, the debate is between practice and knowledge – a recognizable distinction following the standard knowledge-experience binary that shores up dominant Western science. But this is not all. The *dai* is not merely reviled for her practice and its failures or inadequacies; she is reviled for her behaviour, her character, her near-criminality. We have seen, in the previous chapter, the tribal communities that are notified as criminal in the classifications of the 1870s onwards, and amelioration exercises of the first decades of the 20th century; work towards this set of notifications has obviously begun before and has implications for some of these practitioners. Further, any interventions like vaginal examination performed by the *dai* are what come up for strict censure. In the work for women, her role can at most be as tolerated observer; any invasive step is categorically denied her, even though some training centres support therapeutic work of an advanced degree by the *dais*, supplying surgical suture for perineal repair in their kits, for instance (National Association for Supplying Medical Aid by Women to the Women of India, 1928, p. 92). No wonder, then, that the *dai* is considered untrainable – she is being trained to *pull back from her therapeutic role*. The image of the *dai* who attempts a perineal repair with needle and thread after having watched it done once, then, could be read differently from how it is described with despair at ignorance and unsanitariness in the papers by medical women, and referred to by Forbes (1999). The image conjured begs an alternative explanation – of a practitioner who has both skill and confidence, accompanied by a familiarity with the woman's anatomy, and who knows she can replicate what she has seen, although she does it, in the absence of surgical resources or adequate instruction, with 'a dirty needle and thread' (p. 72). It is an image of a desperate practitioner also, perhaps, who has put together these artefacts as the kind of magic that western science appears to be, knowing the power of that magic, and using it to acquire power in an environment where it is being taken away from her. This move was also, seemingly paradoxically, part of the colonizing impulse to bring in science, as Prakash has noted (1999). Her accessing this route to power is what is seen as uniquely corrupt behaviour.

In the same papers are accounts of *dai* practice from different regions – Sind, Bengal, and various parts of mostly the northern regions of the subcontinent. Some of the papers even mention the impossibility of devising a single scheme across such vastly different '[c]onditions and customs' as exist 'in even neighbouring districts' (Wylie, 1918, p. 84). Some of these papers also recognize the aspect of childbirth impurity as 'the rule laid down by caste' (ibid). All these descriptions, however, coalesce, as I mentioned above, into one image, so that what we are left with is the suggestion of a concrete single agent – 'the low caste dai' (ibid, p. 85) – who impedes the progress of reform and redress. This may be extended to the standard forms of othering that have been historically constitutive of modern science. Prakash highlights one of the responses of modern science:

> '[w]hat began as representations of science staged to conquer ignorance and superstition became enmeshed in the very effects that were targeted for elimination. We encounter this intermixture in the museum's evocation of the awe of the visitors, in the exhibition's utilization of a sense of marvels, in mesmeric science's attempt to show magical efficacy, and in the miraculous powers evoked by public demonstrations of scientific instruments.
>
> (Prakash, 1992, p. 163)

Magic lantern use – an example of such visual demonstration of scientific prowess for both the subaltern and educated elite – was, in *dai* training and awareness sessions for zenana audiences, common. Prakash' understanding may be extended to examine the othering of the colonized. The *dai*, in her exaggerated and caricatured descriptions, can become now the spectacle, the identity that may be museumized, or given a new role as observer and facilitator, but not accepted on terms of equality as a practitioner (Prakash, 1992; Visvanathan, 2009).

It is in these contexts, then, that the Dufferin Fund proposes the training of *dais*.

Can she, can't she, be trained? Perspectives from the Victoria Memorial Scholarship Fund

> 'Constant supervision will be required in any work amongst the dais as the "aseptic conscience" soon slumbers in an Indian bazaar'.
>
> (McMichael, 1918, p. 107)

While the *zenana* woman must be saved from the *dai*, as we will see later, the *dai* herself is seen as embedded in contexts into which she is bound to be sucked back, unless and even when supervision is constant. To this end, an array of supervisory positions – inspectresses for schools and factories, *sarkari dais*, hospital midwives, sub-assistant surgeons, and medically trained doctors, is listed. With regard to this practitioner, however, a certain notion of the indigenous as excessive, chaotic, symbolized in the idea of the 'bazaar', continues despite all attempts at 'taming' her. We have seen some of this idea in the workings of the Indigenous Drugs Committee in Chapter 3, where the complaint of impure and ineffective drugs regularly arises with respect to preparations sourced from the *bazaar* or local practitioners. Here, the 'lower-caste *bazaar dai*' symbolizes, in her very mien, this excess, this chaos. All the descriptions in the medical women's papers, the exhortations towards modern medicine by medical men, the earlier missionary accounts, hint at this excess, this chaos. This chaos is of another climate, another soil than that of Empire. Arnold has talked about the tropicalization of the colony and the implications of such a tropicalization for indigenous knowledges. He discusses particularly a period beginning from about the second decade of the 19th century:

> [a]s colonial rule became more assured and feats of canal-building and railway construction ... [a]s India's Oriental identity became eclipsed (though never entirely erased) and as the British regime associated itself more with "modern" science and technology and less with "traditional" learning and indigenous culture, so the identification of India with the tropics grew in strength.
>
> (2006, pp. 135–136).

Arnold is referring to a shift in emphasis, not full perspective, from an Orientalist to a tropicalized view of the subcontinent. This lens may be partly useful to understand the attitude toward the *dai*, and the manner in which she is both named and made abject in the consolidation of the indigenous at the turn of the century – a consolidation that works for colonial governance. The *bazaar*, in particular, the source of her presence, is a product of the casually Orientalist and possibly the tropicalized view of the Indian climate and landscape, where pestilences and fevers abound; this second view gained ground during the early 19th century when India, with its products, drugs, and subjects, 'was all too connected and half-familiar to Europe' (ibid, p. 136). The named *category*, the *bazaar dai* became, I would argue, one of the symbols of this tropicalization. Despite the curbing and structuring of her therapeutic role, then, is the fear of being overrun by this excess and chaos, where 'the hereditary dais ... are looked upon as women gifted with abnormal powers, and the public while having great faith in them are afraid of them also, for they believe that these women when offended can harm them in various ways, being a kind of sorceress', as one WMS practitioner of the Raj Dufferin Hospital at Bettiah puts it (Sen, 1918, p. 127). The answer, for the medical women, is 'midwives from a more respectable class of people ... who can be trusted to do their work conscientiously' (ibid, p. 128). Clearly, this is the route to save the people from the *bazaar dai*, who is both untrainable and must be kept in check. Supervision is also meant to be European, for even good trainees are expected to lapse into old ways.

The Dufferin Fund proposed two modes of training – one, to create a cadre of

> trained midwife attached to a hospital, going out to cases for which she may take fees. On the plea of the hereditary indigenous *dai* being unsanitary, unskilled, untrainable, and her lower caste location being practically a causal condition for this, the Fund proposes that a superior class of women, from the higher castes, be trained to take their place. The other, which should always go on side by side ... is to train the indigenous dai.
>
> (Victoria Memorial Scholarships Fund, 1918, p. 72)

In the latter case, she is under the supervision of a trained nurse or Sub-Assistant Surgeon and gets 'Re. 1 notifying fee if they do it in time for her to be present at the labour, and 8 annas if after' (ibid, p. 73). These indigenous *dais* are also to be encouraged to attend classes that 'can be made very attractive if augmented by a magic lantern for demonstrative purposes' (ibid). Whereas the trained midwife is mostly concentrated in Bombay, Calcutta, and Madras, indigenous *dais* were trained in Bombay 'together with their daughters and daughters-in-law [via] simple lectures ... in the vernacular on elementary hygiene, how to attend normal cases of labour, the need of aseptic precautions, etc' (ibid, p. 72). Such classes were also conducted in Nagpur, Amritsar, Bhopal, Ferozepur, Jubbulpore, and Agra, among other provinces. It was noted that for indigenous *dai* training to succeed, supervision was of the essence, but also 'tact and gentleness' for an agent whose autonomy needed to be stripped, and whose role was to be restricted to the basics. The training of indigenous *dais* is taken up under the aegis of the Victoria Memorial [VM] Scholarship Fund, which works out of Dufferin offices till 1931, when it is taken over by the All-India Maternity and Child Welfare Bureau. The trained daughters of *bazaar dais* are sometimes referred to as the Victoria Memorial dais who will, it is presumed, be successful in course of time. Like the Dufferin Fund, the VM fund too, with funds put aside under Lady Curzon, has both central and local committees – the former with the presence of the Dufferin Fund nominee. The local committee is accountable to the Inspector-General of Civil Hospitals or the Administrative Medical Officer.

But is she trainable? 'Is it worth while', the medical women ask, 'to try to reach her [the indigenous *dai*] at all, or should we leave her alone and set to work to train more promising pupils who will gradually take her place? In places where the calling is not hereditary, as, e.g., in Jubbulpore, the dai might comparatively easily be ousted. But in Nagpur such a proceeding would take generations ... The question would then arise:- Who is to take her place? At the present rate the output of trained midwives yearly being practically negligible, we are simply providing no substitute ... it is only within the last four years that anything practical has been achieved' (Papers continued, Wylie, 1918, p. 87). Prior to this, in the VM scholarships fund report for the year 1913 (29th annual report), the Quinquennial Report on Education in India is cited as saying, '"All efforts to promote female education have hitherto encountered peculiar difficulties"' and that '"In Bombay ... the great mass of Indian womanhood remains almost untouched"' (National Association for Supplying Female Medical Aid to the Women of India, 1914, p. 89). The VM report uses this finding to suggest that, in these circumstances, 'any advance in teaching a particularly illiterate and prejudiced class is a matter of considerable congratulation' (ibid). Given, in this climate, the preference for the hereditary *dai* among 'ladies of the highest family', the *dai*'s 'fear of losing ... practice still prevent[ing] many of the ignorant dais from accepting scholarships, and from attending classes where they have opportunities of learning modern ideas' (ibid) is understood. And yet, obstinacy and the attitude of 'any offer of teaching [being seen] in the nature of an insult' (ibid) carries the day. On the one hand, she is afraid to train for fear of losing livelihood if seen as 'modern'; on the other, she is seen as so powerful that she 'would obstruct the Lady Doctors who would improve their knowledge in every possible way' (ibid, pp. 89–90). It is strange, however, that it is the indigenous category of *dai* that is considered to be riddled with caste prejudice. Is this a case of not feeling up to the task of learning? Or is it a case of holding these women responsible for their own backwardness, as the attitude in the reports seems to suggest? Native prejudice against accepting this woman inside their homes, if mentioned at all, is laid at the door of the *zenana* women's resistance to modernity.

A variety of observations that complicate this position are also available, however. It is reported that prejudice against *dais* trained in European methods seems to be diminishing in certain provinces, like Dacca and Punjab. The 29th annual report of the VM fund for the year 1913 suggests that '*dais* at present under training are all Mohamedan women, fairly intelligent and work satisfactorily' (ibid, p. 99). Benares also reports much success, saying that 'none now remain undiplomaed'. A report from Miss F. Leach, M.D., Dufferin Hospital, of the Cawnpore branch, throws some light on caste relations and the impact of the training on them.

> Owing to caste and other Indian rites and customs, most of those trained dais have absolutely refused to accept posts out of the station or practise privately away from the hospital. They assure me that for the above reasons they prefer being attached to a hospital and being in touch with the Lady Doctor. In this way they can pacify their caste friends and relations, and moreover secure a considerable amount of protection and respect from the public.
>
> (ibid)

Some detailed observations suggest that *Dhanok* and *Basok* women are the indigenous caste *dais* here, and there is lesser demand for them as they are deemed unsatisfactory. The worry also seems to be that once trained, they go beyond Fund control.

The hospital or trained midwife is clearly available in much poorer numbers than desirable, even about 40 years into the Fund's work. Part of the reason would be, as the previous description suggests, the continuing stigma attached to birth attendance that comes in the way of the 'right' kind of women coming forward for training. At any rate, the Victoria Memorial Scholarship Fund, which was instituted in 1901–2 by Lady Curzon, took upon itself the task of training the indigenous *dai*, in an avowed climate of 'extraordinary superstitions caste prejudices and ignorance' (National Association for Supplying Female Medical Aid to the Women of India, 1913, p. 73), focusing primarily on 'cleanliness, and the need of realizing ... when a case requires *skilled* assistance' (Wylie, 1918, p. 87, italics mine); the idea being 'not so much to give a course of instruction to dais, examine them, give them certificates ... but rather to keep in touch ... inspect their cases' (ibid), and so on. Some of this training is conducted in hospitals (Bhopal, Hyderabad Deccan, Lahore, Baroda), some in homes (Hyderabad Sind), so that 'the dais are taught how to meet the difficulties that must inevitably meet them in the Indian home' (National Association for Supplying Medical Aid by Women to the Women of India, VM Fund report, 1923, p. 89). The idea is also 'to get in touch with their children' (Wylie, 1918, p. 88), as Dr Henderson, who has set up a course for the Mang *dais*, states. We find, then, efforts like schools for Mang children in Nagpur, where it was found that Mang women were the primary category of indigenous *dai*, where 'part of the routine is hand-washing and nail-cleansing, in view of their future profession' (Wylie, ibid). Some of the younger generation are also to be considered possible candidates for hospital midwife training, with the possibility of scholarships for daughters of *dais*, so that 'gradually the effects of training would be felt by the whole caste and profession'. This mechanism is deployed in the Victoria Zenana Hospital in the Hyderabad Deccan too (National Association for Supplying Medical Aid by Women to the Women of India, 1923, VM Fund report, 1923, p. 89). For those daughters who would receive such hospital training, it was proposed that they might be outfitted with 'blunt-pointed scissors to cut the cord with, ligatures for the cord, soft linen to dress it, catheters, enema syringes and antiseptic lotions' (Wylie, ibid). For the mothers, simple training in the vernacular is sometimes followed with instructions to outfit themselves with simpler kits – the scissors, clean ligature material, and a vessel for boiling these – made available for them to buy. The Sarkari *dais* may be allowed to pass on some of these accouchement packets to reporting *dais* 'for the use of patients who can afford them' (p. 96). Once the dangerous *dai* has been processed through the institution, then, she may be allowed to perform some form of therapeutic work, although she will still not have a certificate of skill, her role will continue to be in reporting cases, and her autonomy will be contingent on continuing supervision and approval. This is also the time when the push for compulsory registration and inspection is seen, continuing and consolidating in 1911 and thereafter. The Patiala Association annual report, for instance, cites an order 'that has been passed that after the lapse of 12 months no dai shall be allowed to practice in the city who has not the certificate of the Lady Curzon School' (National Association for Supplying Female Medical Aid to the Women of India 1913, p. 68). Local Acts regulating *dai* practice after training are also in place by the 1920s. There are also proposals for lists of registered *dais* in police *thanas*, *tehsils*, ladies' clubs, octroi posts, etc., inviting not only institutional but public and social surveillance on the therapeutic work these women have been doing, and normalizing such surveillance as a facet of civic responsibility. In fact, the Jubbulpore municipality has, at this time, already imposed a licensing fee on all practising *dais,* and a Punjab Central Midwives' Board is set up as part of the work of the Victoria Memorial Fund, to conduct examinations for midwives and their subsequent registration and supervision of *dais*. The structure is well delineated, with a local Training School for *dais* tied to selected women's hospitals, a Central Training School at Amritsar, and the majority of the *dais* proposed to be taught at 'the bedsides of their own patients' (Dr Agnes Scott 1918, Punjab, p. 92). A District Medical Superintendent of *Dais* is proposed, a qualified doctor, exclusively allowed to devote her time to maternity work and supervision of the Health Visitors, with perhaps the role of Medical Inspectress of girls' schools in the district. Dr Scott further proposes that the *tehsil* will have a Head Midwife – fully trained as a 'nurse and midwife, European or Anglo-Indian, acquainted with the language and customs of the people and in sympathy with them' (p. 93).

'Sarkari dais under the Head Midwife' will be in charge of a group of villages and the 'Hereditary or village dais' in them. 'Sarkari dais at first would be drawn from classes other than the indigenous dais and must be, if possible literate and possess a certificate of two years' training in midwifery' (ibid). It is at the tail end of this hierarchy, at the village level, that a hereditary *dai* for a population of every thousand, is to be nominated by the village headman,

> as Reporting dai of that village ...[who] at first would probably be untrained but ... would be the first to be trained ... [would] visit their supervising dai thrice a week to report the cases of the ten hereditary dais for whom they are responsible in the same way that the village Chowkidar has to visit the nearest Police Thana every few days to make his report on the peace, etc.
>
> (p. 93)

This structure is further detailed. Here and in other places including Quetta, Bhopal, Nagpur, a system of attendance, advisory committees, bills for *dai* charges, are in place, along with some stipends during training. This is, in the second decade of the 20th century, in the process of being moved to government funds from the Victoria Memorial Fund.

We see, then, that the hereditary *dai*, who cannot be 'exterminated', is sought to be regulated, supervised, and re-invented as an administrative entity – what we today recognize in the public health system as the link worker – introducing modern hierarchies that sustain traditional caste hierarchies while offering a sense of power over equals – the reporting dai vis-a-vis her non-official local co-practitioners, for instance. The upper-caste Sarkari *dai*, whose job it is to 'get that particular piece of knowledge [some simple matter connected with maternity work] into the dais' heads before the next visit' (p. 94), is both granted superior knowledge status to the reporting *dai*, and continues to be treated as a subordinate. The social status quo is thus dutifully maintained, with the scientistic attachment to hygiene and codified knowledge and the casteist notion of purity and epistemic authority going well together. In fact, before trying to teach the indigenous *dai*, 'it will be necessary to use a certain amount of moral force, together with ... bribes and other inducements' (p. 97), also accompanied by punishment for 'disobeying instructions', some of which may be routed through a government agency, as suggested by Dr Scott. Victoria Memorial *dais* getting scholarships for training are proposed to be made to sign bonds of service for three years thereafter. Overall, there is consensus that St. Catherine's Hospital at Amritsar has been most successful in this rewards-fines approach and must be emulated. By the 1920s, this system of supervision seems to have worked – for the 1923 report, 'the chief thing is that there is a satisfactory increase in the number of cases shown', and that 'the women who employ these dais are beginning to criticise their methods and evidently expect them to attain a certain standard as to their work' (National Association for Supplying Medical Aid by Women to the Women of India, 1923, Baluchistan, p. 95). Several reports also acknowledge the local nature and context-based livelihoods of the indigenous *dais*, agreeing that training should take place in their home districts rather than at the Dufferin centres.

What about remunerations and stipends for post-training work? All the medical women consulted on this agree that some supplemental support from the Fund might be offered to the trained *dai*, on the understanding that she take from the family the same fee as the indigenous *dai*. A fixed salary, it seems, might encourage laziness, so it is not approved. Kits and outfits are also encouraged to be bought, as they would then apparently be more valued. Rewards for reporting are seen as the way to go, with deductions and fines for failure to report, or for neglect. In Quetta, the rules formulated included deductions of four annas for a torn perineum, only three-quarters of payment given for a dead child, half the amount for a miscarriage (Stuart, 1918, p. 119). Several local ad hoc mechanisms of reward and punishment are in place. For those seen to misconduct a delivery or not bring a case in on time, for example, practice is stopped 'for a month or two' (National Association for Supplying Female Medical Aid to the Women of India, 1913, Bhopal, p. 83), with the police helping to enforce the ban. There is, however, another observation. With access to kits, certificates, and other proofs of patronage by the institution, the indigenous *dai* definitely acquires greater power in her communities; she is, in some cases, seen to 'raise her fee'.

The other aspect is, of course, the increased scope of employment for British medical women who have, in the medical service, fought for equality and the freedom to run their own hospitals. Forbes, Arnold, and others have written of the racial and gender hierarchies involved in the setting up and trajectory of the women's medical service. We see, in the accounts by English medical women, suggestions that

> 'it is a good thing that the English doctor should herself have a good deal to do with the training and superintending of the dai as she will carry more weight than an Assistant Surgeon and also as she constantly goes in and out among the houses on her regulation visits the people will grow accustomed to her presence and will not be afraid to send for her in time of need.
>
> (Stuart, 1918, p. 117)

This form of supervision is, of course, proposed for the cities, with the small towns left to the nurse midwives.

It is in the context of this growing scope for newer professional cadres that the description of the dangerous indigenous *dai* may also be situated. For one, while on the one hand, she comes to life in the *aturghar*, with no seeming knowledge of antenatal care, there are occasional descriptions of women who appear in both antenatal and postnatal scenarios; these are not explored further. As for the *aturer dai* – the woman of the lying-in room – the description of her outrageous and dangerous practices by all, including Indian medical women, both consolidate the stereotype and provides grist to competition for livelihood. Indian medical women have become, by the early 20th century, key figures in at least upper-caste middle-class homes as agents of delivery who will be amenable to the status quo, and for them to flourish, the cheaper *dai* must go. Even trained *dais* who 'work without supervision taking abnormal cases and thinking themselves doctors' (Victoria

Memorial Scholarships Fund, 1918, p. 152) are, as per Miss Misra, Sub-assistant Surgeon, Nainital, and one of the emerging professionals of the time, dangerous. Ties to privileged-caste notions of childbirth impurity are expunged from the discussion as an aside. While there are multiple references in the papers to 'friends' and relatives of the woman who insist on interference to get the baby out, or on keeping the lying-in room closed, and on ritual arrangements that may be harmful to the mother, the principle of harm is laid at the feet of the *dai* alone. In a curious paradox, this accountability comes from seeing her as a therapeutic agent, and yet, that is a role that is comprehensively denied to her. Given that the *aturer dai* herself is described as an unclean lower-caste woman, it is little wonder that despite being embedded in the cultural contexts that insist on childbirth impurity and the consequent separation of the event from the rest of the household, she performs the function of the abject both in the emerging therapeutic, and in civilizational pride and the emerging indigenous.

It is in this context that we might ask if the untrained *dai* is being supplanted, or if a dichotomy of untrained and trained becomes the lens through which she can be delegitimized. Following the trajectories of the Fund, it would seem that the indigenous *dai* is seen as difficult to supplant; in the event, her reinvention as a link of sorts, to provide labour to the health apparatus, is possibly seen as the way forward. But how general is this move vis-à-vis other indigenous practitioners? Berger speaks of the impulse of regulation not only *dais* but also of 'other groups who held knowledge useful to the imperial state, as *hakims*, *vaids* and *pandits* who came to be acknowledged as professionals once they became associated with emerging institutional bodies' (2013, p. 95). I suggest that these other agents, while undergoing regulatory practice, were more included and managed the injunctions/regulations, while the *dai* could not, at least in part because these other agents also participated in her exclusion. The role of the Indian woman physician might be a case in point.

Is there any voice, any resistance, from these women to the strict regulations and supervisions sought to be put in place? We see, midway through the working of the VM fund, that in the newly formed provinces of Bihar, the 'hereditary dais, or their daughters, or female relations have not offered themselves for training' (National Association for Supplying Female Medical Aid to the Women of India, 1913, p. 78), forcing the Committee to sanction 'the training of midwives of a better status' (ibid), which is the secondary mandate of the fund. While this is easily put down to the untrainability and apathy of the 'hereditary dais', we might, possibly, see agency or resistance in some of these actions.

Is this woman empathized with in any way in the workings of the Association? There is some recognition in the papers by medical women and annual reports of the Fund, of the caste prejudice faced by these women, and the fear of losing livelihood they experience in case they go for training. This does not translate, however, into a further recognition that caste discrimination operates exactly in this fashion – disallowing epistemic authority to those who have been occupationally kept outside of knowledge systems, while continuing to force occupational exclusivity on them for the polluting work attached to childbirth. In returning to the image of the *dai* who attempts perineal repair after having seen it once, however, we get a first glimpse of the *dais'* access to power and a chance of being party to a new magic in a space, namely the *aturghar*, that was hitherto completely not part of the corridors of power. With the added incentive of payment, it is *perhaps* a ticket out of extreme vulnerability rather than the apathetic resistance to modern science and progress that it has been read as. This is what I suggest as a first step to re-reading this history.

Training texts and reference points

Given the even more active shift toward imparting practical knowledge to indigenous *dais* based on the acknowledgement of their ability to influence a larger part of the population, oral formats are the primary model of training. Apart from magic lantern lectures, there is mention in the VM Fund of a Manual of Midwifery compiled by Lt-Col C.P. Lukis, Director-General of the IMS, that is translated into several Indian languages, with partial funding from the government. 'First Lessons to Country Dais' by Dr Balfour, WMS, 'Care of the Baby' by the same author, intended for girls' schools, 'Hukm Dey and her baby', meant for *dais* and mothers, 'First Aid in Childbirth' by Miss Campbell, apart from numerous pamphlets, also provide resources. Anatomical models for *dai* training, of internal organs, dummy foetuses, and pelvises, are also in use.

Interestingly, the VM fund reports of these years consistently refer to the *Susruta Samhita* as a treatise on midwifery that was in active use till the 4th century AD, going on to lament the caste prejudices of the people that have resulted in the 'barbarous' childbirth practices of the present, and to connect the Fund's objectives to a revival of ancient traditions that 'have received enthusiastic support from all patriotic Indians' (National Association for Supplying Female Medical Aid to the Women of India, 1914, 29th annual report, VM Scholarships Fund report, p. 89). In addition, there are texts like *Garbharaksha* in Hindi that approach the *zenana* in an attempt to negotiate the *dai's* role in childbirth.

The Health Visitors and the medical women conduct most of the training that begin in the provincial centres in earnest after the GOI Act 1919 (Central Provinces, p. 95). In later years, in some of the native states, the indigenous *dais* are fewer in number, with the literate women trainees taking precedence (National Association for Supplying Medical Aid by Women to the Women of India, 1928, 44th annual report, Gwalior, p. 93). More indigenous *dais* are found to be in training in the provinces of Quetta, and Dacca, for example.

Recognition and appreciation

The annual reports or medical papers rarely mention the *dais* as individuals. In the 28th annual report (1913), a *Dai* Hyaten and a *Dai* Halima come up for special mention, as indigenous *dais* sent by their village headmen for training, and returned to their villages with a successful and popular practice. Several successful trainees were also given presents, apart from the certificates at the completion of training. What rests on such a naming of individual women in an exercise of countrywide magnitude? While some of the impulse seems to be of documentation, the engagement with persons, rather than a category, seems to be, in the light of the dominant tone of the reports, more about the individual physician leaving their mark on the reports than of writing the *dai* practitioners into history.

Other funds

Part of the work of supervision is brought in during this part via other funds like the Lady Willingdon Scheme in Bombay, financed through public contributions, working with the Municipal Health Department, under which up to 160 of the indigenous *dais* were given training in the vernacular, listed, and expected to call in for skilled help when required. The Maternity Homes with better trained midwives, paid Health Visitors etc. are also spoken of under this scheme, along with voluntary workers, and Lady Presidents in charge of different sections of the city. Outcomes are not great in this regard, not only in Bombay but under the VM fund in other places too – Ferozepur, for instance, where from 1907 to 1915, 33 *dais* were trained, but 'nearly all of the non-dai class' (Victoria Memorial Scholarships Fund, 1918, Notes on work done in Bombay, Madras, Nagpur, Bhopal, Ferozepore, p. 158), until the Cantonment Magistrate and Deputy Commissioner of the cantonment and city respectively took an interest and ordered the dais to attend. The Lady Reading Women of India fund, set up in 1922, undertakes to support 'Hindu caste nurses during their training, ... [to] be known as the "Lady Reading Nurses"' (National Association for Supplying Medical Aid by Women to the Women of India, 1923, 39th Annual Report, p. 15). Madras reported a better history with midwife training, reporting up to a hundred yearly. It was noticed here that 'non-caste women especially are willing to come to hospital for their confinements ... [providing] plenty of clinical material for teaching' (Notes, ibid, p. 156).[4] Of course, the 'non-caste woman' *dai* is also the competitor to the trained midwife, to the nurse, indeed to the medical doctor, for 'the barber dai acts ayah to mother and baby for a whole month and gets just a rupee and perhaps a cloth or two in return, whereas my nurses cease all attendance on the tenth day', as one Dr Virasingh in charge of a Child Welfare Scheme in Madras is reported as saying in the report (p. 156).

Saving the zenana from the dai

Why do *dais* need constant supervision? Why is it that 'the very best of dais soon revert to old methods' (Victoria Memorial Scholarships Fund, 1918, 73)? From this and other papers by medical women, it seems the case that 'the people do not like new ways' (ibid), but can be persuaded to listen to the medical women where they do not listen to the *dai*. Clearly, then, this all-powerful figure is not so powerful, but more importantly, the contexts of her powerlessness are significant. The *bazaar dais* are, as the papers describe, women of the 'low Hindu sweeper-class' (ibid, p. 69) – a variety of marginalized castes. While it is unclear at what stage of the labour any of these practitioners would be brought into homes before the

Dufferin fund began its work,[5] the availability of privileged-caste hospital mid-wives and health visitors would likely have tilted the scales further against the indigenous *dai* during the time of the Fund. The *zenana* women by now had access to institutional delivery or medical women to attend to their pregnancies within their homes. The practice of *atur*, or the lying-in room away from the main house, was the condition for the entry of the marginalized-caste birth practitioner. If that needed to change, as sanitary reform agendas and the medical women were insisting, the place of the lower-caste *dai* would have to be vacated, for she could not have a place in the main house. The indigenous *dai's* failure to perform as per new instructions, then, may need to be seen in this light. Nor is it likely that advice on newer practices of ventilation, hygiene, and asepsis would be given ear when coming from this marginalized practitioner, and the medical women themselves admit to this in their writing. 'This suggests', they then say, 'the first step in any measure for reform. Let us educate the women ... in those girls' schools ... and in all boys' schools, let us insist on hygiene, simple physiology, and domestic science' (ibid, p. 86). Given that the *zenana* woman is the object of this reform, the birth practitioner – the ubiquitous *dai* – is at most of use in reporting on birth conditions that can then be recorded as data. In order to complete the reform, however, and in keeping with the policy of non-interference in the 'socio-cultural and religious' life of the natives, is the need to separate the *zenana* woman and the *dai* – a class and caste separation that maintained the status quo. This impulse becomes clearer in the training exercises and their reception. The Bible women of the missionary period performed this function of educating *zenana* women; in the Fund period, the Health Visitors or women sanitary inspectors visiting schools took over. *Parda nashin* clubs are sites where 'older and more influential and probably more intelligent class of women' (McMichael, 1918, p. 104) are sought to be reached for this purpose; Mother's Lectures have been in place in Ajmer for the same, with lectures on antenatal care, care of the infant, simple ailments of childhood, and the training of the child. The 1923 annual report states that 'the people in the houses are beginning to demand dais with "bags" [a reference to the kit that is a metaphor for training] so that is a step in the right direction' (National Association for Supplying Medical Aid by Women to the Women of India 1923, 39th annual report, Reports from centres of the Fund, Delhi, p. 94). Fund reports indicate these measures becoming successful during the 1920s, even smaller towns, with lectures on 'Infant mortality and Maternity and Child Welfare' using magic lantern slides etc, and infant welfare associations and child welfare committees being established (39th annual report, Report of the Lady Hardinge hospital, Akola, N.R. Mucadam, p. 30). Classes on first aid in childbirth, a Travelling Exhibition of the Lady Chelmsford League meant to 'show the main facts of Maternity and Child Welfare by means of models, posters, etc., in a form which can be readily understood by the illiterate as well as the educated classes' (39th ... Lady Chelmsford All-India League, report for 1923, p. 110), and National Baby Week, Baby Days, Health Weeks, are in place by 1923. Baby shows begin by 1924, to showcase *healthy-looking* children. Many of the competitions organized under the auspices of the Lady Chelmsford League were 'novel ... for barbers, for dhobies ... [as] a means of encouraging clean and hygienic methods ... The 'sanitary conscience' of the people ... was encouraged by the offer of prizes for the cleanest house and ward in town ... The mother's day, the children's day, the poor men's day [received special attention] so that all classes might be reached' (National Association for Supplying Medical Aid by Women to the Women of India, 1928, The Lady Chelmsford League report, p. 123). It is useful to note this aspect of health performance here.

In addition to the common knowledge of the *zenana* woman being the primary target of teaching, the 'task of teaching the men' too is not neglected. While educated men who have never 'received any instruction on ... vital subjects – ... which mean the death or the life of the race' (Vaughan, 1918, p. 98) are proposed to have this remedied in school life, '[t]he village men' are proposed to be 'taught by lantern lectures', suggests Dr Agnes Scott, WMS Assistant to the Inspector General of Civil Hospitals, Punjab (Scott, 1918, p. 91). As part of this teaching, 'diseases spread by the indigenous dai' are listed – 'puerperal sepsis, tetanus, gonorrhoea' (ibid). The differences in approach towards men and women in this regard are stark. While women, particularly the younger women, are urged to take control over their bodies, men are approached on particular grounds of the need to pay attention to maternal welfare if healthy sons are to be borne, and the vitality of the race maintained. 'Place the subject on its proper basis, the love of the race, the preservation of life and there will be a ready response' (p. 101), says Dr Vaughan, of the Diamond Jubilee Zenana Hospital, Srinagar. A further suggestion is that of popularizing and publicly communicating aspects of midwifery. At least part of the funds and constituency for this work with men and boys is proposed to build on the Anti-Tuberculosis league already in place, and this is an indication of the gendered nature of public health participation prevailing at the time.

Baby shows, health performance, and governmentality

The Lady Chelmsford All-India League for Maternity and Child Welfare was set up in the year 1919, taking up the work of setting up Health Schools, *dai* training centres, and health propaganda. The spirit of voluntarism and charity, as well as 'very special qualities of initiative and resource, ability to take responsibility, tact and sympathy ... likely to be met with among women of good general education and fair social position' (National Association for Supplying Medical Aid by Women to the Women of India, 1928, eighth annual report of the League, p. 106), were seen as attributes of this work. The Punjab Health School is listed as one of the success stories of the time, with Delhi, Bengal, Nagpur, Poona, and Lucknow also having health schools of their own – all linked to the sanitary idea of before. A combination of philanthropy, reform, and commercial interests seems to have been used to get to the wealthy women of the *zenana*. While the reform agendas are most visible in the histories of nationalism and of empire, the agential *zenana* mother is a newer participant in the modernity of this time. This follows similar practices in the UK and the US, with the first baby shows being listed in 1850s America (Pearson, 2008), with the baby being the mother's product, and the mother being evaluated as producer; babies were also, in the 1860s, exhibits in

Barnum's National Baby Shows in New York and elsewhere. In colonial India, the mother was also being evaluated for her national, racial, and social responsibility. 'Any mother attending three of these four lectures [on maternal and infant health] is entitled to enter her child for the Baby Show open to all babies under 2 years ... [with] numerous prizes ... not only for the healthiest, cleanest baby but to the mothers who have well and carefully tended a sickly child' (McMichael, 1918, p. 105). Some of the papers by medical women (Drs. McMichael, Lewis, Leach, Stuart, Women's Mission Hospital, U.F. Ch. Of Scotland Mission, Ajmer, Rajasthan) note that this effort seems to have led to 'whitewashing and thorough cleaning of the lying-in-room before confinement' (ibid). Proposals were also made for Mothers' Clubs, a Mother's Secretary in every city who 'is bright ... and capable ... but not necessarily a Physician' (Dr E.G. Lewis, American Presbyterian Mission, Ferozepur, p. 109) who could initiate public activities like a Mothers' Day that might also raise funds from among the 'intelligent and wealthy Hindu and Mohommedan women who could be taught to think about the "other fellow" and the "other fellow's baby"' (ibid). These public activities, then, were meant to initiate philanthropic interest in 'others' babies'; supporting the production of the 'beautiful baby' image is also expected to have retrospective effects for the management of childbirth itself.

The turn toward the public, who should, it is proposed, 'be educated by lectures to employ active and clean dais, so that the dirty and unfit would be gradually eliminated' (Wylie, 1918, p. 89), is the final nail in the livelihood of these women, while it presents in the shape of reform and modernity. Although antenatal advice is also brought into sanitary reform, it is agreed upon that 'prejudicial influences on infant life are more serious after than before birth' (ibid), and therefore, alongside milk depots, crèches, and hospitals by the municipality, and public lectures and pamphlets, the mother, who 'can be reached only by the dai' (ibid), must therefore have access to an educated *dai*, 'as far as she can be educated, until such time as her place can be taken by more intelligent workers' (ibid). Of course, in making the case for funds required for antenatal and post-natal reforms, scholarships for younger *dais*, etc., the papers talk of these as 'matters not only for medical officers ... but for Government itself' (ibid, p. 90), and therefore, the Empire's responsibility is appealed to 'to put a stop to ... one of the most serious drains upon the vitality of the Empire' (ibid).

Reports from Calcutta, however, indicate that the attempt to manage infant mortality by having newborns brought to the babies' clinic adjunct to the Dufferin hospital for regular examination failed; the only alternative being to employ the Lady Health Visitors to visit all babies delivered by the trained midwives until a period of 3 months. This welfare approach is reported to have been effective for the poorer women. Much thought goes into layers of institutionalization, not only in the shape of positions and posts – of Lady Health Visitor, Visiting Nurse, etc., and regulatory bodies – like a Midwives' Board, as mentioned earlier, but also in the form of smaller maternity hospitals for women who may fear and avoid the big hospital, crèches that double up as infant care centres, vaccination centres, and the generation of simple textbooks like 'Life, Light and Cleanliness' used in the

Punjab Education Department for *dai* training. Some of these texts are also proposed for primary girls' schools, with the awareness that early motherhood follows child marriage in a large part of the population, while attempts to raise the age of marriage also continue.[6] Practices of institutionalization vary across provinces and compete for claims to effectiveness. Throughout all of this, tact in dealing with customs, and tolerance of the harmless ones, is advised. In some accounts by nurses and trained British midwives practising in India, this tact extends to the indigenous *dai* as well, to disarm her fear of loss of livelihood and to get her on the side of the institution.

Who pays

The majority of scholarship around maternal and infant healthcare work has indicated that the state was not interested, and wives of Viceroys followed mission work in taking up the cause of the women of India. It is possible, and has been suggested, that this rhetoric served the colonial administration in helping it seem aloof from all matters pertaining to culture. More recent work has, however, traced both the Bengal-centric nature of this scholarship and the actual presence of the state in supporting and controlling this work (Lang, 2005; Sehrawat, 2013). This presence may not have been limited to sanitary work (Ramanna, 2012) but to institutional healthcare as well. At first missions, then the Dufferin Fund, shifted to government support in the early 20th century. Association reports of the Punjab province, for example, show government contributions amounting to about one-fourth of the Fund receipts and a third of the expenditure by the early 1900s (National Association for Supplying Female Medical Aid to the Women of India, 1913, 28th annual report, p. 9). Grants from provincial governments are highest in the case of Madras, Punjab, and the United Provinces, while the outlay from the Fund is highest in Bombay and the United Provinces. The contributions by the government are also in the form of land for building hospitals or quarters for lady doctors, as documented in the annual reports of the Association for Bengal, Bombay, and the Central Provinces. Appeals to private charities to come forward for maternal health are to be seen. Infant care is also talked about, as mentioned in the section on sanitary reform – 'A fine milk supply at a reasonable cost is undoubtedly of such vital importance, that when, as in Calcutta, private enterprise fails utterly, it ought to be provided by the Municipality' (Sen, 1918, Chapter VI, p. 131).

It is interesting, in this context, to see the work of the Madras presidency and its suburbs, in setting up lying-in hospitals as well as midwifery training. Both exercises seem to have had a different career than those in Bengal or Bombay; the Madras lying-in hospital, set up in 1840 and taken over by the government in 1847, not only shows state control and responsibility much earlier than in other provinces, a midwifery training programme was set up as early as 1854. By the 1870s, midwives trained at Madras were apparently to be found throughout the country (Lang, 2005). These were, Lang notes, primarily Indian, and seemed to have created a critical mass of privileged-caste trained midwives; accompanied by the active promotion of institutional delivery and the strong network of civil dispensaries, maternal healthcare seemed both to be better and to have a stronger state presence.

All through the Fund reports, however, are accounts of shortages of funds that result in vacant posts, professional women of a lesser calibre than desired owing to poor pay and work conditions, and poor infrastructure. Following the Government of India Act 1919 that introduced dyarchy in the major provinces, with health becoming a transferred subject to provincial governments, further withdrawal of government grants resulted in squeezing of budgets, with provincial health work in particular becoming no one's responsibility. There is, in fact, active rebuke from the Government on the practice of supplying women doctors to local fund hospitals, following which the Association put up a statement to the Statutory Commission. As the 44th annual report says, the government responded to funding requests thus: "'the Government of India do not intend to concern themselves further with the question of pay or strength of the Women's Medical Service, and the Association will have to make their own arrangements'" (National Association for Supplying Medical Aid by Women to the Women of India, 1928, Annexure XIV, Statement for the Indian Statutory Commission, p. 85). Local governments, at this point, were appealed to, and some of them came through to support the local and provincial hospitals.

How does this impact *dai* training and stipends? All along, the discussions in the Fund on the need for stipends while indigenous *dais* are in training, or for trained *dais*, veer towards the bare minimum. As the conversations move towards nursing training, the dearth of applications for nursing as well as midwifery training is lamented, with a reference to poor pay as one of the possible reasons. Nowhere in the discussions around the failure of *dai* training, however, is this listed as one of the reasons for that failure.

Success

The annual reports of the Association mention, each year, an increase in the number of in and out-patients, the number of *dais* trained, and the retaining of women doctors trained into the profession via the Fund. Success is also reported, in the early 1900s, in conducting sanitary inspections of 'zenana portions' of homes, and training orphan girls into nursing. Despite the attempt to train a 'superior class' of midwives and supervise the indigenous *dai*, the Victoria Memorial Scholarship Fund also seems to have met with relative failure, as the writing by medical women on the ground indicates. The kits and stipends for attending lectures all seem to have been taken up in the service of an enhanced livelihood by the indigenous *dai*, without the training on asepsis being used. Therefore, the metaphor of untrainability is consolidated. By the 1920s, it is also clear that wealthy women should be persuaded to attend paying wards for delivery, and poorer women should be supported through private charities and municipal outlay. Indian women in the Women's Medical Service, in addition to the philanthropic view, also urge that '[i]f we want to see India great, we must take care of our mothers and babies' (Sen, 1918, p. 134).

From dais to nurses: the restructuring of institutional childbirth

Finding the right type of woman

Before the Lady Hardinge Medical College was approved in 1912, there was no medical college exclusively for women students in India, although the Cama Hospital for Women and Children began in 1886. With the mixed classes at men's colleges, 'women of the right type' were not expected to 'come forward in sufficient numbers', resulting in the necessity to 'recruit from England' (National Association for Supplying Female Medical Aid to the Women of India, 1913, 28th annual report, Annexure II, Scheme for a Medical College and Hospital for Women, and for a Training School for Nurses at Delhi, p. 23). This is the context in which the Association proposed a college and hospital 'in which women will be taught by women to attend on women' (ibid). This was a proposal that is suggested for both doctors and nurses. It is with respect to the impulses around building this nursing cadre, who could then be available 'for nursing in private families as well as in public institutions' (ibid), that we now turn.

The Cama hospital nurses had been lauded as 'a noble band of workers', for 'these sisters and nurses, ... turn every hospital, not only into a medical school, but into a school of constant and daily self-denial. Self-denial and self-sacrifice are at the root of this work' (Kittredge, 1889, p. 62), and this virtue, linked as it is to the Protestant ethos, plays a role in determining the kind of woman for the work. Meanwhile, finding the right type of woman for *dai* training had been a long and tortuous experience for the Association, as we have seen. The privileged-caste women who were approached and encouraged to join would often refuse or leave after being forced to share quarters across castes. The indigenous *dai*, who was the primary target of VM training, was anyway untrainable. The Association is willing, at this time, to support the upper-caste women's demand for segregation from lower or other-caste pupils, while bemoaning caste prejudice, thus going along with this attitude in the avowed interest in the health of *zenana* or *purdah* women. Local prejudice is thus accommodated within and built into governance. But this is not a matter of colonial state governance alone. The entitlements due to the female colonial subject – the *zenana* or *purdah* woman, i.e. privileged-caste, northern Indian – is the avowed framework within which any and all accommodations are made within healthcare. The Association's efforts to accommodate these attitudes, all under the pretext of not interfering in social dynamics, actually consolidate them and use them in order to pick the weakest link in the chain, namely the *dai*, and subject her to regulation. Worries around the right type of woman do not seem to have affected the Association's work in the Madras presidency, however, that reports a steady number of trained midwives since 1887. While caste prejudice is as much a part of the reality here as elsewhere, it is useful to ask whether the idea of the *zenana* or *purdah* woman, born in Bengal and other parts of the North, is even a reality here.

The modern therapeutic regime of which the Fund is an active part, therefore, replicates within healthcare the very social hierarchies it is happy to deplore as barriers to progress, and in contradiction to objectivity and neutrality as aspects of the scientific rigour that is a regular claim in these systems against the indigenous. It is within this framework that the right type of woman becomes a self-explanatory norm. I will explore the nationalist impulses on the woman's question in greater detail in the next chapter.

In the continuing search, and failure, to find the right kind of woman, a series of letters, fairly urgent in their tone (sent on 7th December, with responses being asked for by the 12th), are sent out in December 1912, to prominent Indian men, including heads of publishing groups like the *Amrita Bazaar Patrika* and prominent medical men like Dr Nil Ratan Sircar (his alma mater, Campbell Medical School, was renamed after him after his death), containing a set of five questions, asking if it would be a feasible idea to train upper-caste women as nurses, not midwives, *not dais* (the difference between the two being reiterated again and again), given upper-caste practices of not accepting food or water or liquid medicine from any except their own, and given the practice of *purdah*, as also, the absence of a nursing cadre in traditional or professional form in India at the time. As the letter says,

> It should be clearly understood at the outset, that by nurse the term dhai is not meant. Dhais, we are led to understand, are drawn from a somewhat low caste of women; and of these there is no scarcity. Unfortunately the name of nurse has been applied to dhais, so that now when one talks of a nurse, the Indian mind immediately forms the concept of dhai ... Up to the present so we learn, such stigma attaches to the name of nurse (mixed up as it has been with that of dhai), that women of high caste have refused to enter the nursing profession. This being the case, Indian ladies when seriously ill, must suffer ... Her Excellency is anxious that something should be done whereby the status and position of nurses might be so raised that the better class of Indian lady might be induced to enter the profession, and so aid in alleviating the suffering ... among purdah Indian women ... our aim is not to go outside the highest castes in our search for nurses, including none below Baidyas and Kaisths and other castes from whom Brahmins may take food and water.
>
> Honorary Secretary of the Countess of Dufferin Fund
> (Bengal Branch) (presumed) (1912)

The 'needless loss of life' among women resulting from the absence of such a cadre is mentioned as the reason for this urgent proposal. Responses are varied, from reiterating practices of caste and *purdah* among upper-caste women to claims of modernity that are helping diminish these, and the statement that there is already a traditional cadre which is familial, still in existence although troubled by modernity and the newly 'delicate' modern urban woman who will not exert herself in the care of her sisters in the family. The men talk about certain 'polluting' functions being performed by a woman from a lower caste, outside family. There is the response that disallowing the lower-caste *dai* into the home is largely owing to the rigid caste practices of the *women* of the house; there are responses that talk of nursing training being possible for upper-caste women only if it is done in *purdah*; the 'needless loss of life' argument is, expectedly, taken umbrage to in several responses. Some of the men observe that Indian medical women in rural and peri-urban areas seem to work with *dais* in attending births in homes.

In a year's time following this, the Association reports show extensive outlays for nursing blocks in the premier medical college of the Bengal province, quarters for women doctors being supported by local government, and similar infrastructural support in Madras, Punjab, and other provinces. The annual report of the same year indicates a rise in the number of 'purdah patients' in several hospitals in Bengal, as well as an increase in contributions from the government – all seen as markers of the Association's success. At the same time, training of 'a better class of women as nurses' (28th annual report, 1912, p. 7) is articulated clearly, as the mandate of the VM fund towards the 'treatment of purdah ladies' (ibid), and the separation of *dais* from nurses as stated above. This scheme of nursing training for 'a better class of women', begins in Victoria Hospital, Calcutta. Bombay too reports 26 probationers, including five Brahmins, enrolled for a nursing course at Cama Hospital in the same year. Parts of the north-western provinces also report work done on these lines.

The movement from *dai* training towards nursing has been in process for a while during the VM Fund work. Wherever the Fund reports success in training and retaining the women during the middle period of the Fund, the women have been put to work in the wards to attend all labour cases, given 'instructions in the details of nursing and preparation of food for invalids' (28th annual report, p. 77). In fact, in certain branch reports, women attending childbirth are referred to as 'dai and nurse', or 'nurse dai', as a designation (29th annual report, Appendix VII, Baluchistan branch, p. 74). In the 39th annual Fund report from the United Provinces, it is suggested that the 'idea is to replace these midwives with women Sub-Assistant Surgeons and to extend further the work of medical relief to women by women in rural areas and small towns', with the costs being borne by the UP government (ibid, p. 27). This period, between 1912 and 1914, then, seems to be one where, with the setting up of the Women's Medical Service, and the attention to nursing training, a *newer* therapeutic structure, resembling that of the metro-pole more closely, with women working for women, takes off. Even in the native states, where the state of medical support for women is generally deplored in all reports, women's hospitals or dispensaries are being built, funds are forthcoming from local beneficiaries or government, and gender segregation in wards is becom-ing more of the norm.

Who were the trainees?

One of the institutions where nursing training for Indian women was broached was the Seva Sadan Society in Poona. Established in 1908 by Ramabai Ranade, a social reformer, for privileged-caste widows, the introduction of women of the Sadan into nursing was not a planned move. Women in distress at the Sadan who completed their training at Sassoon Hospital in 1910 made such an impact, however, that both the government, Dufferin Fund, and philanthropic organizations including the Wadia Trust, the Indian Women's Aid Society, and the National Indian Association, came forward to provide scholarships and support the Sadan's proposal for a women's hostel to accommodate not only their probationer nurses but women who came for medical education to the King Edward Hospital. One of the primary factors that drove this choice was the fact that it was 'easy to obtain probationers of the desired class' from the Sadan (Civil Surgeon, Poona, April 8, 1915), since it was also 'necessary that the women to be trained should be of a good class, intelligent and sufficiently well trained' (Monie, August 9, 1916). To retain this reputation, it was suggested that the Seva Sadan nurses retain that identity. The reputation of the institution relied on its association with 'Mrs Ranade and other Indian ladies of position and influence' (ibid). All in all, the tone of the letters and recommendations would suggest that being able to access this number of women of the 'right type and class' – widowed women in indigent circumstances – was almost a blessing.

In January 1922, the Lady Reading Women of India Fund was set up, with, among others, a mandate to establish an Indian Nursing Association in order to raise the standard of training for Indian nurses. The Association set up an institution in connection with the Lady Hardinge Hospital in Delhi to provide Indian nurses for home nursing. The Lady Reading nurses, as they were called, played an important role during an epidemic of plague in Delhi. But the difficulty of finding Indian women for training continued in this effort as well. Two 'very suitable ladies' – Miss Lavinia Mewa and Miss Maula Bukhsh – were selected at this time to proceed to England for training at the Elizabeth Garrett Anderson Hospital, London (National Association for Supplying Medical Aid by Women to the Women of India, 1923, 39th annual report, p. 104).

By the time of the increase in nursing training, government funding had all but dried up, particularly for the provinces, after the dyarchy introduced via the Government of India Act and the Montagu-Chelmsford reforms. Whatever municipal funds were available for nursing training in cities went to support Indian probationers, listed as different from Anglo-Indian pupil nurses who were expected to pay their way (ibid, p. 25). Europeans or Anglo-Indians were preferred for supervisorship, and were expected to be mostly Christians. Nursing was still seen in a continuum with *dai* work, with the Indian nurse followed by the semi-trained and often unreliable nurse *dai*, and of course the indigenous *dai* 'who kills most patients and yet who will be used for some time to come' (Stuart, 1918, p. 116). Scholarships for 'the training of high caste Indian nurses' had been accorded to the Dufferin Hospital in Calcutta by the time of the 1923 report.

Who should be a nurse or trained midwife? We see that the allowance made for Indian women in the profession is mostly from British medical women; whereas the nursing trainers themselves recommend 'Anglo-Indian women of good education for work among the Indian people' (Miss Twiss, formerly Lady Superintendent of Nursing, Medical College Hospital, Calcutta, in Victoria Memorial Scholarships Fund, 1918, p. 151). The Anglo-Indian woman is the next best to the Englishwoman in this respect, and histories of this dynamic have been written about (Charlton-Stevens, 2016; Blunt, 2005). Again, tact is leaned upon as a device to reach the Indian woman and her people. And here too, the right kind of woman continued to get exhortations to enter the profession, whether by citing the example of Florence Nightingale, or by subtle references to nursing as not 'mere physical drudgery ...

[but something for which] intelligent women, women with a certain amount of education ..., women physically strong and active, mentally alert, quiet, dignified, and above all, kind and humble' (J., 1920, pp. 18–19) were required. The reference to the need for a life of the mind may be read here as a signifier of caste. We will take this up again in the discussion around trainability in the next chapter.

Conclusion

The hereditary, *bazaar* or indigenous *dai*, then, who emerges as a fixed identity category in the various exercises of institutionalization and professionalization in the late 19th and early 20th centuries, also emerges at a remove from the *zenana* woman who is the centre of the nation, and thus from nationalist concerns. As a spectacular 'evil witch', to quote Forbes again, this figure emerges from a terrain of practice to be actively labelled for removal from therapeutic work. This work of erasure is performed by the institution, to which the nationalist indigenous has effectively given her over. What we also see through the exercises described in this chapter is the consolidation of the privileged-caste woman as a familial reproductive being and centre of the nation, who largely slipped the net of institutionalized childbirth and healthcare designed precisely for her in the period under question, as several communications between the Dufferin Fund and prominent Indian nationalists suggest, while *zenana* hospitals set up with philanthropic intent were largely accessed by those at the periphery. As we begin to recognize this female colonial subject at the centre of the nation, it might be useful to understand what seems to be the contradiction between the avowed later colonial policy of non-interference in the social and religious life of the natives, and the continuing insistence on the 'right type of woman' for therapeutic work. It would seem that the 'interference' shifts from this woman to those marginal to her. For the *bazaar dai*, then, one sees a combination of nationalist indifference and colonial interference.

This legacy of state under-representation in medical services recurs in contemporary India, albeit under different premises. The fraught place of the *dai* figure vis-a-vis the idea of the indigenous in this period shifts, as the last chapter hopes to trace, in contemporary India, with this reappearance. What happens to the space offered by the failed attempts at creating a cadre of trained *dais*? The somewhat frantic communications between the Dufferin Fund and prominent Indian men at the end of 1912 talk about the possibility of raising a cadre of nurses instead, with this training being proposed for privileged-caste women, the moral vocabulary of class standing in for caste here. Papers by medical women in India are already talking, by this time, of institutional hierarchies in the interest of childbirth care in hospitals, with Indian women physicians being brought in. Scholarship on these Indian women with access to western medical education is available today, as also emerging, particularly with regard to kinds of education being offered to Indian women of the time (Forbes, 1994). I end this chapter with a short exploration of the emergence of a nursing cadre at this time, with the last chapter attempting to trace connections with a much wider group of categories of women health workers at the primary healthcare level today.

Notes

1 I use abjection following Butler's work, that I find best described in their discussion on abjection of bodies in refugee situations – 'They can get counted, there's outrage generally, but there's no specificity … [a] differential production of the human' (Meijer & Prins, 1998, p. 281). Although this is about bodies in the present, it is also about lives, and I find this extension useful, particularly in the stereotyping and working of power that I refer to vis-à-vis this figure in this book.

2 This innovation may also be read in the light of the ongoing discourse, post-1857, around the non-martial character of the Bengali race, and the kinds of attention to women's bodies that followed. I have indicated, earlier, comments on access to light and air for women in order to contribute to strength and vitality for sons.

3 Labour anaesthesia – twilight sleep – does get talked about as a way to popularize institutional delivery, offering painless childbirth, and even a darkened room that simulates the aturghar and offers the Hindu woman the modesty she apparently seeks during childbirth (Campbell, Rainy Hospital, Tondiarpet, Madras, p. 120).

4 There are some references, through these papers, to the poorer women providing research and teaching material; although outside the scope of my discussions, this is a familiar aspect of the public healthcare apparatus and assemblage, as we see even today.

5 The papers themselves suggest that the *dai* was called in only for cord-cutting in cases of normal labour (p. 85).

6 The position on child marriage among the Indian women doctors is an ambivalent one; we have Dr Bidhu Mukhi Bose of Calcutta saying that early marriage is not harmful to the infant as the establishment claims 'because in Bengal where the practice is prevalent children are born healthy' (Victoria Memorial Scholarships Fund, 1918, p. 151, chapter VIII – extracts from papers written by qualified doctors and nurses). There is, here, a routing of the argument through scientificity rather than a civilizational trope – a strategy common to a lot of Indian medical professionals at the time.

References

Books and articles

Alavi, S. (2008). *Islam and healing: Loss and recovery of an Indo-Muslim medical tradition, 1600–1900*. London: Palgrave Macmillan.

Arnold, D. (1993). *Colonizing the body: State medicine and epidemic disease in nineteenth-century India*. Berkeley and Los Angeles: University of California Press.

Arnold, D. (2004). *Science, technology and medicine in colonial India* (The New Cambridge History of India, Vol. 5). Cambridge: Cambridge University Press.

Arnold, D. (2006). *The tropics and the traveling gaze: India, landscape, and science, 1800–1856*. Seattle and London: University of Washington Press.

Balachandran, A. (2008). Of corporations and caste heads: Urban rule in company Madras, 1640–1720. *Journal of Colonialism and Colonial History*, 9(2), https://doi.org/10.1353/cch.0.0014.

Berger, R. (2013). *Ayurveda made modern: Political histories of indigenous medicine in Northern India, 1900–1955*. New York: Palgrave Macmillan.

Blunt, A. (2005). *Domicile and diaspora: Anglo-Indian women and the spatial politics of home*. New Jersey: Wiley.

Brouwer, R. C. (2019). Opening doors through social service: Aspects of women's work in the Canadian presbyterian mission in Central India, 1877–1914. In L. A. Flemming (Ed.), *Women's work for women: Missionaries and social change in Asia* (pp. 11–34). New York: Routledge.

Burton, A. (1996, July). Contesting the zenana: The mission to make "Lady Doctors for India," 1874–1885. *Journal of British Studies, 35*(3), 368–397.

Charlton-Stevens, U. (2016). The professional lives of anglo-Indian working women in the twilight of empire. *International Journal of Anglo-Indian Studies, 16*(2), 3–29.

Chatterjee, P. (1989). The nationalist resolution of the women's question. In K. Sangari & S. Vaid (Eds.), *Recasting women: Essays in Indian colonial history* (pp. 233–253). New Delhi: Kali for Women.

Chatterjee, P. (2019). Women and nation revisited. In P. Ray (Ed.), *Women speak nation* (pp. 19–28). India: Routledge.

Chawla, J. (1994). *Child-bearing and culture: Women centered revisioning of the traditional midwife: The dai as a ritual practitioner*. New Delhi: Indian Social Institute.

Dalmiya, V., & Alcoff, L. (1993). Are old wives' tales justified? In L. Alcoff & E. Potter (Eds.), *Feminist epistemologies* (pp. 217–244). New York and London: Routledge.

Datta, P. (2009). Ranald Martin's *medical topography* (1837): The emergence of public health in Calcutta. In B. Pati & M. Harrison (Eds.), *The social history of health and medicine in colonial India* (pp. 15–30). London and New York: Routledge.

Douglas, M. (1984). *Purity and danger: An analysis of the concepts of pollution and taboo.* Routledge: London and New York.

Findlay, D. (1993, Spring). The good, the normal and the healthy: The social construction of medical knowledge about women. *Canadian Journal of Sociology/Cahiers canadiens de sociologie, 18*(2), 115–135.

Fitzgerald, R. (2005). Rescue and redemption—the rise of female medical missions in colonial India during the late nineteenth and early twentieth centuries. In A. M. Rafferty, J. Robinson, & R. Elkan (Eds.), *Nursing history and the politics of welfare* (pp. 63–78). London and New York: Routledge.

Forbes, G. H. (1999). *Women in modern India* (Vol. 2). Cambridge: Cambridge University press.

Forbes, G. H. (1994). Medical careers and health care for Indian women: Patterns of control. *Women's History Review, 3*(4), 515–530.

Forbes, G. H. (2005). *Women in Colonial India: Essays on politics, medicine, and historiography*. New Delhi: DC Publishers.

Guha, A. (2017). *Colonial modernities: Midwifery in Bengal, c. 1860–1947*. London and New York: Routledge .

Harrison, M. (2009). Racial Pathologies: Morbid anatomy in British India, 1770–1850. In B. Pati & M. Harrison (Eds.), *The social history of health and medicine in Colonial India* (pp. 173–194). London and New York: Routledge.

Jeffery, P., Jeffery, R., & Lyon, A. (2002). Contaminating states: Midwifery, childbearing and the state in rural North India. In S. Rozario & G. Samuel, *The daughters of Hāritī: Childbirth and female healers in South and Southeast Asia* (pp. 90–108). London and New York: Routledge.

Lang, S. (2005, December). Drop the Demon Dai: Maternal mortality and the state in Colonial Madras, 1840–1875. *Social History of Medicine, 18*(3), 357–378.

Lewandowski, S. J. (1975). Urban growth and municipal development in the colonial city of Madras, 1860–1900. *The Journal of Asian Studies, 34*(2), 341–360.

Lukis, C. P. (1913, October 4). Inaugural address on the medical needs of India. Delivered at the London school of medicine for women on October 1, 1913. *The British Medical Journal, 2*(2753), 837–839.

Martin, E. (2001). *The woman in the body: A cultural analysis of reproduction*. Boston: Beacon Press.

Mayo, K. (1927). *Mother India*. London: Jonathan Cape.

Meijer, I. C., & Prins, B. (1998). How bodies come to matter: An interview with Judith Butler. *Signs: Journal of Women in Culture and Society, 23*(2), 275–286.

Neild, S. M. (1979). Colonial urbanism: The development of Madras city in the eighteenth and nineteenth centuries. *Modern Asian Studies, 13*(2), 217–246.

Pearson, S. J. (2008, Winter). "Infantile specimens": Showing babies in nineteenth-century America. *Journal of Social History, 42*(2), 341–370.

Pinto, S. (2008). *Where there is no midwife: Birth and loss in rural India.* New York and Oxford: Berghahn Books.

Prakash, G. (1992). Science gone native in colonial India. *Representations, Autumn, No. 40,* Special Issue: *Seeing Science,* 153–178. https://doi.org/10.2307/2928743.

Prakash, G. (1999). *Another reason: Science and the imagination of modern India.* Princeton and New Jersey: Princeton University Press.

Ramanna, M. (2002). *Western medicine and public health in Colonial Bombay, 1845–1895.* London: Sangam Books Ltd, by arrangement with Orient Longman, Hyderabad.

Ramanna, M. (2008, March 22–April 4). Women physicians as vital intermediaries in colonial Bombay. *Economic and Political Weekly, 43*(12/13), 71–78.

Ramanna, M. (2012). *Health care in Bombay presidency, 1896–1930.* New Delhi: Primus Books.

Sadgopal, M. (2009, April 18–24). Can maternity services open up to the indigenous traditions of midwifery? *Economic and Political Weekly, 44*(16), 52–59.

Sehrawat, S. (2013a). *Colonial medical care in North India: Gender, State, and society, C. 1830–1920.* New Delhi: Oxford University Press.

Sehrawat, S. (2013b). Feminising empire: The association of medical women in India and the campaign to found a women's medical service. *Social Scientist, 41*(5/6), 65–81.

Semple, R. A. (2003). *Missionary women: Gender, professionalism and the Victorian idea of Christian mission.* Suffolk: The Boydell Press.

Semple, R. A. (2008). Ruth, Miss Mackintosh, and Ada and Rose Marris: Biblewomen, zenana workers and missionaries in nineteenth-century British missions to North India, *Women's History Review, 17*(4), 561–574.

Sen, I. (2012, March 24). Resisting patriarchy: Complexities and conflicts in the memoir of Haimabati Sen. *Economic and Political Weekly, XLVII*(12), 55–62.

Snowden, F. M. (2019). *Epidemics and society: From the Black death to the present.* New Haven and London: Yale University Press.

Stone, P. K. (2009). A history of western medicine, labor, and birth. In H. Selin & P. K. Stone (Eds.), *Childbirth across cultures. Science across cultures: Ideas and practices of pregnancy, childbirth and the postpartum* (pp. 41–54). Dordrecht: Springer.

Thakur, H. P., Pandit, D. D., & Subramanian, P. (2001). History of preventive and social medicine in India. *Journal of Postgraduate Medicine, 47*(4), 283–285.

Van Hollen, C. (2003). *Birth on the threshold: Childbirth and modernity in South India.* Berkeley, Los Angeles and London: University of California Press.

Visvanathan, S. (2009). The search for cognitive justice. *Knowledge in Question, 597.* Retrieved from https://www.india-seminar.com/2009/597/597_shiv_visvanathan.htm

Archival sources

From Wellcome Trust Library, London

Balfour, M., & Scott, A. (1935). *The countess of dufferin's fund: Fifty years' retrospect, Indian 1885–1935.* (PP/MIB/C/4. Part of: Margaret Ida Balfour, CBE, MD, CM, FRCOG (1866–1945)). Archives and Manuscripts. London, New York, Toronto, Melbourne, Bombay, Calcutta, Madras: Oxford University Press.

Balfour, M., & Young, R. (1929). *The work of medical women in India, with a foreword by Dame Mary Scharlieb.* (PP/MIB/C/3. Part of: Margaret Ida Balfour, CBE, MD, CM, FRCOG (1866–1945)). Archives and Manuscripts. London, New York, Toronto, Melbourne, Bombay, Calcutta, Madras: Oxford University Press.

Campbell, G. J. (1918). In Victoria Memorial Scholarships Fund. (1918). *Improvement of the conditions of childbirth in India: Including a special report on the work of the Victoria*

Memorial Scholarships Fund during the past fifteen years and papers written by medical women and qualified midwives. (Closed stores K45291). Calcutta: Superintendent Government Printing.

Wylie, M. A. (1918). In Victoria Memorial Scholarships Fund. (1918). *Improvement of the conditions of childbirth in India: including a special report on the work of the Victoria Memorial Scholarships Fund during the past fifteen years and papers written by medical women and qualified midwives.* (Closed stores K45291). Calcutta: Superintendent Government Printing.

McMichael, A. M. (1918). In Victoria Memorial Scholarships Fund. (1918). *Improvement of the conditions of childbirth in India: Including a special report on the work of the Victoria Memorial Scholarships Fund during the past fifteen years and papers written by medical women and qualified midwives.* (Closed stores K45291). Calcutta: Superintendent Government Printing.

Scott (1918). In Victoria Memorial Scholarships Fund. (1918). *Improvement of the conditions of childbirth in India: including a special report on the work of the Victoria Memorial Scholarships Fund during the past fifteen years and papers written by medical women and qualified midwives.* (Closed stores K45291). Calcutta: Superintendent Government Printing.

Sen, Y. (1918). In Victoria Memorial Scholarships Fund. (1918). *Improvement of the conditions of childbirth in India: Including a special report on the work of the Victoria Memorial Scholarships Fund during the past fifteen years and papers written by medical women and qualified midwives.* (Closed stores K45291). Calcutta: Superintendent Government Printing.

Stuart, E. G. (1918). In Victoria Memorial Scholarships Fund. (1918). *Improvement of the conditions of childbirth in India: including a special report on the work of the Victoria Memorial Scholarships Fund during the past fifteen years and papers written by medical women and qualified midwives.* (Closed stores K45291). Calcutta: Superintendent Government Printing.

Vaughan (1918). In Victoria Memorial Scholarships Fund. (1918). *Improvement of the conditions of childbirth in India: including a special report on the work of the Victoria Memorial Scholarships Fund during the past fifteen years and papers written by medical women and qualified midwives.* (Closed stores K45291). Calcutta: Superintendent Government Printing.

Hoggan, F. E. (1882). *Medical women for India.* (b22304642 Persistent URL: https:// wellcomelibrary.org/item/b22304642 Catalogue record: https://search.wellcomelibrary .org/iii/encore/record/C__Rb2230464). Bristol: J.W. Arrowsmith.

Kittredge, G. A. (1889). *A short history of the "Medical women for India" fund of Bombay.* (Reference number: b21017645 Persistent URL: https://wellcomelibrary.org/item/ b21017645 Catalogue record: https://search.wellcomelibrary.org/iii/encore/record /C__Rb2101764). From the John Hay Whitney Medical Library. Bombay: Education Society's Press.

McNally, C., & CORNWALL, John Wolfran. (1903). *The elements of sanitary science: A hand-book for district, municipal, local medical and sanitary officers, members of local boards and municipal councils, and others in India.* Third edition, revised and partly rewritten by ... J. W. Cornwall. (b28990833 Persistent URL: https://wellcomelibrary.org /item/b28990833. Catalogue record: https://search.wellcomelibrary.org/iii/encore/record /C__Rb2899083). Madras: The Superintendent, Government Press.

National Association for Supplying Medical Aid by Women to the Women of India. (1928). [44th] *Annual Report of The National Association for Supplying Medical Aid by Women to the Women of India, (Countess of Dufferin's Fund including the Women's Medical Service) The Victoria Memorial Scholarships Fund [27th annual report], The Lady Chelmsford All-India League for Maternity and Child Welfare [8th annual report].* Calcutta: Govt. of India Central Publication Branch (b31416639. Persistent URL: https://wellcomelibrary.org /item/b31416639 Catalogue record: https://search.wellcomelibrary.org/iii/encore/record/C_ _Rb3141663).

National Association for Supplying Medical Aid by Women to the Women of India. (1923). [39th] *Annual Report of The National Association for Supplying Medical Aid by Women to the Women of India, (Countess of Dufferin's Fund). Women's Medical Service India [10th annual report], The Victoria Memorial Scholarships Fund, Lady Reading Women of India Fund, The Lady Chelmsford All-India League for Maternity and Child Welfare.* Calcutta: Govt. of India Central Publication Branch. (Reference number: b31416585. Persistent URL: https://wellcomelibrary.org/item/b31416585 Catalogue record: https://search.wellcomelibrary.org/iii/encore/record/C__Rb3141658)

From British Library, London

Bhishagratna, K. (1963). *An English translation of the Sushruta samhita: Based on original Sanskrit text, with a full and comprehensive introduction, additional texts, different readings, notes, comparative views, index, glossary and plates / translated and edited by Kaviraj Kunjalal Bhishagratna* (2nd ed., Chowkhamba Sanskrit studies; 30). (Asia, Pacific & Africa 14043.c.53 UIN: BLL01020115875).

Rây, P., Caraka, & Gupta, Hirendra Nath, joint author. (1965). *Caraka saṃhitā, a scientific synopsis, by Priyadaranjan Rây and Hirendra Nath Gupta.* (History of sciences in India publications). New Delhi: National Institute of Sciences of India. (Asia, Pacific & Africa V 16217, UIN: BLL01016297189).

The Christian Vernacular Education Society. (1888). *The Women of India, and what can be done for them.* In Papers on Indian Reform (8415.e.52).

Madras. Murdoch, J. (1888). *Sanitary reform in India.* (Papers on Indian reform). (Asia, Pacific & Africa T 12625, UIN: BLL01013254527). Madras: Christian Vernacular Education Society.

Honorary Secretary of the Countess of Dufferin Fund (Bengal Branch) (presumed). (1912). *Questionnaire circulated by the honorary secretary of the countess of dufferin fund (Bengal Branch) concerning the possibility of training high-caste Hindu women as nurses, with copies of several replies thereto.* (Mss Eur F165/156) India Office Records and Private Papers.

J. (1920, August 1). Nursing – A service. In R. E. Reuben (Ed.), *Hind Mahila (The Indian Woman), 1* (pp. 16–19). (P.P.1122.m.). Bombay: The Udyan Press.

From Maharashra State Archives, Mumbai

National Association for supplying Female Medical Aid to the Women of India. (1914). *Twenty-ninth annual report for the year 1913.* (Rack no. 64, Compartment no. 54, Bundle no. 2). New Delhi: Superintendent, Government Printing.

National Association for supplying Female Medical Aid to the Women of India. (1913). *Twenty-eighth annual report for the year 1912.* (Rack no. 64, Compartment no. 54, Bundle no. 2). New Delhi: Superintendent, Government Printing.

Civil Surgeon, P. (1915, April 8). *To the personal assistant to the surgeon general with the Govt of Bombay, Poona. no. 965 of 1915.* General Department.

Monie, P. W. (1916, August 9). *Government of Bombay, general department, Order no 5420. Training of Indian women as nurses at the Sassoon Hospitals, Poona.* Bombay Castle. (3515, 53).

5 The nation and its women

Re-examining an old preoccupation

Introduction

Debates around the 'woman's question' have inhabited the nationalist discourse, particularly in the context of education, during the late 19th to early 20th centuries and been extensively written about in contemporary scholarship (Chakravarti, 1993; Chatterjee, 1989; Sinha, 2000; Lal, 2008; Mani, 1987). Writings from the period itself have ranged from *A Memorandum on Hindu Female Education* in 1896, to *The Hind Mahila* in 1920, by way of example. This chapter attempts to trace a biopolitics of pregnancy and maternity related to this question. Commentators on education for women and its relationship to the 'national' question provide a myriad of perspectives on this. The missionary, the administrator, the reformer, and the feminist, even, have spoken, in the period I explore, of these questions, and it is some of this material that I attempt to bring together to the already existing scholarship, as well as to my particular questions.

I explore writing in women's periodicals/magazines primarily focused on health, like *Balabodhini* or *Arogya Jiwan*, coming out of central India from the late 1890s onwards, where the focus is primarily on injunctions and prescriptions for behaviour, and codes of conduct, with accompanying notes on *garbharaksha* (care during pregnancy), *nidaan* (diagnosis), care of the infant, etc. These are almost buried amidst much more strident notes on *pativrata* (a woman faithful to her husband), *lajwanti* (a chaste woman); in other words, injunctions on wifely and womanly conduct. The writing itself is slightly before the time of emergence of the 'couple' and the *'ghar'* – the more sharply bounded domestic sphere – and *zenana* education, within which the woman is the arbiter of the infant's future and destiny. Already, however, the move from the earlier, more porous *andarmahal* (the inner portion of a house – this has a much more spatial connotation, reference to living arrangements and domestic transactions with the outside, and relation to other parts of the home, than *ghar* which indicates both home and family) has begun.

I also explore writing by Indian women prominent in public, political life, or in social work, and by wives of the early philanthropists, who speak for poorer and 'harijan'[1] women from the 1880s onwards. Organizations like the Bhagini Samaj, set up on Gandhian principles for the uplift of 'harijan' women, headed by women also prominent in the All India Women's Congress and the Congress Party, are to be found from this time. This writing marks the shifts in women's status from

DOI: 10.4324/9780367824051-5

earlier times to the late nationalist period, speaks the reform language of education, abolition of child marriage, widow remarriage, and abolition of *sati*, and then
exhorts the British to take over childbirth management.

I suggest, following these, an aspect of the emerging therapeutic, that is the
mobilizing of the upper-caste middle-class female self into reproductive responsibility. While feminist literature on the woman's question has acknowledged the
place of the privileged-caste woman in nationalist concerns, a look at the material
here helps place her with respect to the emerging therapeutic in this period. This is
the primary thrust of this chapter.

This involvement of the self in the nation is not, however, a charge enjoined
upon marginalized women, who are encouraged, rather, into giving themselves
up to programmes of upliftment. This includes the *dai* figure, who, despite the
experience granted to her, does not seem to find a voice in the professionalization
of the therapeutic, nor in the anti-caste movements or assertions directed at the
colonial administration from marginalized castes during this period. We have seen,
in Chapter 3, some of this assertion in the 'Memorial on behalf of all Marathi-
speaking untouchables of Bombay Presidency', in 1927–8, which lists, under the
status of medical and sanitary services, that 'unqualified practice ... by Vaids,
Hakims ... should be mercilessly suppressed'. There is no reference to the *dai* even
in this denouncement of the local practitioner, and neither is there any submission
by the *dai*.

The *zenana* and the privileged-caste householder woman

The zenana as category

Feminist historians have traced the emergence of the category of the *zenana* in non-
professional Englishwomen's writings in the 19th and early 20th centuries, as 'the
principal space ... from which Englishwomen could produce new "knowledge"
of the colonized', a space that stood in for 'Indian womanhood' (Nair, 1990, p.
11). This scholarship aligns with the sharp critiques of the homogeneous category
'woman' or 'Third World Woman' that populated Western liberal feminist positions of the 1980s in particular (Mohanty et al, 1991; Nair, 1990; Sunder Rajan,
2000). While Nair focuses primarily on non-professional English women, we have
seen this impulse of 'reading the *zenana*' clearly represented also in missionary
accounts and in papers by medical women in the previous chapter. Here, I put to
work the following critical arguments that flow from Nair's work. One, the *zenana*
is imagined in the image of the 'essentially feminine' English domestic sphere of
the 18th and 19th centuries, and then applied as a universal term to represent Indian
womanhood, despite it being, empirically, found as a form of segregation practised
only in the 'upper and middle classes of north, northwestern, and eastern India'
(Nair, 1990, p. 11). Two, this idea of the *zenana* is mobilized differently across
different phases from the early 1800s to the 1940s – from a dark space needing
upliftment and reform, to a powerful space that actually rules society, to a resistant space that resists colonization, and consequently, its civilizing influences. Nair
marks, for instance, the shift from the reformist impulses of the pre-1857 period to

a more 'peace and order' (p. 12) approach in the late 19th century and thereafter. Three, the immediate historical contexts of the colonizer nation invariably drive the manner in which this trope is deployed – something we also see reflected in otherwise seemingly contradictory comments on the *zenana* woman as ignorant, resistant, or powerful, in Englishwomen physicians' writings and practice in the previous chapter. Despite these different articulations of the *zenana* in the colonial discourse, we see a deployment of the *zenana* trope as universal in the later colonial period, a finding I see reflected in the papers by English medical women. This is used, I suggest, in the regulatory impulses we see in the therapeutic regime of this period, and it is with respect to this shift, too, that the use of the *zenana* as a category in this regime must be understood.

A significant intervention Nair makes is in her marking of the English view of the properly feminine as the analog of the *zenana*, and the accompanying evaluations of it as failing to match up in Englishwomen's writings in the mid-19th century and later. This failure is further enmeshed, in the writings she explores, with the purported failed masculinity of Indian men, for they either take on feminine roles, or fail to be protectors of their race and nation, or both. Also, nothing in their own societal models prepared these writer-evaluators for the matrilineal living arrangements and relationships visible among some castes and parts in southern India, resulting in diagnoses of 'loose morality', presumably tied of course to poor social hygiene and racial strength. Although Nair suggests that this reading is somewhat complicated by the events of 1857, the 'public assertion of English femininity ... [is thereafter used to reinforce the idea of] the "dubious masculinity" of Indian men' (p. 10). It is in this image of the binary gender-segregated model of English society, then, that the *zenana* is constructed, and seen as both impenetrable and necessary.

The obvious companion categories to the *zenana* would be the household and the family. Following the recognition offered by Nair and others that the *zenana* category made sense only in certain northern Indian contexts, we might look at G. Arunima's work on shifts in matrilineal kinship in Malabar (the southeastern coast) from the pre-colonial period to the colonial 19th century, and its final abolition in the 20th century. Arunima traces this in the changing relations of power between 'men and women; older and younger kin; and landowners and their agricultural dependents' (1996, p. 284) through these periods. She marks the shift from a far more fluid set of arrangements, including the separation of property ownership and heading of households by women, and political power often held by men, with householding and kinship not necessarily defined by co-residence. Later, she suggests, with the entry of Anglo-Indian law, co-residence, control over women and younger kin by older men, women being allowed to move away only through marriage, as well as an attempt at community reform through patrilocality, patriliny, endogamy, and nuclear family units, took place. For our purposes, this shows a radical shift to a more uniform kind of Hindu family. Even attention to the histories of this career of the *tharavad* (kin arrangement) tells us that, for one, the *zenana* was hardly a found object that chroniclers, including medical women, would have us believe. Also, forms of gender segregation were more the result of rather than the rationale for intervention. And these were not by any means common across the sub-continent; rather, the colonial impulse was towards standardization. Arunima refers, for instance, to the *tharavad* that was being critiqued by modernizers for its exploitative structure in the late 19th century, being actually 'a product of [modern] "court-made-law"' (p. 300). She also points to the 'Brahmanisation and Anglicisation' performed through Anglo-Indian law 'allowing the customs of Nayars to be compared to [patrilineal] Nambuthiri Brahmins and those of Malabar to Bengal' (p. 285). In other words, Arunima's work shows us a setting up of vastly different kinship arrangements, including the matrilineal and patrilineal, after they have undergone a process of modernization, for comparative evaluation and legal regulation in the late 19th and early 20th centuries. It follows, then, that the ideas of regulation as well as reform of family, parenting, and inheritance, shared by the colonial regime and elite nationalist reformers, flowed from this standardization.

The idea of the 'inner domain' or *ghar* has had, of course, a life of its own in elite male nationalist assertions. Uma Chakravarti (1989) and Partha Chatterjee (1989), among others, have talked about the woman's question in nationalist discourse. Chatterjee, using the case of Bengal, speaks of the 'nationalist resolution of the women's question', with 'nationalism ... assert[ing] a reformed tradition, selectively reinterpreted to conform to the conditions of the modern world ... [with] the key techniques of reform compris[ing] a set of disciplinary rules governing the spaces where women may move, the activities in which they could engage, the image they could project of themselves, and the pedagogical process to which they were to be subjected' (Chatterjee, 2019, p. 22). The spiritual domain, located within the domestic sphere, was here being asserted as the site of this reformed tradition, and resistant to colonial control or entry. Chakravarti, in a more nuanced move, explores the elite nationalist construction of 'woman', with the construction of a 'national identity for women' (Chakravarti, 1989, p. 52), in the early 20th century. The woman can no longer, she suggests as she explores the literary output of the period, be the passive *sahadharmini*, the suitably educated companion for the elite nationalist man as he challenges imperial power. Rather, she must take an active role, be the nationalist man's moral compass, and if necessary shed domesticity to be his public helpmate. It is in this publicness as sublimation that the woman is honoured; it is also in the service of this honour that her sexuality must be controlled. We find uncanny presaging evidence of this argument in Muthulakshmi Reddy's articulation of the role of the 'right kind' of women in the political domain.

And yet, the early 20th century also saw vocal and widespread challenges to this notion of both the fragile woman of home and the forms of control proposed over her. Anandhi S. writes of the Self-Respect Movement and its sharp critique, in the writings and speeches of E.V.R. Periyar and others, of marriage and family as the source of women's oppression and enslavement, particularly the stress on and valorization of chastity in women. Of the many responses to this historical oppression, the Self-Respect Movement facilitated, from 1928, self-respect marriages across caste barriers, for erstwhile *devadasis*, and between widows and activists; it also organized women's conferences that spoke against caste oppression, exploitation of *devadasis* in Brahminical ritual practice, and demanded compulsory education for women, in addition to demanding bans on *devadasi* initiation, child marriage, and other practices it identified as regressive (Anandhi, 1991).

We see, then, in this very small slice of a scholarship that has also moved from the 80s to now, both the varied contexts of nationalist invocations of women's place, as well as particularly the conflicting positions across caste-aware and caste-ignorant politics. I would add to this set of articulations of a layered and complex history the intuitive comments of Inukonda Thirumali, who, exploring the lives of Telugu women during the colonial period, locates this emergence within a process of Brahminization that accompanies a movement from the rural to the urban, resulting in a 'zenana woman' who is socially functional but not biologically autonomous, well in keeping with her imminent construction as frail; this extends, soon, into one who is politically subordinate, and now 'limited' to the home (2005). The movement from the porous *andarmahal* to the sharply demarcated *ghar* now nears completion, with a sharper distinctness and distance between genders but also from the polluting local outside. We might make the smaller claim, then, that for the Empire, the image of family, household unit, and place of women becomes more normatively fixed through these exercises; for this fixing, patrilineal and patrilocal arrangements, familiar from Victorian contexts, wherever they are to be found in the colony, become the unit of comparison. It is clear that they are to be found in the 'reformed tradition' Chatterjee speaks of, in the Brahmanized and Anglicized rendition of the *tharavad* Arunima points to, and in the biologically frail urban woman Thirumali suggests becomes the ideal site of intervention.

To return to Nair's analysis, which also offers powerful pegs to read the *zenana* as a space presented in medical writings. The medical missionary accounts I have already pointed to. As we move into the later, apparently secular articulations of the first Englishwomen doctors who are claiming the scientific in opposition to the evangelical, we see the evaluation of the feminine occupant of the *zenana* space against the standard of the responsible feminine figure of the colonizer's imagination. This responsible feminine figure is committed not only to the household but to its health, taking on the imperatives of sanitation and hygiene in every aspect of it – cooking, mothering, training of daughters. To be properly feminine means all of this in the England of the 1840s onward – in the context of the sanitary movement, and later germ theory. Englishwomen physicians who took this feminine responsibility seriously, naturally, then found not only the *dai*, but the woman of the *zenana*, wanting. They urged the Empire to take charge of this state of affairs; they insisted that supervision by them was the only route to 'the right type of woman'; they presented this insistence on the 'right type of woman' as a feature of resistance to the modern in caste-ridden Indian society; and yet, this dream of rightness and properness was theirs. As a route to livelihood options, yes, but also to keeping the model of gender-segregated heterosexual society intact. They observed caste practice and declared it, unbelievably, to be a problem of the ignorant lower-caste *dai* women they found; they saw no contradiction in offering to protect the rights of *zenana* women against these others. This is where the heteronormative, racist, imperialist, and casteist impulses of a system of which these Englishwomen in medicine were a part are to be found, and where they intersect.

The active role played by *purdah*, or the *zenana* space, in medical language and discourse itself has been traced by Maneesha Lal (Lal, 2006). Examining the arguments for medical intervention by Englishwomen physicians before and during the Dufferin Fund in the late 19th century, as also by Indian medical women up until the 1930s, Lal talks about how, either following the principle of non-interference in cultural and social customs that was the stated cornerstone of Raj policy, or in a convenient acceptance of 'custom', the principle of *purdah* actually worked to organize institutional medicine, practice, medical education, and research along gender segregated lines. The 'women for women' principle in medical education is a natural corollary of the same. Lal also explores how certain conditions like osteomalacia, rickets, and tuberculosis are represented as being causally linked with *purdah* practice, ignoring the obviously multi-factorial nature of these illnesses. Some interesting results of Lal's analysis tie in with Nair's argument about the essentialization of the feminine and the consolidation of the binary. We will see, in the next section, Muthulakshmi Reddy's arguments about the role of women in the public political sphere. What the status-quoist response of Englishwomen physicians to what they claimed was an overarching practice of female seclusion did, perhaps, was also a structuring of the lives of women outside the *zenana*. For Indian women with access to education, professions, and public life, the complaint of neglect of women's health inside the *zenana* gets addressed by a further circumscription and stereotyping of their professional domains to attend to reproductive health, but also curated specific public political opportunities, around sanitary reform, for instance. Following this imperative as moral responsibility is what we see in Muthulakshmi Reddy's exhortations to educated women in the next section.

A further attitude within medical science is evident from Lal's detailing of the *purdah*-disease connection in the writings of Englishwomen as well as what she calls nationalist feminists of the 1920s and 1930s. A certain practice – the seclusion of women – was apparently seen in certain communities – predominantly Muslim – and apparently predisposed women to certain illnesses – namely osteomalacia and tuberculosis, among others (Lal, 2006, p. 104). The absence of sunlight and air in the *zenana* has been lamented since missionary accounts. What seems particular to the 1920s and 1930s, although multiple aetiologies emerge in medical research of the time, is the closer identification of *purdah* with Muslims, accompanied, as Lal notes, by references to a freer Hindu past for women, in nationalist accounts in women's magazines and women's organizational literature of the time (ibid). With the parallel identification of self-governance as conditional to the status of women, and the consolidation of the *purdah*-Muslim connection, the nationalist version of the indigenous as 'naturally' Hindu finds one more pillar. For the specific purposes of my argument, this set of writings not only contributes to the fashioning of dominant representations of Indian womanhood in this period, as has been well documented; it also serves as an extension of the institution, with Indian women in medicine, privileged-caste women in women's organizations or writing on motherhood, coupledom, education, and morality, the women's magazines and journals that emerge at this time, acting as newer stakeholders in this therapeutic regime. We will see, later in the chapter, the discourse around *gharoa chikitsa*, or home remedies, that constituted a more complex aspect of this institutionalization.

A third, related point about the construction of the *zenana* is significant here. Scholars, including Lal, have pointed to the changing nature of *zenana* practice in homes that were adopting privileged-caste norms as a marker of status. This is while privileged-caste women with access to modern education and reform were themselves coming out of seclusion practices they may have been part of. This movement, however, finds no reflection in the medical discourse of the time, both English and Indian. Indian women who emerged were applauded, but privileged-caste women who stayed in were the primary focus of attention, and marginalized-caste women were universally either the object of upliftment or rejection. As far as the marginalized-caste *dai* was concerned, she was the figure that seemingly brought disease into the *zenana*, in both early missionary and later medical accounts. A static figure, neither within the ambit of reform nor nationalism.

A last point on the *zenana*. The easy collapse of terms like *purdah, purdanashin*, and *zenana*, that may or may not have had semantic substitutability in the period being described, and their use as wholly representative of diverse ways of life even within communities, is, as Lal suggests, part of the structuring of medical education, practice, and research by medical women, and we will explore further its deployment in the discourse of Indian medical women.

A brief note on the 'women for women' doctor, again

As suggested in the previous chapter, critical historians of British imperialism have pointed to how the characterization of the *zenana* as an airless trap for the Indian woman becomes the driving force for the entry, institutionalization, and professionalization of therapeutic work for and by women of Empire (Burton, 1996). Burton argues that the *zenana* was a 'crucial ... material and symbolic site ... for those involved in establishing the provision of medical education for women in Victorian Britain' from the 1870s onwards (p. 372). Jex-Blake's suing of the University of Edinburgh in 1872 for its exclusion of women from medical degrees, and her mobilization of the 'neglected *zenana* woman' argument for her cause, are some of the more potent and visible events in this history (ibid, p. 373). In fact, while the announcement of Edith Pechey as the woman doctor for Cama Hospital and the Jaffer Sulliman Dispensary in reports of these institutions does not take into account a history of struggle by these women in their home environments, Elizabeth Hoggan (1882) and other British medical women of the time remark actively on this history. Nevertheless, the helpless *zenana* women become but also remain the rationale for Indian women to not make it to the top; even after ten years of Dufferin Fund work, the hierarchies of European women doctors and Indian hospital assistants remained.

The missionary and the Englishwomen physicians had, before the infamous diatribe by Katherine Mayo and others in the 1920s, already talked about the need to link self-governance to the condition and status of women. As Campbell states, with respect to the need to raise the age of marriage in order to improve conditions of childbirth, 'if some political genius of Indian birth would devise a scheme whereby in each section of the community the attainment of self-government could be made to depend on its ability to do this and other elementary acts of justice to its own weaker members, a useful stimulus to progress would be given' (1918, p. 124, papers by medical women). The women were seen as the path to progress – 'once the women desire better conditions they have power enough to move the men and we will see better homes, better drains, better water systems, better streets, better ways of living and above all better children' (ibid, p. 126). What were the 'women working for women' expected to be like, whether it be in training *dais* or whether in attending to the zenana?

> [W]herever the teaching of *dais* has been really successful, it has been in the hands of educated women with strong personality and winning character. Such were Miss Hewlett of Amritsar, and Dr. Henderson of Nagpur ... It is not an easy thing to instruct people whose minds have never been trained to think, and whose horizon is bounded by the need to earn daily bread and by the customs of the herd ... teaching of such a class of people is generally a failure when left in the hands of a Sub-assistant Surgeon ... [who is Indian, and different from] the hands of the missionary who is prepared to give sympathy and understanding.
>
> (Balfour & Young, 1929, pp. 137–138)

The Indian lady doctor and her response to the zenana woman

Women of India had begun to make it to medical colleges however, and it might be useful to explore the question of women in the nation through the lives and narratives of those who occupied the slippery zone between the institution and its site of intervention, being quintessential outsiders within both spaces. Not only in relation to their compatriot men but also with respect to the colonial medical service, Indian women who entered the medical professions in the later part of the 19th century had difficult experiences at best. Forbes suggests that medicine was one of the earliest professions entered into by Indian women (1994). Memoirs and autobiographical accounts marking some of these women as *singular* to and separate from their times are available, as well as accounts that speak of these women suffering the same evils of child marriage, reproductive morbidity, or widowhood that other women in that time did in India. This approach attempts to place them within the discourse of the nation's women, the locations these women came from, and their choices of practice. My concern here is their relationships with *zenana* women as a category, with particular attention to the exclusions and terms of inclusion that relationship signified in the late 19th to early 20th centuries.

I have, in the last chapter, attempted to indicate very briefly, with reference to scholarship in the field, the diversity of this constituency of the Indian woman doctor, the extent of their forays into the *zenana*, and their relationships to the state and its regulation of women's lives. Here, I would like to raise at the outset a point about the characterization of the *zenana* or the *pardanashin* women who are juxtaposed alongside these physicians. Forbes, in her introduction to the memoirs of Haimabati Sen, talks of her private practice with *pardanashin* women whom she would treat in her own home instead of the district hospital she worked at, if they needed hospitalization. Muthulakshmi Reddy's position on birth control information to be given by the state to married women is known (Reddy, 1930; Kamatchi, 2016). Both of these stances say something about the exclusivity granted to the constituency of privileged-caste women within marriages, but there ends the similarity. For Reddy, who also took an abolitionist stance on the *devadasi* tradition in 1930, it was the sexual morality and racial strength of a young nation that was at stake, as also the protection of the Brahmin woman; for the kind of private practice that Haimabati Sen and several other 'lady doctors' did, it was about the physical containment of the upper-caste woman within the household; whether or not they had a critical stance on this, this containment provided them with a niche clientele. What the colonial institution attempted, and succeeded partially in doing, was to breach the physical boundary or replicate it, by getting women to deliver in *zenana* hospitals or gender-segregated wards, for example. A fixed idea of the *zenana*, then, that often slips between the physical and the metaphorical, may not be adequate to capture this distinction. Further, the differences – in labour economies or gender relations – between the experiences and contexts of the Bombay and Madras presidencies offer a challenge to any attempt to deploy this term universally. And yet, it has been deployed. While this might seem like a minor quibble in the face of the argumentative potential the category offers for interpreting colonial policy, it is important to make this rupture in order to recognize a possible contradiction in the many messages that young women in marriages received as to their role in family and nation building – a contradiction that was a placeholder for the Indian lady doctor. Not to speak of the inaccurate readings that colonial administrators employed in order to predict what 'women of India' needed.

Of the celebrated names in the list of Indian women who entered medicine from the 1860s onwards, it is a few memoirs and autobiographies that tell us something of the contexts within which they took up the profession, as well as their relationships with the women they saw as their constituency. Between these writings and feminist commentaries on their lives, broadly we see that they emerged in the public sphere either as reformers or as nationalists, as mentioned in the previous chapter. This meant that they saw as their constituency women in more vulnerable situations than their own, but also that they asserted a hierarchy – rooted in modern education and professional training – over these women. These women may be separated from themselves by caste or class, but in some cases also by access to modernity and the public sphere. The relationship with these two 'types of women', to recall the over-used phrase of colonial documents, then, was different. The women underprivileged by caste or class could be reformed, made the object of charity, and so on. The privileged-caste women, however, could be sisters for whom these women could serve as role models or eventual equals. That was the kind of feminism that a Muthulakshmi Reddy, for instance, espoused when she said, in her 1930 tract titled 'My Experience as a Legislator', that 'the education which we give to our girls should be such as to render them efficient household-ers, intelligent mothers and good citizens' (1930, p. 177). As does Rukhmabai, the second Indian woman to receive a medical degree, who states, in her famous tract against the *purdah*

[s]urely the work lies in the hands of the younger women who have energy and enthusiasm to work decisively for the immediate abolition of this deplorable custom, which by causing unhealthy conditions for mothers drains the national vigour, and which degrades India in the eyes of the world.

(1929, p. 148)

While each of these women would have some shared experience of caste margin-alization, class locations and a political aspiration towards education as modernity afforded them the separation from marginal constituencies of women, and the virile nation was centre-stage in this aspiration.

Muthulakshmi Reddy also made another significant intervention on the idea of women in politics as householders, as managers of the space (Anandhi, 2008). Reddy saw this as a carrying forward of women's work in the domestic sphere into the public, and as a way of deploying the skills of emotionality, or experiences of conjugality and motherhood, and the unique experiences of oppression faced by women, into political life and practice. In contrast to so many other women of her time, she offered a gendered model of political labour that mimicked, of course, the gendering of the domestic space, but suggested a refashioning of the political domain and offered women as *natural occupants* of such a space.

Which women were these natural occupants? Not the *devadasi*, the other key figure in Muthulakshmi Reddy's politics, for the *devadasi* was too embodied, too backward, too sexual – 'propagators of social evil and carriers of venereal disease' (Reddy, 1964, quoted in Anandhi, 2008, p. 13). Instead, it was women like Reddy, with modern education, who could actively campaign, as she did, for mofussil girls' education, for residential scholarships for Adi-Dravida (a term denoting mar-ginalized castes) and Muslim girls, in the Women's Home of Service, Mylapore, later the Madras Seva Sadan in 1928, insisting that as part of education, 'special scholarships for girls of the depressed and backward communities' were to be made possible (Reddy, 1930, p. 88), insisting that 'a hostel for Muhammadan girls studying in the Hobart Training School for Muhammadan girls is very essential' (ibid, p. 89), referring to the appreciation by one Swamy Sharadhanandaji upon seeing 'Brahmin and non-Brahmin ladies sitting side by side with the Panchama girls and working out the future of India' (ibid, p. 79) in the Mylapore Home, for 'industrial homes' where widows and older women could live and be vocationally trained, for women doctors not only for childbirth attendance but for treatment of venereal diseases. At the same time, Reddy laments the situation where

the local village people have not yet come to realize the value of trained and scientific midwifery as they have been used all these years to the barber mid-wives whose fee varies from four annas to a rupee or a measure of paddy; ...

I would urge the speedy inauguration of the Dais Scheme in every district in this Presidency.

(ibid, p. 90)

Reddy was happy to exhort men of marginalized communities to focus on these concerns, and to push for these in the legislative council. It is in this frame that we might see the roster of celebrated Indian women doctors of this time – as members of the urban privileged-caste elite endorsing a secular modern education for both privileged and oppressed women. Reddy, in this endorsement, was sharply 'opposed to denominational hostels for more than one reason and I feel strongly that housing pupils of one school in separate buildings according to their caste or creed surely would defeat the very object of education' (p. 93); Reddy may have been one of the more vocal opponents of caste segregation in education, although this did not seem to have translated into a larger critique of caste inequality.

This approach of the privileged woman focusing on her 'less fortunate sisters' and insisting on adult education for women worked well, alongside the imperative of social hygiene that found purchase particularly in the Madras presidency and Reddy's own work. Invoking the recommendations of the 'Indian delegation of the British Social Hygiene Council ... regarding revision of the syllabus for the secondary and primary Grade teachers so as to include Public Health and Social Hygiene' (1930, p. 75), Reddy demands government support for bacteriological testing for venereal disease among the poor, including women. Not only is she, in this and in her push for girls' education, seeing herself as vanguard but also making a case for self-governance. Reddy challenges, for instance, Katherine Mayo's position that 'no Indian woman would come forward to be trained as teachers and that the parents would not send their girls to schools' (1930, p. 88), asserting instead that 'it is the absence of educational facilities that is the chief hindrance to the rapid progress of women's education in this Presidency' (ibid); hence the push for hostels for women from marginalized communities.

The purpose and possibility of female education

It is with the recognition of this imperative that we now look at some individual experiments on women's education and professional training credited to some of the more celebrated women of the late 19th century. Muthulakshmi Reddy speaks in 1930, both of the University of Poona as a model that must be emulated elsewhere so that girls may have a knowledge of 'hygiene, physiology and domestic science' and thus become 'practical and efficient' in their daily lives (1930, p. 127), and also of the Poona Seva Sadan as a model institution that trains widows 'and send[s] them to villages as teachers, midwives and nurses' (ibid, p. 129). She suggests that '[w]e want these widows to get educated to serve the country as they have not the choice of marriage' (ibid). This impulse to educate and train vulnerable women or young girls into feminine professions like teachers, midwives, and nurses can be traced back to the late 19th century, and one of the domains it features in is health for women. The 'women for women' rhetoric is available everywhere by now, from missionary accounts to reform language to papers by medical Englishwomen. The nationalist movement has also begun to take female education seriously, seeing in this the potential for self-governance in the face of criticisms of child-marriage, *sati* and other customs identified by the colonial administration. The key point on which this turns is the female colonial subject and the possible terms of her governability, as well as who constituted the centre and margins of this category. Gender-segregated education, however, was not a policy exclusively devised for the colony, as the commentaries suggest. Both in Britain and the US, women's colleges or universities were a feature at the time these conversations were happening in the colony, and by the time the Hunter's Commission report had been completed. Minna Cowan suggests that it is the American model, with women's universities having 'their separate degrees and completely separated life' (1912, p. 220), that could inspire education for women in India.

Scholarship on the point of women's education in the colony is rich, focusing on the need and purpose of such education, its content, and means, and this section is not intended to explore that in detail, focusing, rather, on some aspects of the who and why of women's education. Colonial and imperial accounts of the status of women's education, including the ancient historical periods, are available (Cowan, 1912), where, in fact, insights into the exclusion of women from education being based on their exclusion from caste rites are seen (p. 30). British rule is described as a period of Renaissance, divided into efforts by missionaries, grants-in-aid by the government to voluntary associations from 1854, and a direct government role in women's education since the Hunter Commission report of the Indian Education Commission, dated 3 February 1882. This report notes that only 0.80 percent of school-going age girls were attending public schools. This is the period when, Cowan notes, the suggestion of different curricula for women emerges, with the entry of 'the spontaneous Indian element' (Cowan, p. 35). Basu speaks of privileged women's early access to indigenous *Vaishnavis* and *uttanis* (literate women of faith) who taught women at home (Basu, 2005), and on the introduction of modern English education via missionary schools in the early 1800s. Like reproductive care, education for women too seemed to have progressed initially entirely through non-state interventions and financing. Like healthcare, the 'grand obstacle ... [was seen to be] the universal want of female teachers' (Mary Carpenter, in Basu, 2005, p. 191). Like healthcare, one of the responses was to have gender-segregated education, with 'women's only' higher education institutions like Bethune College in Calcutta and Shreemati Nathibai Damodar Thackersey Women's University (SNDT) in Bombay also being created, and providing curricula exclusively tailored to preparing women to be better wives and mothers – the idea of *zenana* education. Like healthcare, girls' schools were expected to function well only with British supervision, especially the missionary and grant-in-aid ones. Like the healthcare experience, some women pioneers in the field too seemed to have said, like Pandita Ramabai and Muthulakshmi Reddy, that women must not rely on men for their 'salvation', and must find their way forward independently. Scholarship around this history also documents these pioneers, the first women to enter university spaces, and their struggles (Basu, 2005; Forbes, 1999; Chanana, 2001; Bagchi, 1993).

Educability

This literature already demonstrates a division regarding who could attend which schools, and this has relevance for what I call the aspect of *educability* – which women can be taught? Which women are available for vocational training? This is a slight shift from asking the question in the form – what can these women be taught, or why must they be taught, to asking – what is the raw material in terms of educable subjects available for formal education or training, and how might these be administered? In other words, a reference to the governability that accompanies the discourse around the female colonial subject, particularly the adult woman. This focus on the adult has significance in the context of early marriage, which was said to be a common feature in Indian privileged-caste homes that were the focus of colonial administrators, Indian social reformers, and nationalists. Educability emerged both through social location and circumstance. So, while *Vaishnavis* and *uttanis* were available for the religious education of privileged-caste Hindu and Muslim women at their homes in Bengal, the missionary schools invariably attracted marginalized-caste and poor pupils, with their promise of a fee for attendance, free clothes, etc. Modern public education for 'respectable' upper-caste Hindu women had to be championed by social reformers like Vidyalankar and Vidyasagar, who dipped into canonical texts and learned women's figures of pre-Muslim antiquity (Gargi, Maitreyi, Arundhathi, Damayanti, to name a few) to argue that female education was not proscribed in indigenous traditions. In 1896, Dewan Bahadur Manibhai Jasbhai, known in his lifetime for his work on language and education, including the education of women, published in Bombay a text titled 'Hindu Female Education in the Bombay Presidency', following on, and supplementing, the findings of the Education Commission report of 1882. This text assumes significance both through its author and its comprehensive referencing of and location within social reform and nationalism. Although the Dewan Bahadur was writing after medical education for women had been lobbied for and attained, he was writing on the subject of primary and continuing education for Hindu women at large. He begins by talking about the educability of these women, whose 'intellectual activity', as per the 1882 Report, was 'very keen' (Abstract and Analysis of The Report of the 'Indian Education Commission', with notes, and 'The Recommendations' in full, Johnston, 1884, p. 97). Also, as 'a class, their modesty, patience, instinctive charity, and religious feeling' (Dewan Bahadur Manibhai Jasbhai, 1896, p.1) render them eminently suitable and deserving of this effort. His appeal for their education follows his analysis of available numbers that indicates a very small number of Hindu women in higher and secondary education, at least one reason for which is the paucity of 'purely Hindu schools' (ibid, p. 5). In primary education, he says, most Hindu girls are not able to read a printed book, and in private institutions, almost all advanced pupils are non-Hindus. Manibhai Jasbhai also cites the 1882 Report findings that insist that no one other than 'the educated woman' (ibid, p. 3) can perform the task of educating these women. Of course, Cowan and others find the lower numbers of gender-segregated as well as rigorous institutions another cause of these drop-outs (1912, p. 52).

Manibhai Jasbhai presents, by referencing a large number of papers on educational reform and women's education, a by-now familiar set of rationales for women's education – 'no nation can be truly great unless it has educated mothers' (p. 11), 'the influence of a mother on the destiny of her child' (ibid), '"Educate a girl, and you get eventually a cultivated family"' (Pechey-Phipson, in Manibhai Jasbhai, p. 13), and so on. Another, lesser-known argument he brings to the table is from an 1891 paper attributed to a Prof. MacMillan titled 'Heredity and the regeneration of India', where the author claims that 'the mental and bodily power of children is to a large extent determined by the mental and bodily power of their mothers' (MacMillan, 1891, in Manibhai Jasbhai, 1896, p. 11). This argument for maternal heredity influences is significant, both in terms of the onus it puts on mothers, and the focus on caste, nation, and civilization/*race* and fitness – both physical and mental – that is implicit here. We may extend this argument of fitness as flowing from and embedded in caste status. Manibhai Jasbhai goes on to consolidate this argument, citing various medical opinions – '[r]aces tend to take after the woman' (The Right Honourable Sir Mountstuart Elphinstone Grant-Duff, former Governor of Madras, G.C.S.I., C.I.E., quoted in Manibhai Jasbhai, p. 11) or the extent of importance of prenatal influences. 'Home power' (p. 12), as he puts it, is, of course, also seen as the primary socializing influence on the child. Here again, this socializing acquires a slightly different meaning. 'Our Aryan Shastras describe the mother as the greatest of all instructors, *Mata paramko guru* [written in Devanagari script],' (p. 12), he says. This argument of the mother as primary and most revered teacher, and therefore as a knowledge bearer, is new in the discourse of upliftment or victimhood, presenting as it does the mother as not only morally powerful but also as *knowledgeable*. There is no real discussion of *which* mother qualifies as knowledgeable; as belonging to one caste or community. But in the context of canonical texts and upper-caste practices and figures that Manibhai Jasbhai references elsewhere as representative of the nation, as also the idea of knowledge being tied to Sanskritic traditions and Shastras, the 'woman of the nation' becomes delineated as the upper-caste Hindu woman. This is also where the colonial reference to the *zenana* is reflected in a developing nationalist discourse. Knowledge by birth, and the power to perform ritual, as occupational exclusivity in the caste-patriarchal system delineates, is not a domain, however, that Manibhai Jasbhai, or the Education Commission, or the social reformers at that point, enter into.

Yet another perspective Manibhai Jasbhai brings to the idea of the woman of the family is to link with the *grihini* (householder) and *ardhangini* (the feminine complement of the man) as also *dampati* (the couple unit). In doing this, the author steps away significantly from placing the woman alone at the centre of reform discourse or even at the centre of the extended family or community; rather, he puts her down as the more powerful member of the couple unit. In addition to introducing the couple unit as the centre of society and the nation, this approach presents the woman of the family as ready to be formally educated, while presenting a forceful argument for the need for formal education. It is also worthwhile to note that these ideas – of coupledom or of mother-as-primary-educator – are not presented as modern ideas, as later feminist scholarship has suggested, but as available in Vedic and other ancient texts – a recognizable strategy in social reform discourse. To this end, he mobilizes several tropes and practices – *ardhangini*, the practice of naming gods as husbands of their consorts, and so on. Manibhai Jasbhai goes on to find apposite metaphors of femininity in English writing too, ranging from Mary Carpenter, the English social reformer, to Shakespeare, to the utilitarian philosopher Bentham, to Sarah Stickney Ellis' *Daughters of England*, an 1842 text providing guidance on women's behaviour and duties. The idea of a frugal, dutiful wife as 'one who can comfort and counsel her husband' (p. 16), who is available in trials and in misfortune – the ideal companion – is well consolidated in these, and is a natural extension of the Protestant ethos of the England of the time. In fact, various administrative commentaries on the intelligence of Hindu women are put to use here, and Manibhai Jasbhai concludes thus:

> If the benefit of education to an appreciable degree were added to the natu-ral shrewdness, intelligence, and many other good qualities of the Hindu women, we may safely predict a very bright future for our community and a national regeneration on the best and most permanent basis.
>
> (p. 25)

Given that women are established, therefore, at the centre of every society and race, neglect of education for them, just like neglect of their reproductive health, can result only in social 'decay', and '"national progress ... [is] a pretence and a delusion"' (Rai Bahadur Ranganada Moodeliar, educationist, influential in Madras University, and contributor to the Education Commission, quoted in Manibhai, p. 20). With these and several other reformers' words in place from across different regions and presidencies, Manibhai Jasbhai then consolidates his case for women's education.

Following this set of arguments on the educability of upper-caste Hindu women, is proposed not only a gender-segregated but a caste-segregated form of educa-tion for women, so that the pupils might have 'competent teachers, with whom they can freely associate' (a native gentleman of Poona, in a communication to Mary Carpenter, quoted in Manibhai Jasbhai, p. 32) – competence being a familiar metaphor for social caste status. The 'Agra experiment' that Cowan speaks of later reflects this idea, where 'a Jat of good family, in co-operation with the Government ... succeeded in securing "school mistresses of high caste and relatives of rich and influential zamindars"' (Cowan, 1912, p. 40) for female schools. In fact, this casteism seems to have been justified, as appears from the Northwestern Provinces Report on Education, 1875, which notes that '"[t]he villagers ... value them chiefly as a means of support for Brahmans and relatives"' (quoted in Cowan, p. 41). This was, of course, read via the euphemism of 'community', in the framework of interference into women's lives needing to be done in collaboration with the community. The same was asked of women trained to teach at home – the need for 'Hindu Lady teachers, who could *readily be received* into Hindu homes' (Manibhai Jasbhai, 1896, p. 136, italics mine). Furthermore, the question of how to have enough 'caste' teachers – 'If promising caste girls are to be trained at all, it must be in the immediate neighbourhood of their homes' (Hunter's Education Commission – Madras Provincial Committee, p. 134, quoted in Manibhai Jasbhai, p. 143). This is also cited in evidence to the Education Commission of 1882 (p. 28). In a parallel to healthcare, and nearly at the same time, a group of women outside professions began to enter and participate in the discourse around self-governance, nation, and civilization. The proposals made in the Education Commission report included Hindu widows, wives, or female relations of male teachers as suitable for this training. Training colleges, stipends and scholarships, were also proposed to increase the numbers of women teachers from these trainable ranks, so that the educable young women might be attended to. As in healthcare, these trainees were proposed to have English supervision. As Manibhai Jasbhai reports from one recommendation of the Education Commission – '"A zealous female Inspectress, full of European activity and native sympathy, may work wonders in the great work of Female Education" – Rao Bahadur K.C. Bedarkar, B.A., LL.B' (footnote 2, p. 34).

One of the few differences in the approach to healthcare for women is the preference for institutional education rather than home tuitions, although the latter continued to be kept open for further education for those who desired it or could afford to pay. Another difference was in the space made available for sessions on 'religion and morality', and here there is an interesting difference from the canonical indigenous as accessed in nationalist discourse around medicine. 'A Sanskrit Pandita will be maintained in the Institution, and she will deliver Lectures in the Vernacular on broad principles of religion and morality, illustrating the same by citations from approved Sanskrit works, sectarianism or dogmatic religious teaching being avoided', says Manibhai Jasbhai, while citing commentaries that suggest that '"social and moral order can only rest upon a religious basis"' (Cotton, Bengal Civil Service, quoted in Manibhai Jasbhai, p. 38). A difference is made, then, between dogma and an 'underlying ... religious sentiment' that indicates, apparently, the 'stability of the Hindu character' (Cotton, Esquire, Bengal Civil Service, quoted in Manibhai Jasbhai, p. 38).

Role of women, and books suitable for girls

One of the requirements for women's education that Manibhai Jasbhai urges for, citing the Education Commission as well, is the generation of more vernacular literature – 'a healthy general Literature for the Zenana or Household as distinguished from Text Books for Schools' (p. 40). It is here that we find one of the stated contexts for the production of a literature particularly suited for the *zenana*, and of women as a reading public. While this reading public could not, obviously, be controlled in terms of what it read, the ideas of 'self-instruction', morality, leisure, and education via cheaply available vernacular literature drove policy emerging around women's education at this time. Sanskrit, seen as 'the sacred language of our religion' (p. 42), becomes the bulwark where instructions on 'piety and morality charmingly united' (ibid), can be found. In a further alliance with the Protestant ethic, one of the points of education continues to be self-denial, as proposed by Hannah More, among others, and a strong association of religion and morality become the bulwark for women's education, as a means of bringing to 'oriental women, with oriental feelings and traditions' (p. 46) the values of family, the Aryan race, and nation, so as to contribute to the 'future regeneration of India' (ibid). This nationalized character of education for women is seen in the setting up of various institutions for 'Indian girls of good family' (Cowan p. 144) so that they can be given a 'womanly' education, with courses suitable for girls not being an adjunct but a constitutive element of curricula. And it is here that the need for 'Magazines, intended specially for the benefit of our Hindu women' (Manibhai Jasbhai, p. 46), is suggested as a complement to education. It is in this context that vernacular women's magazines already in circulation in the provinces of Bengal and Tamil Nadu are approvingly mentioned by Manibhai Jasbhai.

The right kind of woman reader

Swati Moitra speaks of the emergence of the Bengali *bhadramahila* (a category that could be partially aligned to the *zenana* or *pardanashin* woman in terms of caste-class locations but with the added qualifiers of modernity) in the mid-19th century, and the 'alignment of the *bhadramahila* with the less-than-respectable producers and readers of "street literature," the "contesting" other to the project of becoming modern' (2017, p. 628). This alignment is accompanied by the emergence of a 'women's literature' (Ghosh, 2006, p. 97), and a readership. Anindita Ghosh, focussing on this sub-genre, elaborates on the porosity of the distinction between this and other literature and oral traditions of an earlier period – '[i]n reality, however, 'women's language' or meyeli bhasha was nothing but an integral part of a shared domestic speech system, till it was sought out, segregated, and marginalized for want of refinement by the educated male in the early nineteenth century' (Ghosh, 2006, p. 226). Ghosh explores this idea of *meyeli bhasha* in oral cultures preceding print, tracing this form in 'the imitations of speech patterns and sung narratives – with liberal use of rustic humour, conversational topical digressions, songs, proverbial usage, elements of magic and fable, didactic reiterations' (Ghosh, 2002, p. 4331), and the sharing of this culture among 'a host of little known cultural worlds – of folk deities, low-caste movements, non-conformist religious sects – that ran parallel to the 'Renaissance' activity in urban centres' (ibid). Sumit Sarkar has written about the contexts and influence of *battala* literature as embedded in the 19th-century social upheaval that produced a middle-class salaried immigrant group of workers that patronized the *battolar boi* (the books produced at the Battala presses in north Calcutta; these presses were a world occupied not by privilege but traders and metal workers including *Karmakars, Shils, Lahas*[2]). Ghosh, however, extends this readership to include women and other social groups not necessarily literate – 'itarjan' (lower/mean folk), a poor Muslim Bengali populace, traders, shopkeepers, mill workers, musicians, and domestic workers – a vast and heterogeneous group. This coincided with the practice of communitarian reading in the 19th and 20th centuries. While this interpretation presents a challenge to the 'encounter' model that follows the idea of Western influence in creating a caste-class privileged *bhadralok* group, it also helps us see the early difficulty of crafting the right kind of woman reader until at least the latter half of the 19th century. Ghosh suggests, in fact, that

> Bengali print-language actually escaped much of colonial and bhadralok disciplining, for print had a much more varied and wider penetration than has been previously thought. Despite bhadralok disapproval, the Battala presses did a brisk trade in this ephemeral literature, and enjoyed a large and popular readership.

> (Ghosh, 2006, p. 108)

Biswas notes, in fact, with reference to Rabindranath Tagore, the celebrated Bengal poet and Nobel laureate, how a religious text like the *Krittibas Ramayan* is read in the *zamindar* (landowner) household, well-worn and thumbed, hidden beneath the grandmother's pillow, and read in secret by the poet in his boyhood, sitting on the threshold, in the fading light of day (Biswas, 2000, p. 22). This literature, as part of its reach into the *antahpur*, is seen as empowering, as the celebrated Vaishnavite Rassundari Devi is said to avow – 'In a startling reversal of prevailing revivalist nationalist and Hindu-Brahmanical world views, Rassundari blesses the *kaliyuga* (the evil era invoked as the ill of modernity) for it had taught women like her to read' (Ghosh, 2006, p. 257). Ghosh also notes that 'a lot of women were taught by *Baishnabis*. Despite their low-caste and class origins, and their alleged immorality, the women from these educated devotional sects were often employed to teach women and young girls privately' (p. 253). Rasasundari's autobiography, *Amar Jibon* (My life), is published in 1876.

This experience is not replicated in the same form elsewhere. Ramabai Ranade's autobiography,[3] among other texts, and its oft-quoted narration of a domestic upheaval that accompanied an act of solitary reading[4] in the midst of her everyday chores, shows us the extreme loneliness of home education for some women – here the wives of reformers and otherwise 'modern' men in western India. It was not merely the control exercised actively by men, but the sanction of older women of the family that exercised patriarchal control over these women's lives. Ghosh's (2006, 2008) and Moitra's (2017) reference to a collective readership that emerges in women of the family in Bengal, at the opposite side of the colony, offers perhaps a glimpse of the normative gendered familial sociality that gives women access to language and texts while escaping the vigilance of mainstream society around such practices. Moitra's reading also suggests that, apart from the elite male nationalist impulse to 'educate' women in a particular manner, and into a particular content, the colonial impulse to decode, reach, and regulate the minds of the women of Bengal, Bombay, and Madras presidencies brings forth an audit of the vast amount of printed material available in the vernacular, and an attempt by elite reformers and colonizers to replace some of the licentious texts entering households via street vendors with more sanitized, respectable texts. Ghosh (2006) and Moitra both refer to the account of one Reverend Long, commenting on such an incident, where a request by a privileged woman to her European lady teacher for *Bidya Sundar* – a romance text at once considered obscene and sought to be recovered as classical in nationalist resistance – is rejected in favour of *Sushila'r upakhyan* – an approved publication of the vernacular literary society and one directed at fashioning the 'good woman'. Moitra nuances the earlier scholarship around the emergence of the *bhadramahila* by suggesting that while this *bhadramahila* did indeed signal a more docile voice, the 19th century also saw the emergence of women as an important reading public, and 'the increasing importance of reading as a leisure practice made *available* to women' (p. 639). For all the caveats placed upon reading inappropriate texts, they continued to find their way into the *antahpur* or *andarmahal*, and generate conversations and affect among this reading public, Ghosh (2008) and Moitra (2017) note. We will see, in the section on women's magazines, the workings of this incomplete regulation, in a paradigm that supports the woman's role in the home as healer. The point about readership – particularly communitarian readership – is to point to a certain sociality around the interface between the home and the world that becomes, for the modern therapeutic, a site of intervention.

The moulding of the woman of home and nation

Battala presses are a useful, if paradoxical, entry point into the category of the ideal woman of the nation. The content of *zenana* education has been the subject of extensive scholarship and explored with respect to notions of the ideal woman of the nation. One of the key elements of this debate, and one that is often lost sight of in the discourse, is the age of this woman. Jasodhara Bagchi speaks eloquently of the *khukumoni*, or the girl child beloved of the upper-caste family, who is expected to blossom into the *bhadramahila*, the *grihalakshmi*, or be lost to widowhood, *sati*, or death in childbirth, which is the understated subject of this discourse. This child bride, spoken of via implicit 'idioms of loss' (Bagchi, 1993), is the actual subject of education reform for women of the colony, or the nation too – a reform that is literally developmental, offering 'an elaborate code of socialisation ... for the girl child' (Bagchi, 1993, p. 2214). While male social reformers sought to partly site their exhortations to reform in the *Shastras* – the canonical Hindu texts, women like Pandita Ramabai took a different path, laying the responsibility of the injunctions to keep women in check in the text of the *Manusmriti*, as well as to a motivated reading of the Shastras by corrupt Brahmin priests. The Pandita indicated in this reading the paradox of the 'loving mother of the nation ... [who] is "as impure as falsehood itself" ... is never to be trusted; matters of importance are never to be committed to her' (Ramabai, 1901, pp. 81–82, referring to the *Manusmriti*). The Pandita's sharp critique remained one of a kind, however, alongside a few other women like Kashibai Kanitkar who, in 1889, spoke up against familial control over women's lives and education, offering, as Meera Kosambi puts it, 'the boldest "naming", in nineteenth-century Marathi writing, of the coercive power of men over women' (Kosambi, 2000, p. 430). The Pandita was 'a solitary and largely unsupported Indian woman ... who "named" most eloquently and systematically the problems of the "oppressed Indian woman"' (Kosambi, 2016, p. 1), while the approach to women's education described above took hold, taking either 'ameliorative solutions ... [or the route of] "political reformers" who prioritized political autonomy and ... the need to postpone social reform' (Kosambi, 2000, p. 431) including women's education. The 'right type of woman' sought to be moulded via this education has also been explored in scholarship around texts like Madhusudhan Mukhopadhyaya's 1859 text mentioned above – *Sushila'r upakhyan* (Bandyopadhyay, 1994). Bandyopadhyay speaks of Sushila, the upper-caste woman student who is the subject of this text, as the perfect *Nabina* or modern woman who is both in touch with and separate from the *Prachina* – the woman subject of a more traditional norm. This is a woman committed to *stree-dharma* (a wifely moral) – a conjugal role and value that emerges as ahistorical, decontextualized, and essentially feminine. As such, it recalls, somewhat, the subjective interiority that Tamil magazines for women from the 1890s to 1940s also propose (Sreenivas, 2003). Although this model is referred to in most scholarship as an impulse to be seen in 'nationalist resolutions of the women's question', to refer to the title of the significant and much-critiqued postcolonial text by Partha Chatterjee (1989), writing by Englishwomen like Minna Cowan, committed to the improvement of women's status and education, show that the impulse towards normative femininity finds adequate reference points in school curriculum in Britain in the late 19th century. As Cowan states, 'in Great Britain the leading girls' High Schools have developed a flexibility and variety of curriculum wherein many a "womanly woman" has found her training' (Cowan, 1912, p. 53). And it is in close collaboration between English educators and Indian missionaries, that such gender-specific curricula are proposed, although not always agreed upon, and it is here that the aim to demonstrate to 'the people that the girls who have been to school become superior housewives and mothers' (ibid, p. 54) is articulated, as 'useful information' (ibid). Gender-segregated curricula, however, are not deployed in all provinces, as we see in descriptions of Burma, where both numbers and presence of girls in co-educational spaces is higher than elsewhere, and where the practice of *parda* is not widespread. We see gender-segregated curricula at greater work in the teaching of home science and economics in the 1920s and thereafter. A closer look at the deployment of the category *zenana*, as also the aspects of educability and trainability and their mobilization into governance, show us a gender and caste-segregated model of female education, as I have been tracing in this section. This model, with its more covert caste qualifier, allows us to re-examine some of the findings of this scholarship, and it is to such a re-examination that I will turn in the next section.

Gender and caste-segregated education progressed to eventually take the shape of home science, which, in the 1930s, became the discipline that 'sought to reform women's education and to reorganize domestic life' (Hancock, 2001, pp 871–872). Hancock, in fact, traces the 'strategic alliances' (p. 871) between colonial administrators, Indian social reformers, nationalists, and in particular nationalist feminists, in the emergence of the discourse around home science, domestic science, and home economics that became the placeholder for women to participate in building the family but also in imagining the modern nation and creating professions exclusive to women. Hancock traces this emergence across the late 19th to mid-20th centuries, and the different roles that emerged for different women – mothercraft and family welfare for the upper-caste woman of the family, care professions for privileged-caste widows, political presence and social reform for a small elite. While home economics became institutionalized in curricula between the 1930s and 1950s, continuities from the sanitary reform movement in England and its manifestations in the colony are clear. One of the most stark connections emerging in this consolidation, Hancock suggests, is the purported meeting of tradition and modernity, as the emerging discipline of home science asks its practitioners and teachers to revisit traditional practices around the home with a new eye and find in them the principles of scientific hygiene. This was done on the premise that a particular 'built environment could promote social change' (Hancock, 2001, p. 889) – an impulse that travels into the post-independence Nehruvian principle of development as well.

Educability and trainability

A number of associations follow from Hancock's arguments. One, caste-given principles of purity and pollution align with scientific proposals for hygiene and separation – of the inside and outside of the home, of the family and its outsiders, of the community and those outside. Some of these included the slum improvement work of the women's associations in the mid-20th century, like the Bhagini Samaj, begun in 1916 in greater Bombay and Gujarat, with rural centres like at Udwada that engaged in 'Harijan' welfare and the removal of untouchability, free medical checkups, and the propagation of ideas of health, hygiene, nutrition, sanitation, motherhood, and family planning. Such centres worked for Adivasi communities and aspired to a higher secondary home science institute that would be like a mini polytechnic, thus placing some of these norming technologies in an expert domain. Some included the sanitary reform work of earlier times, or indeed even the differential approach to training Indian women as doctors or *dais*. For one, in all of these, the division of educability and trainability of women along the hierarchy of caste lines is clear. Two, the conflation of upper-caste Hindu practices with the nation. Alongside the eugenic moments in this exercise that called for strengthening the race, this translates also into a racialization of this upper-caste Hindu nation, and an announcement of the familiar and yet new, modern conditions of motherhood that can accomplish this. Three, with the parallel moments legislating who are to be the central women of the nation, like the Devadasi Abolition Bill and its related legislation, including the demand for testing for venereal diseases that are moved by Muthulakshmi Reddy, sexualities outside the realm of the family are marked as imprudent and excessive, in opposition to rationalized reproductive sexuality from within the domain of which a healthy Home Science can operate. Attention to the 'nature of women', and their familial roles, of course, infuses all the commentaries.

Elite nationalist positions on a different content of education for women also join this principle of gender-segregated education, including that by Keshab Chandra Sen, leader of a breakaway section of the Brahmo Samaj, proposing an education 'calculated to make them "good wives, good mothers, good sisters and good daughters"' (quoted in Manibhai Jasbhai, 1896, p. 56), offering '"an artistic, poetic education, with a practical training in domestic duties, elementary

200 The nation and its women

science and the laws of sanitation"'; others remark that "'denationalizing the girls is most dangerous"' (Ruler of Cutch, quoted in Manibhai Jasbhai, 1896, p. 56). While this danger is usually dealt with by teaching in the vernacular, providing privileged women with as liberal an education as will make them able companions and enlighten their homes, while ensuring that 'what is imparted is pure, solid and true' (ibid, p. 62), is what nationalists seek in these times. This was expressed in as harsh tones as an MM Joshi in his 'Ideals of Indian Women' in *Hind Mahila* (1920, pp. 5–11), where he ordered discipline and education for women following the principles of Manu, and inasmuch as it developed their intuition and prepared them to build families and teach 'young boys up to a certain period'; or in a more liberal language of freedom. Funding and organization of girls' schools also followed this dualism of conservative and liberal, with the *Mahakali pathshalas*,[5] for example, established in Bengal from 1893 as 'the orthodox Hindu response to what was viewed as excessive Westernization' (Karlekar, 1986, pp. WS-28) on the one hand, and the efforts from the Brahmo Samaj, or Parsi community-sponsored English-medium institutions in Bombay on the other. I would flag another aspect of this discourse here. While, in the talk about women's education, regional imperatives and impulses are visible, as Manibhai Jasbhai and others active in the Bombay presidency suggest, asking for Bombay to follow examples from Madras, the overarching impulse is one of racialization, addressed to 'Aryan brethren' who are also Hindu and Indian (p. 77). This language, seen as emerging from canonical Hindu texts, is happily married to ideas of Enlightenment, to then speak of 'useful' education and progress that women can be part of. Thus, we also see analogies drawn between prescriptions for maternal health to be found in texts such as the *Charaka Samhita* and a modern English text like 'The Gentlewoman's Book of Hygiene' by Kate Mitchell (1892). The *collaboration* between the racially superior Hindu Aryans and the colonizing British is now verbalized, in place of the defences that a later, more militant nationalism, poses to Western influence. Keshab Chandra Sen, Pandit Shivanath Shastri, and others are part of this thinking. This is made more visible in provinces like Burma, where neither 'womanly' curricula nor vernacular mediums are popular,[6] and where commentators like Cowan note with some sense of failure, that 'only about 25% of the girls were taking Burmese, ... many of them take Latin, ... [s]ewing ... is at a low ebb' (Cowan, 1912, p. 72); in other words, the purpose of female education has been lost (although the nature of gender relations being different in Burma is commented upon).

One of the roles prescribed for (elite and royal upper-caste) women of the nation was as advisors to the field of education for Indian women at large. To that effect, some girls' high schools like the Victoria May Girls' High School in Lahore attempted not only to design curricula primarily designed to prepare young women for their future as wives and mothers but also to have 'a reflex influence on the whole scheme of education', by reserving seats for 'rajahs' daughters and their necessary attendants' (Cowan, p. 145). It was assumed that this proximity would show the elite women how the other half lived, and thereafter 'induce them to act where possible as helpers and advisers' (ibid).

As to what the nationalists were doing, some of the testimonies given to the Education Commission of 1882 also indicate nationalist sentiments, pointing reproachfully to the 'sum spent in awarding grants to schools for Europeans and Eurasians ...' which is double that spent on educating 'Native females' (Extract from Evidence of Nowrojee Furdoonjee, Esquire, p. 310, quoted in Manibhai Jasbhai p. 151). Of course, these were accompanied by injunctions to focus on 'domestic economy, house management, singing' and so on for women (ibid). Organizations like the Arya Samaj were instrumental in this. Native states showed different policies, with Baroda in the Bombay Presidency having strong schemes undifferentiated from boys' schools for the education of women and teachers, Mysore demonstrating the influence of mission schools, the Maharani girls' school with restricted caste entry and teacher training for Brahmin widows, and Travancore with the highest proportion of girls at school by the early 1900s, and an impetus to girls' education by the establishment of a Maharajah's College for girls. Arya Samaj institutions run by widows were also to be found in Ajmer, among other states. Bombay occupies a unique place in this history, with women being far more present in the public domain than in *purdah*, with cultural expression being seen as highly evolved and inclusive of education for women, and with the age of marriage being traditionally higher than in other regions. The particular composition of this city's population also played a role, with the Parsi community being known for its contribution to institutions of healthcare as well as education, and for the education of its women. The famous exemplar of leading Indian members of the Students' Literary and Scientific Society of Elphinstone College starting schools for girls in their houses in 1849 comes to mind; Dadabhai Naoroji, Parsi-Zoroastrian, professor at Elphinstone, moderate Congressman, philanthropist, and the 'Grand Old Man of India', was one of these (Cowan, 1912, p. 165). The Parsi community also adopted a specific educational policy for their women in 1857 – 'a thorough training for life for middle-class Parsi women' (Cowan, p. 174), with the difference from other approaches that it promoted English education. A greater proportion of the private schools for women in this time were also Parsi-run. Schools for girls were proposed by the Gujarati Stri Mandal, founded in 1909 for *parda* women. Co-educational schools are also to be found in Bombay and Poona; mission schools as well. The Public Instruction Report of Bombay showed that primary schools had the highest numbers of pupils from among non-Brahmin Hindus, while higher education showed a higher number of Parsis and Eurasians. Training colleges, mostly government or aided, showed the highest proportion of non-Brahmin Hindus, closely followed by Brahmins and native Christians.

Outside of all of these impulses, and at least 50 years or so before the schools, reformers, and arguments around content named in the extensive scholarship around women and education, however, are to be found figures like Savitribai Phule, Jyotiba Phule, Mukta Salve, Fatima Sheikh, and Tarabai Shinde, among others. These thinkers are curiously missing from the dominant historical and post-colonial commentaries on nationalist discourse on the woman's question, as also from the sociological analyses, till at least the early 2000s. Savitribai and Jyotiba Phule, founders of the Satyashodhak Samaj in 1831, proposed a different version of national history from that which saw either the Mughals or the British Raj as the starting point of the decline of Indian civilization. Marking the 'Aryan invasion', the 'foolish Peshwas', and the Mughals, as at least as much responsible for the exploitation of the 'true natives' (Desai & Roy, 2022, online) and the erasure of their epistemologies, Savitribai and Jyotiba Phule, along with Fatima Sheikh, started the first school for women in 1848 in Pune. These thinkers, marking as they did the origin stories of oppression in pre-colonial times and within the oppressive structures of caste and race, saw in English education and colonial educational structures the scope to develop different curricula, inclusive and collective pedagogies (Rege, 2010), and chose non-gender or caste-segregated curricula for young girls and boys. Rather than using schools as extended sites of gendered socialization for women, they taught mathematics and the sciences, agriculture, and histories of oppression by privileged castes that informed dominant pedagogies. This was the idea of education reimagined as *Trutiya Ratna*[7] – '(third eye) that has the possibilities to enable the oppressed to understand and transforms the relation between power and knowledge' (Rege, 2010, p. 93). The Satyashodhak schools, open to oppressed castes but also to non-Bahujan (non-oppressed caste) students, widows and orphans who had historically been kept out of education or access to knowledge, challenged the exclusive rights of Brahmin men over knowledge production. Satyashodhak thinkers also went on to revise wedding ceremonies, following a recognition of Hindu marriage rituals as a way of perpetuating caste oppression and gender inequality, much akin to Self-Respect marriages proposed in the Self Respect Movement in southern regions about a century after. Strangely, or not, perhaps, although Savitribai and Pandita Ramabai, as well as Ramabai Ranade, along with the male social reformers, shared at least some historical time, and definitely geographical space – western India, particularly Bombay and Pune – we find no records of reference to the work of these reformers in the later much more celebrated and known reform work. It could not but be so, because, apart from entrenched caste hierarchies and historical denial of knowledge space to the communities Savitribai and other Satyashodhak members were speaking from and for, the nationalism they adopted also did not follow the 'binaries of western modernity/Indian tradition, private caste-gender/public nation' (Rege, 2010, p. 93). The neat proposal of indigeneity following these binaries, then, was not made available in their formulations.

Shailaja Paik, writing of a later time, speaks of 'the "interlocking technologies" of education, caste, community, gender, sexuality, and family' (2016, p. 14) that formed the contexts and sites of intervention for Dalit women in colonial western India and in the creation of 'a new Dalit womanhood' (p. 15). Dalit male reformers, suggests Paik, in demanding access to public institutions and spaces for communities historically excluded, also engaged with a discourse of modernity and English education in order to do so; and further engaged with the emancipation of women of oppressed caste locations as a route to the emancipation of these communities. While Paik recognizes a certain ambivalence in the messaging of these reformers with regard to the 'place of women', as also with regard to middle-class respectability particularly expressed through changes in Dalit women's changing attire, practices, etc., as a movement towards mainstreaming – a movement that many scholars have marked as Sanskritization (Srinivas, 1956), she highlights the powerful appeal that B.R. Ambedkar makes, for instance, to oppressed-caste women, for '*nischay* (resoluteness), *dhadaadi* (bold and dauntless), and *dhamak* (willpower and daring) ... to rethink their attitudes towards education, motherhood, public roles, and employment' (p. 25). Such transformation was exhorted 'for *sudhaaranaa* (improvement) and *vikaas* (development or progress)' (p. 15). Paik also traces Ambedkar's consolidation of Phule's work in 'making the development of *svaabhimaan* (self-respect), dignity, and modern citizenship (*naagarikatva*) the core of education and pedagogy' (p. 16). Paik goes on to explore the writing and work of 'ordinary Dalit women' like Manoramabai, Anusuya Kamble, and Anusuya Shivtarkar (p. 16, 22) in the early 20th century in accessing secular education as a transformative tool for themselves, family, and community. The most stark difference between these positions and those of a Ramabai Ranade or a Muthulakshmi Reddy was that these reformers were not interested in 'merely a "recovery" of women' (p. 17). Also important for the present discussion, gender as well as caste segregation in schools and colleges was actively resisted by these thinkers. As for Reddy, her own social location as the daughter of a *devadasi* mother and Brahmin father, or her political awakening, was never invoked in her autobiographical writings; in fact, she refers to herself as 'neither a politician nor was I interested in politics of the country' (1930, p. 4).

Which brings us to feminist recastings of the nationalist question. Although I do not go into women's or other movement histories with transformative agendas here, it would seem, following the variety of elite and non-elite reform, nationalist, and imperial positions traced here, that the mid to late 19th century offered a wide and heterogeneous, even conflicting, set of positions on education for women. And yet, as the century draws to a close, we see a dominant picture emerging – of the kind of woman who is to be provided access to primary and some secondary education, the content of education, and the bifurcation of higher education and skill training among the privileged and the marginalized.

Women's magazines and socialization

Women's magazines of the late 19th to early and mid-20th centuries have been the subject of intense scrutiny and scholarship, tracing this space as a contributor to norm-building for women privileged on grounds of caste and class, and by extension, the source of guidelines on gender roles for all. These magazines have also been spoken of as continuing a community of women from an earlier pre-print era. The literature also suggests slight differences in commentary on the norm, with the 20th century showing, in many ways, the emergence of a unique subjectivity, an interiority, as well as a political voice. I am more focused on the earlier output and examine, in this section, two broad kinds of literature that circulated in these magazines. One, the exhortations to women of the nation – whether to follow appropriate norms of domesticity and perform domestic forms of nationalist resistance. Two, the mobilization of this space towards a home-based nationalist therapeutics.

Needless to say, these dovetailed in obvious ways. This examination helps, I suggest, to name, once more, the subject of the *zenana*, her place in a newly emergent middle class that also carries caste privilege, the internalization of the Gandhian nationalist principle of self-reliance for the emancipation of widows, and a particular reconciling of learning and householding that also foregrounded the indigenous.

The scholarship around women's magazines and their role in the socialization of women have examined the contexts of Bengal, Maharashtra, and Tamil Nadu, among other spaces, in the work of Sreenivas (2003), Moitra (2017), Bagchi (1993), Lahiri (1998), Sen (2004), and Karlekar (1986), among others. Closely linked to the question of education for women, these magazines, alongside various small print publications, addressed women as readers, writers, householders, and indigenous therapeutic agents. The core question for most of the scholarship has been to examine whether these publications produced and reinforced norms of docility, 'appropriate domesticity' (Sreenivas p. 61), or created a counter-public or at least a resistant form of femininity that incorporated the idiom of loss of autonomy (Lahiri, 1998; Moitra, 2017). Some of this scholarship also examines the production of a feminine interiority related to conjugality (Sreenivas, 2003), as well as desire as a 'natural' impulse not always dictated by marital status. I am more interested in the various exhortations to a national imaginary that these magazines and their parallel advice publications presented. In terms of the value of education, perspectives on women's education linked the idea of education as a route to self-reliance and Swadeshi, particularly in the early 20th century, via employment as nurses, teachers, doctors, or social workers. Rachel Berger (2013) writes about the domestic guides or *grihalakshmis* that emerged in the late 19th century onwards, which consolidated the home science that was being taught in schools into a more 'native' image. Specific kinds of nationalist action – like *arandhan* (a refusal to cook) or *raksha bandhan* (a tie of solidarity)[8] – were, in the first decade of the 20th century, spoken of, in magazines like the *Bamabodhini Patrika*, as forms of political participation (Lahiri, 1998) uniquely possible for (caste-privileged) women of the home, thus offering a politicization of the private feminine sphere. It is in this framework of politicization that the advice literature on childbirth, childcare, and home remedies of the late 19th and early 20th centuries, contained in magazines directed uniquely at women, may be seen. The magazines that explored home therapeutics also included exegeses on the making of the home, care of newborns and children, and prescriptions for acquiescence to the husband. I will now focus on the advice literature in magazines that forms a significant but as yet relatively underexplored domain within which indigenism finds a place.

The *Arogya-Jiwan* advertised itself as a monthly medical journal focusing on various Ayurvedic treatments and was published in Lucknow and later Allahabad in the 1890s. Another monthly publication was *Balabodhini*, which actively advertised itself as dear to women and was published in Hindi from 1874 until at least 1877. Both of these publications carried similar kinds of prescriptions – for pregnancy, childbirth, admonitions on the use of Tantric practices (seen as deviations from Vedanta or classical text-based practice), nutrition, and care of newborns – with the difference that *Balabodhini* appeared under the genre of the women's monthly magazine, and *Arogya-Jiwan*, while not explicitly stating its readership, devoted itself almost entirely to concerns around pregnancy, with a few scattered items around recipes. Serialized discussions around pregnancy care (*garbhadan chandrika*) that actually focus on fulfilling the sensate desires of the pregnant woman – be it music or a particular vista – are available in *Arogya Jiwan*. Desires are also evaluated for the effects they will have; thus, visions of well-being and beauty are expected to beget a *rupvaan putr* (a handsome son, October 1890, p. 43). This publication recalls very much the 'modern Ayurvedic text' that Mukharji refers to that we saw in Chapter 3. Other topics covered include *Streerog chikitsa* (treatment of the diseases of women), where '*mithya achar aur mithya vichar*' (impure thoughts and actions) invite *pitta* (bile) into the woman's sexual organs, giving rise to various diseases (November 1890, p. 57). *Balabodhini* is advertised as *streejanon ki pyari hindi bhasha se sudhari* (presented in Hindi, the beloved language of women), with a list of names of women glorified in the Hindu everyday – Sita, Anusuya, Sati, Arundhati – for propriety, docility, knowledge, and such values. It began publishing in 1874 in Kashi, continued until at least 1877, and focused on questions of care in pregnancy and childbirth. Mukharji's pointer to everyday technologies being referenced as a marker of Ayurvedic technomodernity can be seen here, in the casual insertions of references to pulse rates in adulthood and infancy. *Balabodhini* also focuses on the *sutika griha* or birthing room, and the care of the newborn, interspersed with articles on *saticharitra*, or what constitutes *dharma* for a woman – obedience to the husband, as indicated in the *Bhagavad Gita* (June 1874, p. 68).

An 1892 text titled *Garbharakshahidayatnama* (care during pregnancy/guidebook), written in narrative dialogic form and focusing on the value of having a trained *dai* for childbirth in the home, presents a different set of circumstances and tackles a series of stereotypes and myths – around the *dai*, the quack or '*nawaqif hakim*' (ignorant hakim), care during pregnancy, and practices of childbirth. Nutrition and hygiene are touched upon. More significantly, it takes on questions of son preference, caste discrimination, and community othering, thus setting itself apart from other texts of the time. The dialogic form of this text is to be seen in other texts of this time too. For instance, a woman-authored serialized text on *Sati Chitra* (delineation of a chaste woman) titled 'Grihini' of 1918, by one Srimati Subarna Prabha Som, published by the Majumdar Library, Chitpur, Kolkata (this library and others flourishes well into the 20th century). Interesting about this text, which has one section on pregnancy, childbirth, and care of the infant, amidst a whole set of sections on marriage, chaste behaviour of the woman, service of the husband, and household responsibilities, all couched in extremely moral language, is the fact of the dialogue being between Manoranjan and Mrinalini – presumably a Hindu man and woman based on their names – even in the sections on pregnancy, childbirth, breastfeeding, and so on.

Moitra suggests that this volume and kind of material is a feature of the print era that produces a community of women somewhat in continuity with the *antahpur* in 19th-century Bengal. While the print era brought with it other material from the Battala presses as well, including novels and erotic romance literature like *Bidya Sundar* – popularly derided for its non-respectability – this oral, sensual culture of reading and consuming, up until then fairly unique to women, supported by women vendors hawking these and a variety of other products to privileged caste homes, finds a somewhat uneasy companion in a fairly regulated genre of advice literature, and a more obvious complement in *gharoa chikitsa* (home remedies) texts – also addressed to the home, also generated in the street, but companionate to modern medicine and offering a new, advanced role to the women of the nation. While still unregulated, this genre, with its casual invocation of both the modern and the indigenous, offered to women of the home the unique opportunity to belong to the nation while belonging to the home, with a legitimacy afforded by the appearance in print of the many *totkas/nuskhas* ('simples' or medicinal herbs) that were otherwise being dismissed at best as old wives' tales, and at worst as regressive and harmful. A reorganization of the relationship between family and nation, then, is in evidence here, supported by new social ties being built between women of the *zenana/antahpur* and women of the outside. This form of belonging is more implicit than the far more strident figure of the middle-class woman who emerges as the agent of reform via both women's education and this culture of reading and writing in the early 20th century. We have seen, in the writing of Ramanna, the reference to the trajectory of several Indian medical women who also became active in organizations like the All-India Women's Conference or the Association of Medical Women of India. We see reflections of this voice in the magazines too, like *Bamabodhini* in Bengal or *Penmati Potini* in Tamil Nadu. It is this middle-class figure who becomes the face of politics for women in the nationalist and early post-independence periods as well, an impulse that we see as late as the *Towards Equality* report of 1974. Muthulakshmi Reddy's strident support of *devadasi* marriage as an exit from improper professions is a classic example of this impulse, and I have examined this in the previous chapter. Some impact of Dravidian nationalism is also evident in demands for women's equality within and outside of marriage.

Women of the nation as home healers: *gharoa chikitsa*

As mentioned above, a genre of non-recurring publications on *griha* or *gharoa chikitsa*, mostly individually undated, were available from about the late 1800s, with 1867 being the year the Press and Registration Act was passed, so that all publications had to mandatorily be registered in catalogues from then on. Some of the dated publications are from the first two decades of the 20th century. These range from short pamphlets to several hundred pages, and names range from *Griha Chikitsa* (1905, Mathura) to *Grihini* (1918) to *Homeopathy Matanujayi Garhasthya Chikitsa Pranali* (1870); multiple titles often appear under these names, and they claim allegiance to Ayurveda, homeopathy, plant remedies, or *totka,* sometimes combining aspects of all three, and often borrowing from metaphors of biomedicine. Women of the home are constantly invoked in this literature written by men who retain epistemic authority. This material sits alongside a variety of other publications by *Kabirajes*, on *nadipariksha* (examination of pulse), etc., subaltern doctoring braided traditions that Mukharji speaks of (2016), but without an explicit conversation between them. Some of these publications seem almost exclusively directed towards women of the home, some to an unnamed audience presumably of the family. The 20th century sees a surfeit of smaller publications on *totka, gharoa chikitsa*, and so on. With the coming of colour prints, all the texts have illustrations of women of the family attending to the sick. A few of these also have men as addressees, particularly when speaking of *guptarog* (secret/taboo illness) – a familiar euphemism for sexually transmitted diseases presumably affecting men. Advertisements for the *guptarog* remedy in fact appear in women's magazines, as Berger notes, referring to a women's magazine, *Madhuri*, of 1940, where a product is advertised as a treatment for gonorrhoea. Berger suggests that morality is replaced with medicine in these ads, with a focus on the man's 'sexuality and virility' (2013, p. 101). I would suggest that this would more likely seem like another way in which it was the responsibility of the respectable and educated woman of the home to serve as the moral compass and 'save' her man, by redressing whatever follies he may have committed, and healing him as proof of her effectiveness as a wife. In that sense, addressing it as a medical condition was precisely the condition of putting aside, not erasing, moral judgement, but urging the devoted wife to take charge of his health for the sake of the family, strong children, and a strong nation. We see that while women were exhorted to take on the responsibility of the health of the family, via attention to hygiene, nutrition, and home economics in the women's magazines genre, the *griha chikitsa* publications also performed the function of familiarizing a lay public with the vocabulary, in addition to acting as reckoners for family physicians. These have continued into the present day. Here there is no debate on what is indigenous; rather there is a claim to what is accessible. Mukharji makes reference to some of this literature, as also to literary texts metaphorically evoked by these, suggesting that 'women who possessed the knowledge of the medical properties of wild herbs now come to use it in the service of ... male bourgeois heroes ... and [to] eventually be domesticated as obedient housewives, mothers and grandmothers' (2009, p. 207).

Following the arguments of Moitra, Arnold, and Mukharji, several movements around the 'indigenous' come to light in this literature. Mukharji speaks of the early Orientalists whose reference points were Sanskritic in accessing the East, and even of later botanists like Hodgson who 'had written of their access to the plants within a socio-cultural milieu' (Mukharji, 2009, p. 195), and were more committed, perhaps, to a cartographic naming of plants, while colonial botanists of a later time began to rely more on scientific classificatory naming and were influenced by tropes of contamination and confusion in the use of vernacular names. Mukharji speaks of the shifts in the work of O'Shaughnessy as he builds the Pharmacopoeia for India, and his preference for 'elite, learned collaborators as representatives of the indigenous botanical traditions' (p. 199). We also see, at this time, a shift from naming collaborators as equals to referring to native or plant collectors from among marginal castes, as Arnold points out. I have discussed, in Chapter 3, with respect to the meetings of the Indigenous Drugs Committee, the element of 'procurability' rather than nativeness that marked the meanings of 'indigenous' at this time when aspects of cost and commercial use had become clear players in the debate around drug procurement. Gyan Prakash and others speak of the hybridization of Western science in colonial contexts; Pratik Chakravarti explores the social history of Western science in India, tracing a movement from a metropolitan to a colonial to a national and then nationalist science. Mukharji explores the 'braiding' of, and perhaps resistance to, compartmentalized identities of colonial and indigenous sciences. For the purposes of my argument, it is useful to follow this movement to see how a selective realignment with elite collaborators in the therapeutic regimes emerging at this time results in what I would call the subalternization of the local practitioner, who can now be dismissed as deceitful. Parallely, with the symbolization of the privileged-caste woman of the home, and the recuperation and, in fact, centralization of this symbol powerfully within the discourse of nationhood, the 'mothers and grandmothers', as Mukharji indicates, become the torchbearers for home remedies, as a female *maternal* botanical tradition – powerful but supplementary. This tradition is not necessarily authored by these or other women, but they definitely carry the responsibility to 'know' it, and articulate it within the simpler world of the home while being a wisdom that can also be challenged within scientific traditions. There is, however, a more empathetic dynamic between this maternal botanical tradition and the institution of biomedicine, an empathy born of shared social locations and a vision of the nation, than the subaltern practitioner can hope for. *Jakhan daktar nei hather kache*, reads one of the *gharoa chikitsa* titles, translated as 'When the doctor is not readily available'; this is not a relationship of conflict or opposition. It is in this context, then, that we might read some of the texts on *gharoa chikitsa*.

We see here a fairly unregulated space – of braided, respected or otherwise, popular material – that stays in print almost till today. While most of this literature takes on some of the language of women's magazines in terms of exhortations to proper behaviours within family and so on, and speaks of home-based therapeutic work, it also offers space – in vocabulary and approach – to non-classical, non-elite practices of healing and pharmacy. Some of the content also refers to remedies preparable within the home, and at low cost, as also sometimes of greater efficacy than many '*mulyavaan davayiyaan*' – expensive drugs (*Gharelu chikitsa*, 1626, Allahabad). These medicines – *chune hue abhootpoorna vividh nuskhon ka apoorv sangrah* (a selected collection of various amazing hitherto unheard of remedies) – are, of course, proposed in the text after *anek suvikhyat daktar, tatha anubhavi stri-purush* (several well-known doctors, and experienced men and women) have endorsed their efficacy. While this text does not name an author, the ones in the 19th to 20th centuries are authored by different practitioners, and add the endorsement of ancient *rishis* (sages). Most stay within the domain of plant medicine, stressing their naturalness, and seek to fill a gap rather than replace or contest pharmaceuticals. Some of these celebrate a single species, indicating its multiple medicinal uses, for example, an undated series with titles on *Rog Arogye Batgach* (the value of the banyan in illness and health), or *Rog Arogye Pepe o narkel* (the value of papaya and coconut in illness and health); several of these are authored by men with the title of *Kabiraj*. Mukharji (2016) has written in some detail about the *Kobirajes* who produced texts in the period after the 1870s, detailing the preparation of *pachons* (digestives), *totkas* (simples), and so on, thus offering a glimpse into the braided traditions of this time. My concern is with the role and place of women in these traditions – as practitioners or as women outside the home – and with the manner and extent to which women were either considered able to mobilize these textual resources towards familial health, as also the ways in which the relationship of this mobilization with high indigenous traditions played out. While this aspect of my argument is largely conjectural, it is worth pursuing in the context of the overwhelming force of postcolonial scholarship that concerns itself with the nation and its women. This argument focuses almost entirely on the 'woman of home', in other words, the elite privileged-caste woman. While the space that was home to this woman might well have served as the space for racialized cultural difference to be established in the elite nationalist political vocabulary, this woman was also in touch with, following Moitra's argument, other women, and also had access to a variety of literature apart from the socialization available in ideal texts like *Sushila'r upakhyan*. It would seem, then, that therapeutic indigeneity was a very different order of beast, and while gendered, a more fragmented space, than the nationalist political creation of the indigenous as radically other. Are we then saying that there was a narrowing of this space via majoritarianism or regulation, or that this space has never really narrowed, but remained heterogeneous, if not syncretic?

Bottola medicine vis-à-vis gharoa chikitsa, or the messy indigenous therapeutic?

Following the recent explosion of academic interest in *Bottola* publications and their relationship with the domestic space in the late 19th and 20th centuries (Ghosh, 2008; Moitra, 2017; Sarkar, 1992; Chaudhuri, 1990; Biswas, 2000) in Bengal yield some further speculations on unregulated therapeutic practices during this time. If, alongside poor Muslims, immigrants to the city, the lower echelons of salaried employees, boatmen, and others, different classes of women, including those of the upper *bhadralok* or middle-class, had access to printed material through communitarian reading cultures and non-classical language forms, some of the therapeutic material generated in this print culture was bound to enter the domestic space via oppressed-caste women and other vendors, alongside popular material written and published by doctors. We find, in the lists of vernacular publications and *Bottola* books, references to a wide set of genres. Biswas (2000), putting together a collection of difficult-to-source *Bottola* publications, says, '*emon kono bishoy nei ja chilo bottolar kache ajana ... chikitsabidya ... sedik theke sadharon bangalir kache jeno ek kholamela bishyobidyaloy*' (p. 22, there was no issue unknown to or unexplored in the Bottola, including the science of therapeutics ... it was like a public university for the ordinary Bangali). This included *Panchalis* (narrative tracts in verse) on dengue, drains, and famines – in other words, natural disasters, administrative reform measures, and epidemics. While these were probably social commentaries, given what we know of other such tracts, there would surely be references to healing as well. *Gharoa chikitsa*, then, surely could not have retained a 'purely' privileged-caste flavour, while elite nationalist attempts to create a 'caste' indigenous therapeutics, in collaboration with the administration, on the grounds of 'upper' caste as the well of knowledge, were well in place.

Another space and set of practitioners who did not get spoken of in the postcolonial histories of medicine are street practitioners. Alavi highlights the role of *fakirs* as 'dispersed authority referents', not necessarily agents of 'anti-colonial political activism' (2008, p. 338). She also speaks of the creation of 'medically aware communities' in the mid-19th century via the proliferation in print of *materia medicas* in the vernacular, or of translated lists accompanied by *nuskhas* or prescriptions. Many of the purported authors of these texts were British medical men, where the refraction through translation that they did from Arabic or Hindustani was invisible. Extending from Alavi's arguments, the emergence of Hindustani or Hindevy as the preferred language of these texts would seem to have resulted in the emergence of a public sphere around this literature – that combined chemical jargon with recognizable lay processes. Alavi tellingly speaks of the standardization, the manner in which this writing 'transformed local knowledge through the laboratory to a form distinct from that of the habitat where it had been collected' (p. 140), and sees these processes as being consolidated in the growth of dispensaries and the consequent institutionalization of Western medicine. I am here, more interested in asking the question of street medicine, the place of this outside of this institutionalized therapeutic sphere, the porosity of this interface, and the relationship, if any, to the more fragmented versions of *gharoa* or *gharelu chikitsa* directed at women of the privileged-caste home. Explorations of modern Ayurveda have already suggested that these relationships were fraught, and the compartments not watertight, as Girija, in her exploration of the relationships between forms of *naattuvaidyam* and classical Ayurveda, suggests (2021). Through her and other scholars' work, including Berger and Mukharji, there is no real clarity on Ayurveda's hold over the public, although the idea of Hindu medicine did occupy a great deal of space in the discourse, and Ayurveda was seen as quite attached to institutionalized religion. Scholarship does speak of therapeutic practices like *chandshi* from the 18th century (Mukharji, 2012) and bone-setting in the present (Lambert, 2012) that have escaped codification, regulation, and active criminalization. My question, of the relationship of these with some of the fragmented texts around *gharoa chikitsa*, however, remains at the level of conjecture, until more materials come to light.

Trainability, educability – Ramabai and Ramabai

We return to the question of the possible caste division of occupations within the 'women working for women' frame. I approach this question through the distinct kinds of work towards women's emancipation performed by Pandita Ramabai and Ramabai Ranade in western India at the cusp of the 19th to 20th centuries. Both these experiments were directed at women outside of marriage and family; both had responses to the caste question. Both are being put in place once teacher training institutions, or what were called Normal schools, started across the subcontinent in 1885. One of these women is today revered in the mainstream; the other is considered historically significant but is received ambivalently otherwise.

The supply of widows

Educability and trainability were, during this period, well mapped onto the binary registers of knowledge and skill. If the upper-caste woman within the marital unit was educable, various women tied to the family unit but at its margins were trainable into care professions, and it is on this premise that we see the work of various institutions and homes for widows in the late 19th century. The British administration found, also, this constituency to be useful based on their own experience back home concerning the 'complications which the element of married women's work introduces into the labour market' (Cowan, 1912, p. 186). Widowed women were, therefore, an excellent choice of labour. Nursing was one such area of respectable work. We have seen, in the last chapter, the parleys for nursing training for widowed women of the Poona Seva Sadan. Vocational or skill training was seen to be a useful future for these women whose sexual and reproductive life had come to an end. We see, in the exhortations towards nursing as a service in women's magazines of the 1920s, a reference to the need for both intelligence and skill for good nursing. Given the accompanying discussion of the need for the right kind of woman for nursing as a service, this may be read also as a subtle reference to caste privilege and occupation, to delineate the profession as one of intelligence and empathy rather than 'mere physical drudgery' (Joshi, 1920, pp. 18–19). The call to the upper-caste woman is clear here, in the juxtaposition of mental and physical work – a gendered as well as caste-based dualism. This call finds an echo in the search for teachers too, where widows 'may with proper training and care become a main source of supply' (Cowan, 1912, p. 58), or where the physical travails involved in travelling 'many successive nights … in bullock carts, in trains, and on horseback to reach inaccessible parts' as teachers and inspectresses of schools are seen as 'hardly … work which a woman should do' (p. 95), and yet must be taken up by women, while 'retaining her Sita-like devotion and her gentle bearing' (p. 96). The symbol that Florence Nightingale had become, it would seem, was very much on the minds of this and other writers, along with what they chose to see as Indian women's contexts.

Pandita Ramabai's Sharada Sadan, started in 1892, is one of the most-referenced examples of homes for widows, who were given 'the opportunity of a self-supporting, self-respecting life, and a vision of … self-sacrifice' (Cowan, p. 181). It is useful, at this point, to examine Pandita Ramabai's own context and motivations in setting up this institution. With her declaration, in her 1888 tract *The High-Caste Hindu Woman*, of the life and plight of the upper-caste woman through life, and in particular when widowed, the Pandita, highly educated herself but primarily through the informal labours of her parents, stood tall in calling out both casteism and the hypocrisy and corruption of Brahmin priests in laying down principles of morality for the rest. Ramabai's prescription for bringing widows back into the mainstream of social life drove her impulse to educate and train them into self-reliance. For this to be achieved, Ramabai pushed for native women teachers as a starting point. Re-marriage is not, for Ramabai, the one panacea for widows, unlike the position taken by male reformers in this time. Her particular concern is for the high-caste Hindu woman, and in challenging the shackles of caste norms that keep this woman within the system of marriage and family. While she proposes education for the woman in marriage, she is able to find, in the constituency of high-caste widows, both willingness and an opportunity to come out of the terrible conditions of their singleness via self-reliance, and laments the absence of institutions that can train them to 'be independent of their relatives and make an honest living for themselves' (Ramabai, 1901, p. 133). The high-caste woman is, in Ramabai's arguments, doomed to remain a 'virgin widow' despite all the reform talk of re-marriage, and therefore one of the worst victims of Brahmanical patriarchy. This widow, in the missionary institutions already functioning at that time, is neither able to maintain caste lines nor resist the pressure to convert, and therefore, in what seems like a contradiction to her views on caste as an oppressive institution, but what may have been her backing down from a direct challenge to the same, the Pandita suggests that '[h]ouses should be opened for the young and high-caste child widows where they can take shelter without the fear of losing their caste, or being disturbed in their religious belief' (p. 137) and, in 'order to help them make an honorable and independent living, they should be taught in these houses to be teachers, governesses, nurses and housekeepers … and other forms of hand-work, according to their taste and capacity' (ibid, pp. 137–138). Such an institution is also, therefore, best achieved by finding 'women-teachers for the Hindu zenanas' (p. 134). The Pandita also makes moving recommendations before the Hunter Commission in this regard. The Sharada Sadan, opened by her in 1889, is a step in this direction. As she speaks further of the content of the education in these institutions, one also catches a glimpse of 'womanly' education at par with that being prescribed for women within marriage. Later, in 1895, Ramabai opens the Mukti Mission, a more evangelical Christian organization, where her ambivalences regarding conversion as salvation for the upper-caste Hindu woman appear, but the impulse towards education and training remain the same. Ramabai, a figure who could neither be accepted nor ignored in the reformers' pantheon, positioned as she was from the perspective of the *zenana* woman they all sought to save, and a critical reader of canonical Hindu texts, separated, as did many other women of the time, Hindu nationalism and female autonomy, and called for active societal and public space for those whom other reformers were happy to treat as *purdanashin*.

The Pandita's efforts, both in Sharada Sadan and the later, more controversial Mukti Mission at Kedgaon, were met with much criticism on account of her own conversion and her relationship with Christian evangelism. It is in the form of this criticism, and its authors, that we see Ramabai Ranade's resistance following her husband's resignation from the board of the Sadan. Ramabai Ranade, the Pandita's contemporary and cherished acquaintance, helped run, since 1909, the Bombay and then Poona Seva Sadan, which actively worked towards educating and training Hindu widows in nursing, among other professions. Along with D.D. Karve's Home for Widows set up in 1896, that later evolved into the first women's university in India, the Sadan's success 'hinged upon … ideological adherence to women's essentialized wife-mother roles, in an inversion – or subversion – of the Pandita's insistence on women's self-reliance implicitly predicated upon gender equality' (Kosambi, 2000, p. 440). These were institutions that, alongside the iconization of educated upper-caste Hindu women in that time, served as a foil to the ideals of self-reliance and autonomy that the Pandita had stressed. These institutions, and the training they offered, were more in the manner of self-denial – an acceptable trope for the widow of the upper-caste household. They offered a patriarchal exit route without disturbing institutions of marriage and family, indeed offering a way out for the male reformers who had rashly proposed widow remarriage prior to this.

Were the widows to actually taste freedom through employment? Various conservative elements took charge of making sure that Indian women were not 'de-nationalized' through education, and one route this took was through the training of teachers. The Arya Samaj was one of the organizations that took this line, with a teacher training school in Dehradun, apart from its many girls' schools across the country. The other was Annie Besant's school for Indian girls in Benares, unfunded by the Government, that, in 'connexion with the Hindu Central College, ... pose[d] as a definite revolt from the anglicizing tendency of Government and mission schools' (Cowan, p. 133). The students seemed to be 'almost all of the Brahman caste, [and it was supposed that] ... here one might find a solution of the curriculum problem and a constructive theory of Indian education ... [with] the teachers ... free to saturate the instruction throughout with the ethical elements of a religion acceptable to the parents' (ibid, p. 134). This school and this form of education seemed to continue for some young married women too, and it is here that the complementarity argument of education for women was to be realized. As Cowan notes, however, this was more a case of exclusive access to modern education for upper-caste Indian girls than a nationalist Indianization – a practice that complicates, or at any rate particularizes, Chatterjee's claim of the home and the world, to the more elite and upper-caste women.

The use to which young 'parda-nashin' widowed women – upper-caste women, in other words – could be put was, however, fraught with obstacles. Speaking of Bengal, Cowan notes that, despite having been through some schooling prior to marriage, followed by a period of marriage and widowhood, 'their brains have remained fallow for six years and the problem of their training is a difficult one' (Cowan, 1912, p. 154). These obstacles are fewer in the case of Brahmo Samaj women, and even fewer with Christian women who constitute the bulk of teachers, who are to teach in the vernacular. Cowan notes about Bombay that 'at first the girls of the lower castes went, as they still go in many villages, to the boys' schools; in other places separate schools gradually sprang up wherever there were enlightened Indian members of the Municipalities to welcome the official suggestion' (p. 182). The government role remained largely in coordinating and directing, as regards girls' schools.

If trainability was the feature of the marginal woman who could still be useful to the family unit, it was also a placeholder for skill training for those who were not, by caste location, naturalized occupants of knowledge communities. There is scholarship on the *Ekalavya* destiny of young men of underprivileged castes, who were disallowed entry into the portals of higher education. For women, the training in care vocations following missionary school education became a model, albeit one not actively spelled out; they could now *naturally* occupy the domain of care and skill. The Report of the Education Commission notes that despite experiments to train Vaishnavite women as teachers, based on a history of them being a strong presence in the Bengal *zenanas* at the turn of the century, the 'only native women who can be induced to regard teaching as a profession ... seem to be native Christians; the wives of schoolmasters ... and, under certain conditions, widows' (1882, p. 538). The last-mentioned constituency begins to become visible over time, with the report itself citing the example of the Female Training College at Ahmedabad. A few years down the line, the

> sources of supply for teachers in Indian schools of all grades are women from English-speaking countries, Anglo-Indians or "country born" English girls from the Hill schools, members of the Brahma and Arya Samaj, Indian Christians, Parsis, married women of some education from the Hindu non-Brahman community and lastly "women who have learnt to read and write at home".
>
> (Cowan, 1912, p. 57)

In a diverse, under-prioritized, and chaotic pool, then, the non-Brahman Hindu woman, presumably still of a privileged caste, too finds a place.

The Isabella Thoburn College in Lucknow, which supplied teachers across North India, was primarily attended by Christian girls, although it had hostel provisions for Hindu and Muslim students as well. It followed the government code for its curriculum; therefore, Indianized teaching was not an option, unlike some other missionary schools that attempted – what was called 'an experimental attempt to give some conception of the Hindu environment of religious thought to the students' (Cowan, p. 139). The principle of earn and learn was also in place in some schools, with lace-making being one of the skills put to use in exchange for learning English; this was seen as a better route than mandatory English education, which could be a route to denationalizing. In the lament about poor educational conditions for women in reports of the 1890s to the early 1900s, the problem is put on the schoolmistresses. Cowan, for instance, notes that 'the majority of students in training are lower-caste Hindus' (p. 185); it is unclear whether this translated into casteist pedagogic practices that undervalued these students.

Conclusion

I have attempted, in this chapter, to delineate the layered character of the discourse around women's education and responsibility for nation-building in the 19th to 20th centuries, and the place and role of the Indian medical woman in this discourse. I have attempted to trace a parallel history of caste and gender segregation alongside racial segregation, participated in by both colonial administrators and

elite nationalist reformers. The organization of institutions follows this segregation, although it is never complete, and through this, I trace a certain biopolitics
of pregnancy and motherhood, a therapeutic vocabulary that is enmeshed with
these segregations. In tracing the tenuous connections between these segregations
and an emerging disaggregated indigenous, I mark sites like the privileged-caste
home that become the centre of the nation, and of the dominant indigenous. Yet,
the boundary work on the epistemo-political category of the indigenous remains
incomplete as well. Outside of this space, those outside of privileged marriage and
family are denied knowledge but encouraged towards skill building. We see, then,
extensions of caste-based therapeutic occupations available to both oppressed and
privileged communities of women.

Notes

1 A term introduced into popular usage by Gandhi, as his way of repatriating those considered untouchable in caste-ridden societies. Harijan literally means 'people of/dear to
Hari', Hari being one of the many names of the god Vishnu of the Hindu trinity. The
term has been sharply criticized for its ascribed character, and the failure of 'Gandhi and
the upper castes … [to] genuinely integrate the Harijan category into their consciousness
despite its divine association. Thus, this term lacks discursive capacity' (Guru, 2004, pp.
260–261).

2 Ghosh writes of the history of emergence and flourishing of the Battala presses, that
emerged in the northern parts of Calcutta, as different from an earlier time when other
presses had been concentrated in the Tank Square area of the city, referred to in some
scholarship as the 'White Town'. By the latter half of the 19th century, with the printing
hub shifting to the Black Town, and 'native entrepreneurs … [from] a displaced scribal
population from the higher Brahmin and Kayastha castes, who had made their way to
the commercial centre of Calcutta for better opportunities, in the 1850s and 1860s, these
[newer print entrepreneurs] were mostly men from lower-caste groups such as smiths
and artisans … Bengal Library Reports from 1867 onwards, show that men from non-
scribal lower castes were prominent in the business' (Ghosh, 2006, p. 122).

3 Titled, tellingly, 'Himself', as it details her life in the marital home, always in reference
to her celebrated social reformer and judge husband, but also in the shadow of the older
women of the family.

4 The act of silent, solitary reading of that modern evil – the newspaper – as opposed to
the communal listening to, or reading aloud of, a religious text or primer.

5 'Purdah girls arrived at school in closed carriages and horse-drawn buses, which were
provided by the pathshala to be instructed about 'the strict observance of Shastric
injunctions in matters of domestic life and about patibrata dharma, devotion to their
future husbands' (Engels, 1999, p. 167, quoted in Chanana, 2001, p. 49).

6 Whether this is in the interest of 'nationalizing' or retaining racial and national hierarchies, is the question.

7 'Phule in the first modern Marathi Play *Trutiya Ratna* draws complex linkages between
religious-cultural and educational authority' (Rege, 2010, p. 93).

8 The history of these two strategies is unconfirmed, but one of the origin stories is that
of a call given by Rabindranath Tagore, celebrated Bengali Indian poet and Nobel
Laureate, to mourn and protest October 16, the day the partition of Bengal took effect.
Arandhan and *Raksha bandhan* were apparently ceremonies performed on the day to
mark this (Das, 2016).

References

Books and articles

Alavi, S. (2008). *Islam and healing: Loss and recovery of an Indo-Muslim medical tradition, 1600–1900.* London: Palgrave Macmillan.
Anandhi, S. (1991, May–June). Women's question in the dravidian movement c. 1925–1948. *Social Scientist, 19*(5/6), 24–41.
Anandhi, S. (2008). *The Manifesto and the modern self reading the autobiography of Muthulakshmi reddy* (MIDS Working Paper no. 204). Madras: Madras Institute of Development Studies.
Arunima, G. (1996). Multiple meanings: Changing conceptions of matrilineal kinship in nineteenth-and twentieth-century Malabar. *The Indian Economic & Social History Review, 33*(3), 283–307.
Bagchi, J. (1993, October 9). Socialising the girl child in colonial Bengal. *Economic and Political Weekly, 28*(41), 2214–2219.
Bandyopadhyay, S. (1994, January–February). Producing and re-producing the new women: A note on the prefix 'Re'. *Social Scientist, 22*(1/2), 19–39.
Basu, A. (2005). A century and a Half's Journey: Women's education in India, 1850s to 2000. In B. Ray (Ed.), *Women of India: Colonial and post-colonial periods, history of science, philosophy and culture in Indian civilization (general editor Chattopadhyaya, D. P.)* (Vol. IX, Part 3, pp. 183–207). New Delhi: Centre for Studies in Civilizations.
Berger, R. (2013). *Ayurveda made modern: Political histories of indigenous medicine in Northern India, 1900–1955.* New York: Palgrave Macmillan.
Biswas, A. (Ed.). (2000). *Bottolar boi: 20 scarce books from the 19th century.* Kolkata: Gangchil.
Burton, A. (1996). Contesting the zenana: The mission to make "lady doctors for India," 1874–1885. *Journal of British Studies, 35*(3), 368–397.
Chakravarti, U. (1989) Whatever happened to the Vedic Dasi? Orientalism, nationalism and a script for the past. In K. Sangari & S. Vaid (Eds.), *Recasting women: Essays in colonial history* (pp. 27–87). New Brunswick, NJ: Rutgers University Press.
Chakravarti, U. (1993, April 3). Conceptualising brahmanical patriarchy in early India: Gender, caste, class and state. *Economic and Political Weekly, 28*(14) 579–585.
Chanana, K. (2001). Hinduism and female sexuality: Social control and education of girls in India. *Sociological Bulletin, 50*(1), 37–63.
Chatterjee, P. (1989). The nationalist resolution of the women's question. In K. Sangari & S. Vaid (Eds.), *Recasting women: Essays in Indian colonial history* (pp. 233–253). New Delhi: Zubaan (Kali for Women).
Chatterjee, P. (2019). Women and nation revisited. In P. Ray (Ed.), *Women speak nation* (pp. 19–28). New Delhi: Routledge.
Chaudhuri, S. (Ed.) (1990). *Calcutta, the living city: The past.* India: Oxford University Press.
Das, S. K. (2016). *Contai Massin the Swadeshi movement (1905–1911).* Karatoya: North Bengal University.
Desai, M., & Roy, R. (2022). Intersectional coloniality in 19th century India: The sociological praxis of Savitribai Phule and the women activists of Satya Shodhak Samaj (Truth Seeker Society). *The American Sociologist, 53*(3), 395–413.
Engels, D. (1999). Beyond purdah? Women in Bengal 1890–-1930. New Delhi: Oxford, Paperbacks.
Forbes, G. H. (1994). Medical careers and health care for Indian women: Patterns of control. *Women's History Review, 3*(4), 515–530.
Forbes, G. H. (1999). *Women in modern India* (Vol. 2). Cambridge: Cambridge University press.
Forbes, G. H. (2005). *Women in Colonial India: Essays on politics, medicine, and historiography.* New Delhi: DC Publishers.

Ghosh, A. (2002, October 19–25). Revisiting the 'Bengal Renaissance': Literary Bengali and low-life print in Colonial Calcutta. *Economic and Political Weekly, 37*(42), 4329–4338.

Ghosh, A. (2006). *Power in print: Popular publishing and the politics of language and culture in a colonial society, 1778–1905*. New Delhi: Oxford University Press.

Ghosh, A. (2008). The many worlds of the vernacular book: Performance, literacy and print in Colonial Bengal. In R. Fraser & M. Hammond (Eds.), *Books without borders. v. 2. Perspectives from South Asia* (1st ed., pp. 34–57). Hampshire and New York: Palgrave Macmillan Ltd.

Girija, K. P. (2021). *Mapping the history of Ayurveda: Culture, hegemony and the rhetoric of diversity*. London and New York: Routledge.

Guru, G. (2004). The language of Dalitbahujan political discourse. In Ghanshyam Shah (Ed.), *Dalit identity and politics*, pp. 97–107. New Delhi: Sage Publications.

Hancock, M. (2001, October). Home science and the nationalization of domesticity in colonial India. *Modern Asian Studies, 35*(4), 871–903.

Hoggan, F. (1882). *Medical women for India. By Frances Elizabeth Hoggan, M.D.*

Kamatchi, M. (2016, January). Muthulakshmi Reddy: The first medical woman professional in South India. In *Proceedings of the Indian history congress* (Vol. 77, pp. 612–623). Indian History Congress.

Karlekar, M. (1986, April 26). Kadambini and the Bhadralok: Early debates over women's education in Bengal. *Economic and Political Weekly, 21*(17). WS25–WS31.

Kosambi, M. (2000). A window in the prison-house: Women's education and the politics of social reform in nineteenth century western India. *History of Education, 29*(5), 429–442.

Kosambi, M. (2016). *Pandita Ramabai: Life and landmark writings*. Oxon and New York: Routledge.

Lahiri, P. (1998, January). Womens' magazines In Bengal, 1905–11. In *Proceedings of the Indian history congress* (Vol. 59, pp. 665–675). Indian History Congress.

Lambert, H. (2012). Wrestling with tradition: Towards a subaltern therapeutics of bonesetting and vessel treatment in north India. In D. Hardiman & P. B. Mukharji (Eds.), *Medical Marginality in South Asia: Situating subaltern therapeutics* (pp. 109–125). London and New York: Routledge.

Lal, M. (2006). Purdah as pathology: Gender and the circulation of medical knowledge in late Colonial India. In S. Hodges (Ed.), *Reproductive health in India: History, politics, controversies* (pp. 85–114). New Delhi: Orient Blackswan.

Lal, R. (2008). Recasting the women's question: The girl-child/woman in the colonial encounter. *Interventions, 10*(3), 321–339.

Mani, L. (1987). Contentious traditions: The debate on sati in colonial India. *Cultural Critique, 7*, 119–156.

Mohanty, C. T., Russo, A., & Torres, L. (Eds.). (1991). *Third world women and the politics of feminism* (Vol. 632). Bloomington and Indianopolis: Indiana University Press.

Moitra, S. (2017). Reading together: "Communitarian reading" and women readers in Colonial Bengal. *Hypatia, 32*(3), 627–643.

Mukharji, P. B. (2009). *Nationalizing the body: The medical market, print and Daktari medicine*. London and New York: Anthem Press.

Mukharji, P. B. (2012). Chandhir Chikitsha: A nomadology of subaltern medicine. In D. Hardiman & P. B. Mukharji (Eds.), *Medical marginality in South Asia: Situating subaltern therapeutics* (pp. 109–125). London and New York: Routledge.

Mukharji, P. B. (2016). *Doctoring traditions: Ayurveda, small technologies, and braided sciences*. Chicago: University of Chicago Press

Nair, J. (1990). Uncovering the Zenana: Visions of Indian womanhood in Englishwomen's writings, 1813–1940. *Journal of Women's History, 2*(1), 8–34.

Paik, S. (2016). Forging a new dalit womanhood in colonial Western India: Discourse on modernity, rights, education, and emancipation. *Journal of Women's History, 28*(4), 14–40.

Rajan, R. S., & Park, Y. M. (2000). Postcolonial feminism/postcolonialism and feminism. *A Companion to Postcolonial Studies, 1,* 53–71.

Ranade, R. (1938). *Himself: The autobiography of a Hindu lady* (transl. and adapted K. V. A. Gates). New York and Toronto: Longmans, Green & Co.

Rege, S. (2010, October 30–November 12). Education as" Trutiya Ratna": Towards Phule - Ambedkarite feminist pedagogical practice. *Economic and Political Weekly, 45*(44/45), 88–98.

Sarkar, S. (1992, July 18). 'Kaliyuga','chakri 'and 'bhakti': Ramakrishna and his times. *Economic and Political Weekly, 27*(29), 1543–1566.

Sen, K. (2004). Lessons in self-fashioning:" Bamabodhini Patrika" and the education of women in Colonial Bengal. *Victorian Periodicals Review, 37*(2), 176–191.

Sinha, M. (2000). Refashioning Mother India: Feminism and nationalism in late-colonial India. *Feminist Studies, 26*(3), 623–644.

Srinivas, M. N. (1956). A note on Sanskritization and Westernization. *The Journal of Asian Studies, 15*(4), 481–496.

Sreenivas, M. (2003). Emotion, identity, and the female subject: Tamil women's magazines in colonial India, 1890–1940. *Journal of Women's History, 14*(4), 59–82.

Thirumali, I. (2005). *Marriage, love and caste: Perceptions on Telugu women during the colonial period.* New Delhi: Bibliophile South Asia.

From Internet Archive

Johnston, J. (1884). *Abstract and analysis of the report of the Indian education commission.* London: Hamilton, Adams & Co. Central Secretariat Library, Government of India. Source URL: http://192.168.1.42:8080//handle/123456789/6551

Mitchell, K. (1892). *The gentlewoman's book of Hygiene* (Victoria Library for Gentlewomen) (W. H. Davenport, Ed.). Digital Library of India. https://archive.org/details/dli.granth.84817/page/n3/mode/2up

Ramabai, S. (1901). *The high-caste Hindu woman.* New York and Chicago: Fleming H. Revell Company. Digitized from the library of Harvard University.

Reddy, S. (1930). *My experience as a legislator.* Madras: Current Thought Press. http://www.new.dli.ernet.in/handle/2015/102742

Bengali texts –

Mukhopadhyay, M. (1859). *Sushila'r Upakhyan* (Vol 1). Digital Library of India http://www.new.dli.ernet.in/handle/2015/289169

Som, S.P. (1918). *Grihini.* Digital Library of India. http://www.new.dli.ernet.in/handle/2015/324329

From Wellcome Trust Library, London

Balfour, M., & Young, R. (1929). *The work of medical women in India, with a foreword by Dame Mary Scharlieb.* (PP/MIB/C/3. Part of: Margaret Ida Balfour, CBE, MD, CM, FRCOG (1866–1945)). Archives and manuscripts. London, New York, Toronto, Melbourne, Bombay, Calcutta, Madras: Oxford University Press.

Campbell, G. J. (1918). In Victoria Memorial Scholarships Fund. (1918). *Improvement of the conditions of childbirth in India: including a special report on the work of the Victoria Memorial Scholarships Fund during the past fifteen years and papers written by medical women and qualified midwives.* (Closed stores K45291). Calcutta: Superintendent Government Printing.

Cowan, M. G. (1912). *The education of the women of India.* (b28068634. Persistent URL: https://wellcomelibrary.org/item/b28068634. Catalogue record: https://search .wellcomelibrary.org/iii/encore/record/C__Rb2806863. Closed stores K43836). Edinburgh and London: Oliphant, Anderson & Ferrier.

From British Library, London

Balabodhini. (May–September 1874, July, August 1876, January 1877). Kashi. Sri Harishchandra Press.
Joshi, M. M. (1920, August 1). Ideals of Indian women. In R. E. Reuben (Ed.), *Hind Mahila (The Indian Woman), 1* (pp. 5–11). (P.P.1122.m.). Bombay: The Udyan Press.
Manibhai Jasbhai. (1896). *A Memorandum on Hindu female education in the Bombay presidency.* (V 9099). Bombay: Bombay Gazette Steam Printing Works, Fort.
The Arogya-Jiwan: A Monthly Medical Journal. (July 1890). Vol. 2 (1). Lucknow. India Office Library. (August 1890). Vol. 2 (2).
September 1890. Vol 2 (3).
October 1890. Vol 2 (4).
November 1890. Vol 2 (5).
December 1890. Vol 2 (6).
January 1891. Vol 2 (7).
February 1891. Vol 2 (8).
March 1891. Vol 2 (9).
April, May and June 1893. Vol 2 (10, 11, 12).
Rukhmabai. (1929). Purdah. In E. Gedge & M. Choksi (Eds.), *Women in modern India. Fifteen papers by Indian women writers* (Asia Pacific & Africa T 10740, General Reference Collection 08416.bb.47., UIN: BLL01001382286). Bombay: Missionary Settlement for University Women.

6 Indigenous therapeutics in the present, the recalibration of the expert domain, and the place of the *dai*

Introduction

In the marking of *dais* as unfavoured practitioners in the battle for control over privileged-caste women's bodies and lives, post-independence India policy continued to attempt to train and mobilize them into primary care. The Health Survey and Development (Bhore) committee report of 1946, (popularly known as the Bhore committee report) with its emphasis on primary healthcare and preventive health work, and continuing in the earlier vein of frustration at the inadequacy of maternal health services in India, recommends the continued 'utilization of the service of the hereditary class' (Bhore Committee 1946, vol. I, p. 171) of *dais* till such time as modern medical systems are available for all, and insists on four trained *dais* to be attached to each Primary Health Centre as a short-term measure before the long-term primary health care programme could be put in place.[1] The Mudaliar committee, in 1961, notes the prejudice against new and modern systems, and thus advocates the training and continuing use of *trained dais till trained midwives* can replace them. The Population Policy draft of 2000 speaks of using the services of the *dai* 'to fill in gaps in manpower at village levels' (p. 33). Mira Sadgopal speaks of the *dai* now having been reduced to the role of a link worker (2009), with a devaluing of her knowledge or the knowledge model she represents. While this history and policy perspective is well-charted, the continued re-calibration of the indigenous within this discourse, the active codification visible in, for instance, exercises like the Ministry of Ayurveda, Yoga and Naturopathy, Unani, Siddha, and Homoeopathy that was set up in 2014, with earlier iterations since 1995, that are not only visible as standardization procedures but also a re-invention of tradition and the nation in what I call a continuing engagement with the idea of expertise, is what this concluding chapter is concerned with. I would suggest that this re-calibrated indigenous, situated in a time of hypernationalism and epistemic consolidation of caste hierarchies in the present, also fashions itself as an expert domain; and to that end, marks its outside as inexpert. This outside space remains a collection of older and newer categories that can now be rendered flatter and homogenous;[2] here, the *dai* is actually the abject of the 'caste' nation while the others – like the *anganwadi* worker, or the accredited social health activist – are unskilled but trained outposts of the state.

DOI: 10.4324/9780367824051-6

The emergence of a dominant indigenous

We have seen in Chapter 3, in the voices of popular and celebrated Indian male doctors in the late 19th and early 20th centuries, the lament around the high mortality among women and infants in childbirth, and the consequent loss of potential warriors to the nation and race, sometimes referenced as Aryan, sometimes Hindu. Somewhere along the line, this lament also becomes about the loss of indigenous traditions that have been allowed to die at the altar of a self-degrading national community. This rhetoric also engages with the need to bring an engagement between modern medical practice and these traditions. In postcolonial literature, this question of the indigenous is not presented in so many words, but it does come back in the form of difference and resistance. Via frameworks of hybridity to examine imperialist, colonial, and Orientalist impulses, postcolonial scholars and critiques of colonial science have spoken of the manner in which nationalists attempted to reiterate rather than return to the idea of an ancient past, thus accessing difference via anteriority rather than origin. I have, in Chapter 2, examined the encounter framework and how it hosts this question of difference, and the manner in which more recent histories of colonial medicine and empire critically revisit this idea of an encounter between pre-existing systems. Mukharji, for example, in his exploration of *daktari* medicine, and elsewhere in exploring *Chandshi chikitsa*, speaks of the impossibility of tracing either a linear history or a coherent singular account of a tradition or system or a practitioner lineage, rather, suggesting a rhizomatic understanding, following Deleuze and Guattari (1987) . Helen Lambert, too, traces groups of practitioners who study pulse or fix bones in Rajasthan, to argue that there is not here a coherent system to be 'found' that can be called medicine, and that this is the precise condition of its survival through imperial and later regulatory practices (2013).

What implications does this have for the majoritarian articulation of the indigenous today? How have these origin stories been presented? How does the 'staging' of encounter operate in contemporary self-descriptions, and relate to its 'Other' in collaboratively extruding some actors? I will, in this section, briefly go over some of the histories with reference to the material I have covered in previous chapters, particularly in late colonial contexts, and thereafter go into contemporary healthcare in order to understand some of the continuities.

The unparallel histories of Unani and Ayurveda

Rachel Berger (2013) speaks of the emergence of Ayurveda post the Montague-Chelmsford reforms of 1919 as a significant therapeutic domain that was ready to be appropriated into systems of regulation, and in post-independent India as 'a universal, "national" medical tradition, properly modernized and fit to be governed, while Unani was marginalized from state planning and cast off as the cultural practice of a minority community' (p. 4). While this articulation leaves something to be desired about the shared histories of constitution of Ayurveda or Unani, Berger helps us understand the complex local socio-political and developmental terrain within which this domain emerges as a significant player within healthcare delivery and policy. I am more interested in the *production* of the subaltern as abject and the canonical indigenous as norm, via these exercises, and to that end, Berger's and other scholarship around Ayurveda and Unani histories is useful.

Berger, like other scholars, presents Ayurveda as a moving rather than static entity, as also one whose historical trajectories within the national imaginary are determined more by local biopolitical impulses than a grand or cohesive nationalist push. Tracing this local biopolitics via the Montague-Chelmsford reforms of 1919, the dyarchy and the delegation of health within the provincial domain in the 1930s, the emergence of print technologies, and the Hindi and Bengali public spheres, Berger reads the history of Ayurveda within 'the political possibilities of Indian governance outside imperial determination' (Berger 2013, p. 6). In so doing, Berger makes a strong case for a conversation between public health agendas, Ayurveda, and, on the cusp of independence, rural development, and aligns with the work of Arnold (1993), Harrison and Pati (2009), Sivaramakrishnan (2006), and Alavi (2008), who, in different ways, suggest the impact of and exchange between public health agendas, social contexts, and practitioners. This position, Berger suggests, challenges the 'enclavist' argument of indigenous practice having persisted in silos during the colonial period (Ramasubban 2022). By introducing the crucial period of the early to mid-20th century into the history of Ayurveda, Berger both opens up the apparent homogeneity of the colonial period and medicine and marks significant moments in the history of what appears today as a coherent system. The idea of the encounter, of course, is also challenged in this historical tracing. Berger is ultimately interested, however, not in the systems debate, but in 'the ways in which systematization was imposed upon Ayurveda as a way of easing its coherent entry into formal politics' (p. 36). Berger also makes a strong case for the nationalist imagination of Ayurveda as a rational space that then makes a claim to modernity. As an impact of dyarchy, Berger sees 'entrenched and expanded separate electorates for Muslims, landlords, and scheduled caste candidates, thus recasting the political process as one that would be representative of the community and not the nation' (p. 108), and the 'sharper lines between vaids and hakims' that grow in the 20s–30s. For my purposes, it is in this making of modern Ayurveda, rather than Ayurveda made modern, that the emergence of the canonical indigenous may be found. To that end, dyarchy may be, as Legg puts it, 'effects of reference rather than structures or frames' (Legg paraphrased in Berger p. 111, Legg 2009, 2016), and it may be useful to think through multiple and uneven axes of power rather than the local/provincial being more important or influential than the national, but that is somewhat beyond the scope of this discussion.

Reading Seema Alavi's (2008) detailed social history of Unani within the context of empires and ethos, from the pre-colonial to the colonial, provides a counterpoint to Berger's account of Ayurveda, although the periodizations are different, as are the lenses somewhat. While speaking of the ultimate Islamization and marginalization of Unani in India, Alavi, like Berger, is clear that the claims in earlier histories of the 19th century that saw the colonial state as all-powerful and native populations as entirely marginalized, do not hold. Alavi is interested in tracing a different modernity, professionalization, and most importantly, in tracing the role and hold of earlier elites in the many changes in Unani's history.

The interesting distinction between these histories is the origin claims of each. While Unani claimed a national particularity and suitability to the people and climate (*ab-o-hawa*) as different from colonial medicine, this did not, Alavi suggests, take the route of a 'narrow anti-colonial territorial nationalism' (Alavi 2008, p. 292). Rather, Islamic universalism and Indian Muslim communitarianism provided additional reference points that emerged through Unani's history in the 18th century and later, as reflected in the shift from Persian to Arabic as the language of medical texts, references to Prophetic medicine, and cultural referents like Sufi healing and astrology, resulting in Unani attempting to claim a global civilizational origin and history. Ayurveda, on the other hand, in its modern making, was claiming the very anti-colonial territorial nationalism rejected by Unani, while seeking to lay claim, in its more fundamentalist avatar, to *akhand bharat* – the undivided nation – as the spatial source of multiple knowledges, including medicine.

Both these traditions of healing, then, challenge the idea of the absolute power of the colonial state. While one claims territorial origin through undivided extension, the other claims civilizational connection, not continuity. Berger has tentatively explored the context of colonial political reform that also carves native populations into recognizably different categories and indicated how, with the coming of separate electorates and the political fallouts of this, communities of belonging separate more sharply. Following Berger, as we look at the accompanying demands of modern knowledge classificatory impulses, and the sharing of power between the traditional elites and colonial administrators, a collaborative relabelling of Unani, from being seen as an equal stakeholder, to an esoteric, immobile, dogmatic set of practices, may be seen to have begun in the middle and late colonial periods. The Islamization of Unani, rather than a matter of seeking a civilizational connection, was perhaps now read as a fundamentalist exercise, to be rejected in favour of both a secular and an undivided nation.

It may be useful here to recall the debates and conflicts within the Indigenous Drugs Committee in the early 1900s and the parliamentary debates around the same that have been explored in Chapter 3. The question of what constituted the 'indigenous' remained a source of conflict here, with Sir George Watt, pharmacologist, member of the Indigenous Drugs Committee, and Reporter on Economic Products to the GOI, insisting on 'indigenous' being defined as also produced in India rather than native to or only available here; Kanai Lall Dey, also a member of the Indigenous Drugs Committee, and others were regularly overridden on these and other aspects of the therapeutic value of medicinal plants native to Indian soil. Interlocutors like Pandit Madan Mohan Malaviya, founder of the Akhil Bharatiya Hindu Mahasabha that broke away from the Congress, kept bringing the issue back to Parliament, speaking of the value and need for education in indigenous medicine. This translation of Ayurveda into the political sphere as a representative of native political ambitions for self-governance, which Berger too speaks of, is a translation that does not seem to happen as powerfully in the space of Unani. While there is, as Alavi suggests, patronage by royal elites who become welfare managers for the colonial administration, and the persistence of Unani as an ethos and way of life well after the loss of Mughal patronage, as well as its travel into popular Urdu texts via British medical men's translations with the coming of print technologies, Unani does not seem to become the metaphor for nationalist impulses, for the exact reasons of origin claims that Alavi has described.

Both Berger and Alavi offer insights into the role of language in the consolidation of identities around Ayurveda or Unani. I have looked at the kinds of medical writing that emerged during this time, in some detail, in Chapter 3. To briefly recall that discussion, Alavi's rich discussion of the movement from Persian to Arabic to Urdu as the host language for Unani reflects the changing political fortunes of this therapeutic practice in the post-Mughal era. Berger speaks of, in addition to the format of 'formalized' texts which 'would print a Sanskrit sloka followed by both a translation and explanation of it in Hindi immediately below' (p. 83), thus claiming the authority of Sanskrit, a practice of replacing Urdu or Persian words with Sanskrit in these texts. This would have contributed to the 'natural' mapping of formal modern Ayurveda and Sanskrit, while allowing Devanagari Hindi to emerge as the language of the popular. If this impacted, as Berger, King (1994), and others have shown, both oral and print cultures in at least the north-central Indian provinces in the early 20th century, the emergence of Hindi as the 'natural' language of the nation, imagined largely in these spaces, would follow.

The home and the world: writing, selling, debating the indigenous

Mukharji, Berger, and others have indicated forms of social behaviour that emerged as aspects of modernity in the 19th and 20th centuries. These may be seen in the debates staged between western and *kabiraje* systems in Bengali medical journals like *Bhisak Darpan* (Mukharji 2009), in a polemical focus on the nation and tradition in various public speeches given by Indian men trained in British medicine, or soirees and club events where the regular intellectuals would debate. The *adda*, or café, where questions of political importance or social relevance were discussed among men, has remained active today, while being recognized for the hierarchies, feudalisms, and exclusions that constituted them – somewhat akin to critiques of Habermas' public sphere (Fraser 2021, Garnham 2007). I suggest that this debating behaviour served as an aspirational sign of civilizational maturity, and nationalist medicine and vocabulary were a site for this aspiration. Who served as claimants for nationalist medicine? Berger has spoken of the

> representation of the relationship between Ayurveda and Unani as one of symbiotic co-existence but careful separation, and [how] the expansion of services based upon this ideal, served to reify a 'historical' vision of the Indigenous Medical Systems that had actually only existed from the 1920s on and had in fact been created by the Board of Indian Medicine.
>
> (p. 145)

Secularism, in this schema, becomes about 'adequately identifying community-based divisions' (p. 145), a practice employed by the provincial Congress government of Uttar Pradesh in the 1930s. I offer another speculative argument here. If, following Berger, we assume that indigenous medicine was a primary object and site of control and intervention by the Congress governments in the dyarchic model, what happens when, with the Nehruvian development model assuming centre-stage in the approach to independence, this gets left behind? Does a Sanskritic Ayurveda become the concern of marginal professional associations like the Akhil Bharatvarshiya Ayurved Mahasammelan, formed in 1907, and also left out of the processes of professional recognition and control over populations by the colonial government? Does this result in a period of greater esoteric status for this practice? How does Pandit Madan Mohan Malaviya's insistent focus on the teaching of indigenous medicine in Parliament appear in this context? With the perceived distinction between Muslim and Hindu bodies, and the purported suitability of Unani and Ayurveda to these respectively, with the perception of Unani colleges and organizations having received greater patronage from the imperial government, does the argument of a Hindu or Aryan race under threat gather ground?

Meanwhile, the home remained another important site of nationalist medicine. Through the many publications on *gharoa chikitsa*, written mostly by male *vaids*, but with also a few, perhaps exceptional texts by women like Yashoda Devi, starting in the late 19th and early 20th centuries, an expanded public discourse of caste and community in relation to a national imaginary was being built, also supported by caste associations. I have reflected on this in Chapters 4 and 5 of this book; I reiterate here the caste aspect of this vocabulary, and the manner in which middle-class privileged-caste women of the household occupied the centre of it, were invited into an empathetically considered component of the inexpert domain, as satellite vehicles of a nation both under threat and in the making, were offered shelter and shown affective concern so that they could protect their children and families, as also reposed confidence in that they could do this well enough. The *vaids* whose names were attached to these texts, then, became household names, as the woman of this privileged-caste household found a role and enhanced status for herself. In the developing discourse of the demarcation between nation and the foreign, then, the home remedy became a function of the nationalist indigenous. Berger has spoken of how Ayurvedic dispensaries and practitioners were accessed by the public as a nationalist practice; I find this argument more applicable in the case of *gharoa chikitsa*.

What of *bottola* medicine, and its possible entry into the privileged-caste home? Anindita Ghosh speaks of the 'abusive language' attributed to 'women of a lower order' that colonial commentators document in early Bengal; and it is this representation that 19th-century male reformers are attempting to unseat in their framing of the woman of the home (Ghosh 2006, p. 235). The *gharoa texts* that emerge in this and a later time, then, would seem the perfect foil that would support the reform agenda, offering a movement from the 'ignorant' to the responsible and educated health manager of the family. Whether *bottola* medicine does get finally unseated from its place in the privileged home is an open question.

Regulation and a place for the indigenous practitioner

Berger speaks of the Board of Indian Medicine that was set up in 1921 with the intent to standardize the curricula and practices of indigenous practitioners in dispensaries, as health became a provincial government subject. She notes that *vaids* began getting more prominent positions on the Board, or at least outnumbered *hakims*. Alavi traces this history more attentively, marking within it the resistance to earlier registration acts by *vaids* and *hakims* both, who then were constituted into a committee that advised the colonial government on both Ayurveda and Unani needing to be brought under both hereditary familial and state control. This recommendation was accepted, thus creating a collaboratively shared governance mechanism with a place for the indigenous practitioner. It is in this non-state location of expert power that the beginnings of today's Ayush may be found. Berger further traces the use this indigenous practitioner was later put to in northern and central parts of the subcontinent, 'in the collection and ordering of data about the population, thus increasing their institutional value outside of the health infrastructure as well as within it' (p. 139). The dispensary, moreover, became the site for the trial of new pharmaceutical drugs produced in the laboratory (p. 139), thus consolidating the chemical over the herbal within the indigenous drugs industry. This network, clearly drawn and outlined, created 'an intellectual and economic network of educational institutions, merchants and practitioners that the government considered to be the legitimate portion of the indigenous pharmaceutical industry of the UP' (p. 141).

A separation, and an othering

In both histories of Unani and Ayurveda, we see hints of separation and community-building. With the shifting of patronage, the coming of print culture, and the contests over authoring of practice via textuality and with the codification that take over from handed-down knowledge, a sharpening and exclusivity were underway. But with the coming together of Arabic as the language of Unani, meant to increase expert family control vis-à-vis the public, the separation of *mulk* (nation) and *qaum* (community) via the seeking of continuities with global Islam, provincial biopolitics, separate electorates, and the rise of the perceived threat to the Hindu polity, the once-powerful *hakim* becomes increasingly, and somehow, the frozen-in-time, esoteric, poorer cousin within indigenous systems; ghettoized as narrow community practice, while Ayurveda takes off as the vessel of a resistant medicine, a nationalist medicine. As Berger and Alavi have traced, the introduction and the increasing presence of *vaids* over *hakims* in these spaces, in a climate of increasing communalization, bring these multiple discourses together.

The communalization and caste implication of dirt in the emerging middle classes of Punjab have been reflected on in detail by Anshu Malhotra. Malhotra speaks of the 'colonial period in Punjab [that] witnessed the establishment of the myths of Muslim fecundity, virility and masculinity (Malhotra 2003) at a time when the religious communities in Punjab were beginning to be embroiled in questions of health, vitality and numbers' (2003, p. 232). As I discussed in Chapters 4 and 5, this translated into the childbirth discourse, with the Punjabi elite feeling the need to protect and separate the privileged-caste woman's body from the *dais*, a

> large proportion of [whom] ... were Muslims belonging to the Jhinvar or Machchi caste, a caste of water carriers, fishermen, palanquin bearers and basket makers ... The perceived notion of low-caste dirt could at times envelop Muslims as well, creating a powerful myth of Muslim 'dirty' habits, especially at fractious times of communal tension.
>
> (Malhotra 2003, p. 232)

Malhotra remarks on the expressed need to produce strong sons, in particular, in this discourse (a capacity ironically seen in the very same communities that were being sought to be removed from the childbearing moment) that led to the bringing in of privileged-caste women into *dai* training and nursing in Punjab. The celebrated midwifery training institute of Dr Aitchison in 1866 marks this impulse. I have detailed some of this work in other parts of northern India in Chapter 4, and here emphasize the impulse of separation and othering based on metaphors of dirt, that are visible with respect to both Muslim and marginalized-caste *dais*.

And a place for quackery

I have briefly reflected on the practitioner who fails to make it to the category and status of professional, in Chapters 3 and 5, with respect to caste hierarchies and the claims to professional status for oppressed caste communities, the links between *bottola* medicine, the street practitioner, and *gharoa chikitsa* in Bengal, as well as parts of northern India. Girija, in her account of the extrusion of *naattuvaidyam* as 'folk medicine' in the construction of modern *Aryavaidyam* in the region that is now Kerala state, presents in compelling detail the process of reorganization of epistemic authority and the production of the quack in the 20th century. Exploring the practice of 'interactions and collaborations' (2021, p. 56, 51) that was the trend before this period, Girija talks about specific domains – like *balachikitsam* (treatment of children) and *vishavaidyam* (broadly, treatment for poisons) – that were acknowledged as specialties of the *Velan, Mannan,* or *Kanian* castes, considered lower castes and subject to social prejudice but recognized for their knowledge and skill. *Dhanwantari,* an influential magazine started in 1903 in the region, sought to bring together the wisdom of privileged-caste Vaidya men and the marginalized-caste *vaidyas* in an effort to visibilize non-textual forms of knowledge; up until 1907, Girija notes, neither conflict with biomedicine nor between these multiple sources of knowledge and practice was a feature. Visibility, rather, with borrowing across traditions, was the aim. With the 'reformation debate formally started around 1907' via a questionnaire on the pages of *Dhanwantari* (p. 49), the *Velan, Mannan,* or *Kanian* castes continued to be recognized as plant collectors, 'collecting herbs, cleaning them, preparing medicines and treating patients' (p. 56), a practice unavailable to the 'Brahmin vaidya in the nineteenth century', for whom 'the marketplace, the field and the forest were spaces that caused spatial pollution' (ibid). But the fact that these marginalized castes used and wrote vernacular texts for reference, or relied on oral traditions, and the fact that they had occupational diversity, doing other kinds of historically delegated caste-based work like clothes-washing and so on, became the grounds on which 'many practices such as *adivasi vaidyam, nattuvaidyam*, etc., were bundled together as folk practice by the mid-twentieth century' (p. 54). By this time, reference to Sanskrit texts, incorporation of knowledge from non-textual traditions into modern forms of therapeutic writing, the 'reformulation of the practices of upper-caste vaidyas as a classical tradition' (p. 55), all contributed to a closing and sharpening of boundaries between textual and non-textual, Sanskrit and vernacular texts, privileged and marginalized caste practice; and the birth of both a classical tradition now to be called proper *Aryavaidyam*, separated from a heterogeneous set of practices called *naattuvaidyam*, which had even begun with an aspiration to regional identity (p. 53), and 'folk' medicine, along with home remedies, being recognized as quackery. It is in this category of quack that we see the *dai* figure being placed, as I discuss with respect to the *bazaar dai* in northern India in Chapter 4.

Lambert approaches the 'therapeutic configuration across diverse elite and subaltern domains of therapy' (2013, p. 109) somewhat similarly, suggesting 'conceptual continuities … in order to point to the discontinuities in therapeutic traditions' (p. 121). Lambert explores bone-setting and some other practices in 'subaltern' settings, in a continuum across 'practitioners ranging from laypeople who have acquired a very limited familiarity with one form of therapy that they may provide informally for family and neighbours on request, to quite specialised folk healers who have inherited or acquired esoteric knowledge and reputed skills in a specific form of therapy and who may have a large clientele. In neither case does the therapy constitute a full-time occupation' (p. 120), and never does it claim the status of a system. Lambert interprets the contemporary survival and relative invisibility of these practices as a possible result of being outside the realms of governance and regulation in the later colonial period. This outsideness is of course what the colonial and independent state have read as remoteness – a distancing that also facilitates the abjectness and dispensability of marginalized populations.

What of the women? Girija speaks of women of the *Velan* and *Mannan* castes who were 'skilled and competent *dais*' until the mid-20th century (2021, p. 53), and alongside her own reading of *balachikitsam* as a specialty of these practitioners, as also other scholarship that locates oral transmission of healing and therapeutic traditions shared by women and men of marginalized caste locations, suggests a shared rather than a gendered knowledge domain. With the fall from grace of home remedies, seen as the recourse of the 'lay person who had access to indigenous medicinal knowledge through print media' (p. 45), and the creation of a demarcated inexpert domain composed of these lay persons, including women of the home, and 'folk' practitioners, as Girija suggests in mid-20th-century Kerala, we find perhaps a consolidation of the speculation I offer in Chapter 5. The distancing of these persons and these texts and practices from a more regulated, standardized, universally legible practice of modern Ayurveda (p. 54), we may now read, following Girija, as a consolidation of the boundaries of the nationalist indigenous; the 'remoteness' of places where the *dai* is now to be 'found', her absence from present-day national policies on midwifery, the Sanskritized 'classical' wellness regimes in the public healthcare system, the export of this regime as the singular voice of the nation-state.

But to expand on the category 'woman-of-the-home'. Does this figure occupy as distanced or remote a location as the folk practitioner or the *dai*? Girija points out that oral cultural wisdoms were appropriated into textuality in the early 20th century, and following Berger, this may have meant the emergence of nodes of power that visibly constituted a recognizable Ayurveda that could collaborate with state power. This also means that the origin myths of the dominant expand and become the primary historical record of this period. Post-independence, this collaboration would become at first more difficult, with the modern secular state feeling the need for distance from 'unproven' traditions, and then more 'natural' with the populist critique of secularism preparing the soil for Hindu majoritarian positions and, by association, therapeutic practices that had by then become associated with Hindu communities. I will go into this in some more detail in the last section of this chapter. For the amorphous collection of practices attributed to the *indigenous* or the *bazaar dai*, however, access to the label of indigeneity was associated more with ignorance, illiteracy, and lack of hygiene – those old motifs. As far as the fate of this figure in the expert domain was concerned, some clues might be found in what Berger has called eclectic medical guides with the body at the centre, coupledom as the goal, and the author as expert. I have also discussed, in Chapter 5, the *gharoa chikitsa* texts that highlight both the possibility and the responsibility of the woman of the household as legitimate extensions of the re-articulated Ayurveda as indigenous, in fact, as the creation of a category of inexpert that could serve as extended sites of institutionalization of Ayurveda. The authority invested in this particular category of 'woman-of-the-home', privileged in terms of caste, and perhaps *zenana* education through reform, and thus, woman of the nation as well, depended on the extrusion of the *dai* figure who had, since the beginning of the colonial era, been seen as invading this ideal household and who now needed to be removed. It is in these contexts, then, that the indigenous as a symbolic, nationalist entity is constructed. The *vaid* is a part; Hindu privileged-caste communities are a part; the woman of the privileged household is an important part. The *hakim* has by now become suspect as *qaumi* rather than *mulki*. The *dai* is a danger and must be disallowed from occupying any part of this image. Alongside the quack, then, the *dai* can be rendered abject, actively erased from the history of authentic or useful indigeneity, or as knowledge worker, while still very much a presence, deskilled and renamed as traditional birth attendant (TBA), in the organization of healthcare, as we will see in the next part of the chapter. The active injunctions against the *dai* that we see in some of these home guides are an indication of this.

What of the *vaittati* or privileged perinatal family consultant? And the natural childbirth vocabulary as emerging in the present? Both these spaces, one presented as traditional, the other corporate, are today visible in the logic of childbirth therapeutics, as a container for critiques of industrialized institutionalized childbirth, and I will explore these in more detail in the last section of this chapter.

The categories of those pushed out from therapeutic visibility, and yet active as contemporary remnants, of course, do not end here by any means. Plant collectors, variolators, the *madrasi* doctor, and the native *daktar* (Mukharji 2009) – a whole series of liminal identities – that appear within the colonial context to begin with, do not entirely disappear with time. As Mukharji, Lambert, and others have noted, these practices may continue to be found while the identities disappear with regulation, having been named for that purpose in the first place. As far as the canonical indigenous is concerned, they may be *remembered* for their folksy connotations. Since they pose little or no risk to regulated therapeutic spaces, like the *dai* may do with respect to the body of the woman, they can be allowed to live. The steady historical extrusion of the *dai* as a knowledge worker from the space of the indigenous is what we will see in the next section on the organization of healthcare post-independence, and this may have implications for the parallel process of the consolidation of caste hierarchies – what survives as knowledge, and what as service.

The ritual practitioner – an other world

Contemporary anthropology, some of it feminist, has offered a strand that explores the domain of traditional healing via cosmology. Tracing links between some of the contemporary oral traditions among *dai* women and the Ayurvedic worldview, scholar-activist Janet Chawla reads an epistemology of gender relations centred around the *Purush-Prakriti* model, where the earth and the female body are analogous sources of fertility, of an inner self. While being critical of this dualism, Chawla continues to find value in what she terms the 'dais' imagery of the female body' (2002, p. 147). Chawla holds this imagery at the centre of what she sees as traditional resource and knowledge, and an alternative understanding of the female subtle body that emerges through this imagery, in her work with *dai* women in the northern Indian states of Bihar, Delhi, and Rajasthan as part of the MATRIKA project in the early 2000s. These women are also understood, in Chawla's argument, as holders of collective oral knowledge that is caste-based and learned through apprenticeship.

While seeking to overturn colonial-era stereotypes of the 'dirty dai' and modern forces of mainstream development and biomedicine that have resulted in their marginalization, and marking the figure as a ritual practitioner, Chawla's arguments are fraught with problems. Her mobilizing of metaphors of holism and interconnectedness in a near-Orientalist fashion, her understanding of cultural difference as essential and incommensurable, her acceptance of esoteric-sounding language as evidence of stable difference, her uncomplicated reading of various practices as related to or even found in Ayurvedic texts while also reading caste oppression in Brahminism are some of them. I mark this strand of thinking, however, in order to pay attention to the attempt by Western or Western-turned feminist scholars to find easy connections between contemporary practices among women in extremely vulnerable livelihoods and a homogeneous worldview, namely contemporary Ayurveda, that seems to offer textual origins for these practices. All this, while acknowledging caste and gender hierarchies and Brahminical practices that disallow knowledge worker status to the *dai*.

Chawla's explorations do offer some unintended consequences, however, when she reflects on UNICEF's contention that 'nobody could identify, precisely, who was (and who was not) a *dai*,' (2002, p. 151) – a contention also borne out by other authors in the same collection (*Daughters of Hariti*, 2002) who speak of common and specialist knowledge of childbirth and the sharing of birthing labour among kin and other women (Unnithan-Kumar 2002, pp. 109–129). We might recall both the colonial production of the category that I noted in Chapter 4, and the contemporary looseness of the category in the face of extreme precarity of women's informal labour in the context of the organization of healthcare. Chawla's tentative hypothesis around *narak ka samay* (a time in hell) that *dais* in northern parts of India speak of, as a reference to the inner (secret?) world of the body might find references in a shamanic mobilization of secrecy that is different from the blackboxing that is a constitutive feature of biomedicine. And here there might be some clues, however speculative, to alternative worldviews. Chawla's other hypothesis – that 'ritual uncleanness is the language of Brahmanic sacerdotal and textual tradition and that women's work of birth involves different forms of sacrality and ethno-medical rite and practice' (2002, p. 158), seems to build on re-reading *narak* as fertility and the 'inner world of the body' (p.160), and is the most provocative, challenging as it does the argument around caste abjection, but we do not really find convincing evidence of the same.

Chawla recognizes, in addition to other scholars (Pinto 2008, Gopal 2017), the steady erosion of the *jajmani* system with changing patterns of patronage in the colonial era, as a result of which caste oppression continued while caste-based occupational income, like that of the *dai's*, diminished. We might add the shift in discriminatory practices that occurs from an earlier developmental-political era to the present one – a shift from marking of the *dai* as non-knowledgeable to marking her as a non-legitimate actor in healthcare.

I have attempted, in this section, to draw together the strands of movement across the 19th to 20th centuries that mark the emergence of what I term a canonical indigenous. The making of a modern Ayurveda and its natural home in the Hindu nation, the sharp separation from practitioners rendered subaltern in this history, including the *dai*, while the woman-of-the-home emerges as an extended site of this new therapeutic, are part of this movement. I now attempt to explore the journeys of these in the independent nation-state.

Healthcare organization/regulation, segregation and the *dai* in independent India

Health planning

As Chatterjee (2000) and others have noted, the early years of independence saw development articulated as planning in the context of a young nation. Health planning followed the same principles, as did the curriculum of Preventive and Social Medicine, later Community Medicine, in allopathic medical graduate coursework

232 Indigenous therapeutics in the present

since 1955. The first of many committees constituted to assess the status of health conditions and the organization of healthcare services on the cusp of independence was the Health Survey and Development Committee, appointed in 1943 and headed by Sir Joseph Bhore, popularly referred to as the Bhore Committee. It had 24 members, three of them women. Sir Bhore himself had been a part of the Civil Services since 1902. The Bhore Committee proposed, as some of its first recommendations, the integration of preventive with curative health services, the preparation of 'social physicians' via training in preventive medicine, and the improvement of service to rural populations. The vertical organization of healthcare linking the village unit to the referral hospital, and the setting up of the Primary Health Centre, or PHC, was one of the first suggestions. The implementation of these recommendations was evaluated by the Mudaliar Committee in 1959, which advised in its 1962 report the setting up of an all-India health service on the lines of the Indian Administrative Service (IAS). The Chadah Committee in 1963 mooted the idea of multi-purpose health workers (MPHW), a terminology that persists today. MPHW were the basic health workers who would be tasked with additional duties of public health, family planning, and census, 'in addition to malaria vigilance' (Park 2015, p. 874). This combination of functions was quickly revised by the Mukerji Committee of 1965, which requested the delinking of family planning and the allocation of separate staff for it. Meanwhile, the idea of 'integrated health services' rather than segmented departments was defined in the Jungalwalla Committee in 1967, and in 1973, gendered allocation and segregation of healthcare work was suggested by the (Kartar Singh) Committee on Multipurpose Workers under Health and Family Planning. The Kartar Singh Committee suggested that

> the present Auxiliary Nurse Midwives ... be replaced by the newly designated "Female Health Workers", and the present-day Basic Health Workers, Malaria Surveillance Workers, Vaccinators, Health Education Assistants (Trachoma) and the Family Planning Health Assistants ... be replaced by "Male Health Workers".
>
> (Park 2015, p. 875)

This was followed, in 1974, by a 'Group on Medical Education and Support Manpower' popularly known as the Shrivastav Committee, set up by the Ministry of Health and Family Planning, to 'devise a suitable curriculum for training a cadre of health assistants so that they can *serve as a link* between the qualified medical practitioners and the multipurpose workers, thus forming an effective team to deliver health care, family welfare, and nutritional services to the people; (2) to suggest steps for improving the existing medical educational processes to provide due emphasis on the problems particularly relevant to national requirements' (ibid, p. 875, italics mine). One of the most important recommendations of this committee was access to primary health care within the community, and to this end, it suggested immediate action for the

> creation of bands of para-professional and semi-professional health workers from within the community itself (e.g., school teachers, postmasters, *gram*

sevaks) to provide simple, promotive, preventive and curative health services needed by the community' (ibid). This would ensure that 'the health of the people is placed in the hands of the people themselves.

(ibid)

It is useful to understand the language and recommendations of these committees in the context of the nation and indigeneity, although the latter is comprehensively kept out of the deliberations except to relegate it to the domain of the provincial/regional, just as colonial-era planning had done. From the Bhore Committee onward, the rural, named as such, is seen as the starting point of and ideal location for preventive and primary healthcare; in keeping, it would seem, with the Gandhian stereotype of India that lives in its villages and the geographic distribution of populations. Rural development would be achieved, and village health best served, by training to build a cadre of 'social physicians' (Park 2015, p. 873) – and here the core idea of Preventive and Social Medicine (PSM) as a discipline is born. The proposal for social physicians is in keeping with the ideal of a welfare state and in alignment with a call to voluntarism as part of the nation-building exercise. This idea develops later, in association with the Alma Ata declaration of 1978, which refocuses the efforts of global healthcare on health as a precondition and preventive mechanism, into a 'social engineering' project within PSM, recognizing social contexts of illness as the necessary sites of intervention. This moves, of course, very quickly into a focus on social behaviours rather than social contexts, especially in the context of chronic illnesses, but that is a separate debate.

While the Indian systems of Medicine and Homeopathy (ISMH, as they were then called) were recognized as a major source of succour for rural populations, they are not included in these planning documents or in PSM curricula as part of healthcare planning or social physician culture. There is, however, a call for the 'deprofessionalization of medicine' (Park 2015, p. 11) in the organization of primary healthcare. Multipurpose workers, community health workers, village health guides, *anganwadi* workers, practitioners of indigenous medicine, and trained *dais*, are seen as forming a 'lay network' that is encouraged to comprise 'village "health teams" [that] bridge the cultural and communication gap between the rural people and organised health sector' (Park 2015, p. 890). As 'deprofessionalisation', this exercise would seem to be in sharp contrast to colonial efforts to professionalize healthcare organization; as a way to expand sites of institutionalization, however, continuities may be seen.

We see, then, an invitation to the expert practitioner, now clearly defined as trained in allopathic medicine, to find a way to work with a variety of 'lay' people and groups. This laity is categorized into several ad hoc, informal categories, seen as 'culturally connected' to the target population. The adhocism of this categorization is evident in, for example, the allocation and reallocation of multi-purpose health workers, already a definitionally flimsy and informal labelling, into and out of family planning work. What we do see is an expansion of the inexpert domain, somewhat similar to *gharoa chikitsa*, to include a variety of experienced and local but 'non-knowledgeable' members of the local populace.

What of the indigenous medicine practitioners, health assistants, or trained *dais*? Locating these practitioners in the domain of the 'lay' may mean deskilling and neglect by the system, or it may mean a reconstitution of paraprofessional link workers. None of these locations constitute knowledge work; while the 'link worker' position granted to the health assistant is confusing given the unclear parameters of training or job roles (Rao et al. 2013, Kumar 2016), practitioners of indigenous medicine are treated as sharing cultural roots with patient populations and therefore experienced, and trained *dais* as a component of PHCs. How are these roles separated? Is it likely, given the interface of a techno-scientific system and a social hierarchy, that those hierarchies will be reproduced as these informal categories?

Task shifting

A great deal of the conversation around deskilling is today located in the task-shifting debate. While the involvement of the 'laity' is an exercise that was part and parcel of the involvement of the community in primary healthcare in India in the 1950s, as we saw above, as also in the 'barefoot doctors' exercise in China and village health volunteers in Thailand in the 1950s (Campbell and Scott 2011), task-shifting was first named as such by the World Health Organisation (WHO) in 2006 in the context of HIV/AIDS work involving peer supporters and educators. Under the call to 'test, train, retain', the WHO proposed work with HIV volunteers in communities as not only the best equipped to engage with peers but also to counter stigma and manage resource-poor settings. WHO defines task shifting as 'a process of delegation whereby tasks are moved, where appropriate, to less special-ized health workers' (2007, p. 3). WHO also recognizes, and there is ample critical scholarship on, the principle of task shifting, apparently studied in low and middle-income settings where 'auxiliary personnel' became the necessary stand-ins for more trained health workers, allowing 'doctors to use their time and expertise for people with more complicated diseases ... [so that] many other people benefited by receiving treatment closer to home in local health centres rather than having to travel to hospital' (ibid, p. 6). This was also proposed for management and fol-low-up of chronic conditions. Task-shifting has also been spoken of in maternal health (Deller et al, 2015), and persons with lived experience of drug use (Olding et al., 2021) where communities take charge of dose control. All of this strenuously emphasizes the principle as one of collaboration with the community rather than delegation, triage, or stop-gaps.[3]

The moral/ethical impulses in task shifting still hark back to Alma Ata, which critiqued what it called 'medical elitism' and the pushing of the biomedical model as the answer to all problems (Campbell and Scott 2011), as well as the contin-ued ignorance of social determinants of health in this model. It is in this con-text and that of the need to 'fill in gaps in manpower at village levels' (National Population Policy 2000), that we might locate the emergence of the ASHA worker, or Accredited Social Health Activist, within the National Rural Health Mission (NRHM), in 2005. The idea for the ASHA first began with the considerable success achieved in Chhattisgarh state, a region with predominantly tribal communities, by the *Mitanin* programme, a deployment of the Community Health Worker programme, since 2002. Seen as embedded in the community, the *Mitanin* (lifelong friend) was considered a community advocate and organizer, selected by block-level health workers – Auxiliary Nurse Midwives (ANM) – through community consultations and meetings. Health was defined in a structural sense, taking into account social determinants, and the *Mitanin* was seen as a volunteer-activist who would bring these questions into health planning and delivery. The *Mitanin* was specifically deployed in primary health concerns of women and children, including nutrition, immunization, institutional delivery, and maternal and neonatal care, as well as gender-based violence. The *Mitanin* was not paid a salary; she was primarily an extension of the community rather than of the healthcare system, and as such, the former was where her loyalties lay. Therefore, she emerged as an advocate for other women in both family and community. Qualitative studies done about a decade after the intervention began showed increased awareness of rights and entitlements, including food schemes, gender-based violence, the value of collective action to ensure accountability in local governance as well as community (Nandi and Schneider 2014). The women were not usually of the village elite, however, and attrition was high, the authors note. At any rate, it was this notion of women promoting the empowerment of other women within existing frameworks that translated into the nationwide ASHA programme in 2005. The 'women working for women' colonial governance formula continues here, somewhat.

The ASHA worker continued to carry the value-ladenness and essentialization of women's care work that the *Mitanin* did, but evaluations of the programme have shown up significant shifts. ASHAs are a key component of the NRHM, now the National Health Mission (NHM), and are poorly paid by the state, in a mobilization of the voluntarist ideal. Evidence of this moral pressure can be seen in a quick look at the ASHA's tasks:

ASHA will be pivotal for convergence of services at grass root level in coordination with the ANM, AWWs and *Gram Vikas Panchayat Adhikari*. She will be trained to advise rural community about sanitation, hygiene, contraception and immunization etc. She will provide treatment of minor ailments like diarrhoea, minor injuries and fever; she will also accompany patients to health facilities. She would also be expected to deliver Directly Observed Treatment Short-course (DOTS) for tuberculosis. She will be a depot holder of health products like ORS, IFA, chloroquine, Disposal Delivery Kits, Oral Pills and Condoms etc. She will act as a key informant and link person in an outbreak of health-related events.

(Nandan 2005, p 168)

Further, she is expected to provide inter-cluster links, so that representatives of different community groups (like *Bal Parivar Mitra*[4]) can be brought together and managed. These are expectations of the *Mitanin* taken to a whole new level, with the ASHA expected to be the anchor for family, community, other community representatives, and other women. ASHA as a word translates as hope; clearly, she is expected to bring hope and light to the community – following on her 'natural' nurturer role. Being paid by the state, however, means that her formal account-ability is to the healthcare system; further, incentives for institutional deliveries or other top-down targets consolidate the very division between the system and the community that she is supposed to bridge, with the community understood as an unruly constituency that must be managed rather than as a cultural root or anchor for the ASHA. As Nordfeldt & Roalkvam (2010) have noted, community targets like vaccination are expected to be ways of accessing the modern, and ASHAs are expected to be facilitators of this – 'the main governing technology in this trans-formation of reason, achieving the proxy targets set forth concerning mother–child health: hospital birth deliveries, vaccination and family planning/sterilization' (p. 333). If she fails to do this, the ASHA, already in precarious labour and social conditions, is literally caught in the middle; target-based remuneration hauls her towards her employer, and she ends up blaming the community for not turning up. Although the Alma Ata declaration focused on culturally appropriate primary health care, which meant community health workers who were embedded in and responsive to the community (Scott et al. 2019), what this programme has achieved has been largely a delegation of responsibility and accountability for any failures, with the community. Meanwhile, evaluations of ASHA programmes routinely mark the local *dais* as offering opposition to the ASHA's work (Kohli et al. 2015). The riot of local language vocabulary that informs these scheme documents – ASHA, *Bal Mitra, Mitanin,* all referencing naturalized relations and gender socialization – is just about the only embeddedness in the community that is in evidence here.

Filling a gap

Two outcomes emerge from this framework. One, with the implicit articulation of community as ungovernable – a reiteration of colonial positions – the 'use' to which community can be put is only as a stopgap, a stand-in, and this is in fact one of the stated recommendations of the 1946 Bhore Committee about the role of trained *dais*. Scholarship in the field has also pointed to this adhocism, both critically and favourably (Thakur et al. 2017). The community health worker, here the ASHA, although 'accredited', is still seen as a link, not a knowledge worker. Task shifting is well in place here, in the frame of delegation, not collaboration. It is a measure of the success of this delegation that we see today ASHAs organizing themselves much more visibly as workers on par with other government employees, seeking formal labour rights and protections (Scott et al. 2019, Bhatia 2014), with no vis-ible demand for recognition as knowledge workers or community advocates.

Critical scholarship in the field has also explored the contexts of healthcare pro-grammes within which ASHAs are placed. For one, Srivastava et al. (2015) point to how community participation mirrors social hierarchies. Thakur et al. (2017), reflecting on an earlier period, have already noted that 'India's Second Five-Year Plan (1956–1961) described the role of auxiliary health workers as activities that supplemented the contributions made by doctors (GOI, 1986). But their training and role only confined them to focus on family planning, immunization, registration of pregnant mothers at the hospital and awareness regarding antenatal checkups' (p. 179). This target-based approach continues today, alongside the exhortation to voluntarism. Bajpai and Saraya (2013), in a sharp critique of the NRHM, speak of a failure to recognize social hierarchies or ensure employment and food security – essentials to promote health in rural contexts. The authors also point to the NGO-ization promoted in NRHM, with public-private partnerships being 'a convenient alibi to outsource a variety of services' (p. 242), and 'names like "Janani" in Bihar and "Yeshaswani" Trust in Karnataka, … a byword for innovation' (ibid). Further, rights were replaced by the metaphor of activism, which actually translates into a voluntarism expected of the vulnerable. The panacea that NRHM offered to rural health, therefore, has failed, they note. Scott and Shanker (2010) refer to entrenched hierarchies in healthcare provider circles that constrain ASHAs, despite their valorization as change agents, from informing medical professionals of the reasons why women skip institutional deliveries. This is yet another example of deskilling accompanied by prejudices against the ASHAs as non-expert and less privileged women; this ensures that even the respect due to community embeddedness is not met. With the movement from NRHM to the National Health Mission, none of these circumstances or working conditions have changed.

The dai disappears

The second outcome – that which pits the *dai* and the ASHA against each other – is to be expected in this scenario. The studies that have documented the changing relationship between ASHAs and the community (Scott and Shanker 2010) have noted the opposition by *dais* to ASHAs, with the latter trying to coax women towards institutional deliveries even if care is poor there. And once the poor standards of care at government facilities are seen, the ASHA loses credibility in the community. But the weight of the institution behind these interventions invariably results in the gradual effacement of the *dai*, not because of the institutional power vested in the ASHA, but because of the consolidation of discourse around the institutional management of childbirth, including regulatory governance mechanisms like the issuance of birth certificates only in cases of institutional delivery, etc. This is not a linear case of replacement, however. As Ghoshal (2014) and others have noted, modernity and development continue to have to contend with the 'staying power' of the *dai* in her village communities. Extending the core arguments posed by Mukharji, Lambert, and others on the survival of the local, we may also see that the village *dai*, while rendered abject within modern biomedicine, continues to evade and thus survive, barely, on its margins. Azher (2017) offers the argument of 'professional niche differentiation' to speak of this survival, suggesting that this is why 'local dais have survived despite government interventions that distance them from their occupational domain, and how successfully dais have navigated the process of professional niche differentiation to increase local health outcomes' (p. 135). Azher suggests that *dais* in Rajasthan continue to perform 'vital roles as health educators and care coordinators' (p. 147).

And is brought back in

I would like to offer a different way to think about this disappearance, or tenacious persistence, of the *dai*. As the spectre haunting public and maternal health, this 'demon dai' figure (Lang 2005) occupied the colonial imagination, as we have seen in Chapter 4. What of today? While neutralizing and recasting this signifier via the trope of training into modern medicine has been one route, it might be useful to explore what happens to this figure with the entry of non-governmental players into healthcare. While some of this work emerged as an extension of people's health movements and civil society organizations working in underserved and remote areas to mobilize local resources into maternal care, and some in the work of anthropologists reiterating the spiritualism of the East via the *dai* as ritual practitioner, the space of 'culture', frozen in time, has become a fresh fertile ground for an academic romanticization of the care worker, or 'care coordinator', to use Azher's term. Some, although not all, of this exploration, relates to feminist scholarship around the ethics of care; more often, it consolidates the trope of feminine care, without actually naming it as such. Rather than see this as professional niche differentiation between the ASHA and the *dai*, I would name it as a niche differentiation between the state and the non-governmental sector. A new layer in the healthcare sector that speaks of rights and entitlements, is on the side of the community, and also facilitates formal negotiations with state structures, makes one wonder if this manages and contains protest vocabulary rather than making possible transformation. The semi-institutionalization of *dai* practice that occurs in these organizations, with a stated attempt to validate some of the practice via biomedical standards, and a sense of social vulnerability and stigma faced by the women, has had uneven results. In some cases, it has succeeded in keeping alive the ongoing critique of biomedicine (Sadgopal 2009, Jeeva project initiated in 2007). In others, the feminine imagery in marginal religious traditions is emphasized (Chawla 2019, Matrika project) in an attempt to recuperate marginalized tropes of the female body, tropes that are available in *dais*' oral histories. And in some others, there has been an attempt to see *dai* work alongside community health workers (Azher 2017, Barefoot Doctors). At any rate, these initiatives have succeeded in keeping the figure alive in the imaginary of the village.

To what end, though? Nowhere in any of this work are *dai* traditions presented as an alternative, independent knowledge model. When alternative knowledge models are indeed discussed, they have occupied the domain of feminist philosophy (Dalmiya 2002, Alcoff and Dalmiya 1993), located elsewhere from this materiality. Nor are these oral traditions discussed, except in very loose ways, in relation to canonical knowledge systems like Ayurveda or Unani. The only real shift, then, from colonial practice, that we might see is the supplemental move to uplift the *dai* woman. She is an entry point for reform work, today as yesterday; and the origin claims are to Gandhian principles, the Marxist ethic, or the Sarvodaya movement. In that sense, the *dai* woman finds re-entry of sorts into community in these initiatives. As far as the healthcare apparatus is concerned, she continues to be the abject, shadowy figure who must remain segregated and stigmatized.

Midwifery

And so we arrive at the true contemporary midwife. The Ministry of Health and Family Welfare set out under the National Health Mission, in 2018, Guidelines on Midwifery Services in India. Following the protocols of the International Confederation of Midwives, 2015, and the requirements of the Sustainable Development Goals, a midwife was defined in these guidelines as

> a person who has successfully completed a midwifery education programme that is duly recognized in the country where it is located and that is based on the International Confederation of Midwives (ICM) Essential Competencies for Basic Midwifery Practice and the framework of the ICM Global Standards for Midwifery Education.
>
> (Guidelines 2018, p. 2)

Identifying poor intrapartum care as one of the major causes of maternal deaths, and 'lack of trained service providers or over medicalization of the delivery process' (p.1) as the major reasons for poor intrapartum care, the document traces histories of Sweden and Sri Lanka, both of which had difficult access to doctors owing to remoteness and homebirth practices, respectively, but were able to institute trained midwifery programmes and bring down maternal mortality. Following some of these principles, the document marks midwifery as a shift from 'fragmented maternal and newborn care focused on identification and treatment of pathology, to skilled and compassionate woman-centric care' (p. 3). Problems identified in the 'history of midwifery in India' include the lack of separation of roles, absence of career progression, absence of regulations, and proper training. It is in this context that the new guidelines are proposed, and this care is located in the profession of nursing, with proposed midwifery colleges, universal curricula in accordance with standards laid down by the International Confederation of Midwives, remuneration at par with higher educational spaces, licensing and registration, continuing clinical and theoretical involvement, supervisory and monitoring hierarchies, strengthening of connections with international bodies, a national midwifery task force with regional components. Local symbolic flavour (easy to embed in public memory and poll campaign promises, and possible to mediatize) in the shape of acronyms that also form words is once more in place – LaQshya or Labour room Quality Improvement Initiative, for instance (pronounced as *lakshya*, which translates as goal). The guidelines were followed in 2020 by the National Nursing and Midwifery Commission (NNMC) Bill, which aims to supersede the 1947 Indian Nursing Council Act as well as the many state-level laws that were instituted since the 1930s and 1940s (Mayra et al 2021). Prior to these steps, nursing training included a six-month component in midwifery, apart from a 3-year diploma in General Nursing and Midwifery; women trained in both courses were allotted to obstetric wards in public hospitals. Auxiliary Nurse Midwives (ANMs) in primary healthcare also received some training as paraprofessionals bordering on link workers.

While the fate of the bill is unclear at the time of writing, with the latest session of Parliament having failed to see it tabled, formal feedback, as well as several academic and public domain critiques that have been voiced, indicate that this is an exercise in centralizing control while attempting to streamline reporting mechanisms. Several nursing associations have opined that the proposed bill not only challenges the federal system, not taking into account the high numbers of nursing professionals from certain states and therefore the need for proportional representation, but also fails to consider those from disadvantaged backgrounds who will now have to appear for a standardized entrance exam. Regulation continues to be male, bureaucratic, and doctor-led. Representational diversity, of course, continues to be absent (Mayra et al, 2021). With privatization and increasing technologized control over childbirth by doctors, this also becomes a source of competition between nursing and medical professions over childbirth. For our purposes, here, it is also useful to examine the premium placed on a competency-based curriculum in the proposed legislation. Competency-based curricula focus on observable skills and behaviours, taught and monitored via a heavily textual and codified, universalized standard. In doing this, the possibility of building perspective, context, and conceptual knowledge invariably takes a hit. While this approach offers more room to align with universalized medical training, it is the community-directedness or situated learning that is bound to suffer, and here we see one more way in which the nurse-midwife – a more bounded category of health worker – can now be distinguished from the non-trained, community-embedded, experientially learned *dai* woman. Is this a version of professional niche differentiation, as Azher would suggest? Hardly, given that the *dai* has systematically by now been written out of the modern as well as traditional text. Even the critical literature on regulation and precarity of professions speaks of workers' rights, ethics of practice, and education; not necessarily of experiential learning.

In 1912, the push towards creating a nursing cadre had been in the context of the comprehensive failure of the *dai* training programmes conducted by the Dufferin Fund. Among social reformers, including women like Pandita Ramabai and Ramabai Ranade, nursing had a career of its own, with reform agendas bringing privileged-caste women into the profession, constructed as respectable and empowering for widows and other 'saved women'. In early independent India, however, with the shift in focus to community involvement, nursing was subsumed into the allopathic system, with some attention paid to training *dais* to improve childbirth conditions; this continued in fits and starts till the mid-2000s, often led by non-governmental organizations working in rural development. With this new proposed legislation and the clear provision of a professional cadre of nurse-midwives on international parameters, however, the rendering obsolete of the *dai* figure is almost complete. It remains to be seen how this goes forward. It is interesting that nowhere in the 2018 policy guidelines or the law is there even mention of the *dai*, although reference is made to home birth practices in Sri Lanka and far-away Sweden.

I would suggest that this push towards internationally recognized midwifery, without a whisper of earlier histories, might say something about the management of gender in the nation today. While every aspect of the health apparatus in India today has been touched by the metaphor of the indigenous, childbirth, or more precisely, maternal and infant mortality and morbidity are markers that, having garnered international attention, have become the site where the indigenous is immediately connected to neglect. This may have something to do with colonial stereotyping, and the nationalist state responds with its own resolution of the 'woman's question' – the *dai* is listed under cultural barriers to ASHA work, for instance (*Reaching the Unreached*, Brochure for ASHA, ASHA modules, National Health Systems Resource Centre, https://nhsrcindia.org/practice-areas/cpc-phc/community-process-asha). The *dai* is also listed as a resource traditionally accessed by marginalized communities – the 'unreached', defined in the brochure as 'scheduled castes, scheduled tribes and minority communities', 'women headed households', 'daily wage labourers', 'families living in distant hamlets', 'families with disabled children', 'migrant families'. Each of these unreached locations is also a non-normative one. It is the ASHA's task to 'persist', as part of an eight-fold 'path' prescribed to her in the training module so that the pregnant woman from such an 'unreached' location can be brought into the fold of institutional delivery. It is clear, then, that the *dai* belongs neither with the modern nor with the 'caste' nation; the only places where she remains are those which have not followed the norm and are rendered vulnerable therefore; members of the normative nation and its margins must both be saved from her. Also important for the present discussion, the *dai* woman has no place in the continued construction of indigenous knowledge as Hindu, even though the Dalit ASHA worker is still acceptable as a link worker. The exercise of regulation and alignment with global professional standards and requirements, then, is well integrated with the continuing exercise of this caste segregation.

It might be useful here to mark a departure from the metropole's history in terms of midwifery and nursing. Histories of British midwifery carry voices of the midwives from early on. Writings by these women, whose prescriptions range from conception to the prevention of miscarriage to the improvement of breast milk, interspersed with other kinds of remedies or unrelated 'recipes', are available from the 1700s at least, although these are neither common nor standardized. Models of modern midwifery include training and medical supervision, some of which are resented by the midwife women, as visible from the profuse correspondence. Herbert Spencer, Fellow of the Royal College of Physicians, and obstetric physician, delivers in 1927 a series of lectures on the history of British midwifery between 1650 and 1800, and shows the monopoly over midwifery among women practitioners until the forceps begin to be introduced in 1733; the Chamberlen brothers are the key actors in this history. The presence of men provokes massive protests from women practitioners of midwifery. Spencer, in a full chapter on the conflicts between doctors and midwives, notes, of this moment that perhaps marked the turning point in the power that women held over men in the profession, that

'midwives had long inveighed against men practicing a branch of medicine which they regarded as peculiarly their own; made vehement assertions, but gave no evidence of their special qualifications; accused the male practitioners of destroying the child with their instruments (of the life-saving character

of which they were ignorant), and indulged in the most scurrilous and shame-
less attacks upon their rivals.

(1927, p. 146)

Spencer goes on to note that the 'lampoons and diatribes against the man-midwife
form an interesting and amusing chapter in the history of British Midwifery; but
by the end of the century the opposition of the midwives had died down' (p. 149).
There is some evidence of conflict between nursing and midwifery practice as well.
There is a great deal of legislation between the 1890s onwards till 1918, meant
primarily to support and protect the rights of the midwives. While we do not see
this being used as a model in the Dufferin and other Fund work, there is a fair bit
of correspondence on nursing training between nursing institutions in England and
the Indian Nursing Council in the 1950s and 1960s, particularly on the lines of asking for support with curricula, as also the possibility of sending students to England
for nursing training.

The indigenous today and the modern nationalist

A policy and politics of therapeutic indigeneity

In this section, I attempt to explore a bit more the widening gap between the dominant and marginal indigenous in therapeutic discourse in independent India. Berger
speaks of the shift of ideas of preventive medicine as social hygiene into urban
planning in the 20th century, and its reintroduction into state-led health planning at
the cusp of independence (2013). We see, in the teaching of preventive medicine in
medical curricula, this health planning echoing the dream of a young nation, wel-
fare-bound, and with the 'community=rural=primary health care' hyphen firmly
in place. Decentralization was the motto proposed for achieving universal health
coverage in these early years, and the rural was the primary unit. For a discipline
that followed the principle of planning as development, including health planning,
the 'indigenous systems of medicine' appeared, for preventive medicine work, as
a sector that needed to be developed, primarily because these systems were seen
as the fallback for a rural populace that did not have access to 'modern curative
and preventive health services' (Park 2015, pp. 900, 915). While this is seen as
reflective of indigenous practitioners (automatically understood as Ayurvedic)
being 'local residents and … very close to the people socially and culturally' (p.
915), the text itself does not entertain, while going over the history of health planning in India, any discussion on the fraught debates around indigenous medicine in
colonial and post-independence India, and certainly not on the possibility of these
systems posing an alternative. While this may be an expected position in an allopathic medicine textbook, it is also indicative of the socio-political discourses that
produce a text like Park.[5] The text, then, is nowhere near prescient on the present
discourse around indigenous medicine.

Is there a present discourse around indigenous medicine, though? Berger notes
that '[w]here the Indigenous Medical Systems had sufficed as a category of analysis and a subject of reform in 1921, from 1938 the particular contexts of Ayurveda

and Unani started to dominate policy reform' (2013, p. 127). By independence and shortly after, as we have seen, modern western medicine was the cornerstone of health planning, and indigenous systems of medicine, while named, failed to find a place in state health systems. In order to understand an emerging discourse of indigeneity in this latter period, the language of the Chopra Committee, or the Committee on Indigenous Systems of Medicine, is useful.

R.N. Chopra was a professor of pharmacology at the School of Tropical Medicine at Calcutta, hailed as the father of modern pharmacology in India, and is celebrated for his work on the anti-hypertensive drug developed from *Rauwolfia serpentina*. At the School of Tropical Medicine, he was a pioneer in conducting experimental 'research investigations into the merits and demerits of the Indian indigenous drugs which had been used for centuries in ancient Indian and folklore medicine and to explore avenues for finding suitable Indian substitutes for imported drugs' (Chopra 1965, p. 3). His position was

> to make Indian pharmacology self-supporting by enabling her to utilize the locally produced drugs economically, under standardized laboratory conditions and (b) to discover remedies, from the claims of Ayurvedic, Tibbi, and other indigenous sources, suitable to be employed by the exponents of western medicine.
>
> (p. 6)

Chopra authored several treatises on indigenous drugs of India. The Chopra Committee itself was constituted in the context of public criticism of the Bhore Committee recommendations that almost dismissed indigenous systems of medicine, and the health ministers' conference in 1946 mooted a resolution to use scientific methods to evaluate indigenous systems and include Ayurvedic and Unani practitioners in health planning; the resolution refers to a wide array of practitioners, including 'doctors, physical training experts (*Ustads*), sanitary staff, masseurs, nurses, midwives' (Chopra et al. 1948, p. 7).

Released in 1948, the Chopra Committee report begins by examining the work of several previous committees set up by provincial and other governments between 1923 to '47 to investigate the status of indigenous systems of medicine, including Ayurveda, Siddha, and Unani. This included the governments of Madras (1923), Bengal (1925), United Provinces (1926), Burma (1928), Central Provinces and Berar (1939), Punjab (1941), Bombay (1947), Assam (1947), Orissa (1947), Mysore (1942), and Ceylon (1927 and 1947). Observations of these committees ranged from the scientificity of these systems to the failure of adequate coverage of medical relief in the country to the presence of household medicine that was largely understood as based on Ayurvedic medicine. Their recommendations highlighted the need to promote and make these systems through state recognition, support, and practitioner registration in order to bring relief particularly to rural areas and to keep quacks at bay (Madras, 1923), registration of pharmacies dispensing indigenous medicine, the need for modernization of Ayurveda, the setting up of state-funded training colleges for the study of Indian Medicine that would also teach the basics of Western medicine, scholarships, libraries, separate councils, 'free professional association between practitioners of the Indian and European systems of Medicine' (Chopra et al 1948 p. 28), and active support from 'Western trained doctors' (p. 29) while encouraging independent practice, permanent government posts, the use of the vernacular in training, promotion of research in Ayurveda and Unani colleges, Ayurvedic dispensaries to be set up at districts and towns and taluks, and publication of textbooks. Some of these recommendations had already been acted upon by provincial governments in the twenty years or so preceding independence. This included the setting up of councils, schools of Indian medicine at Madras in 1925, grants to the Board of Indian Medicine, and gardens to grow medicinal herbs under state management. Burma and Ceylon showed more active steps in this direction, with a Commission on Indigenous Medicine in Ceylon appointed in 1946, making recommendations for the teaching of Ayurveda and Siddha while discontinuing Unani. Some of the recommendations also reflected, through their focus on the medium of instruction proposed – Urdu or Arabic, for instance – the attempt to purify or retain the perceived purity of these systems. Aspects of language seemed important – Persian, Arabic, or Urdu for Unani, Sanskrit and Hindi for Ayurveda, even prescribing instruction in the 'mother tongue', in Bombay. The stated goal for some of this was to eliminate unqualified or quack practitioners and to enable issuance of certificates of illness, death, and legal witnesses. The Chopra Committee felt that the goal of synthesis between Indian and Western systems of medicine had not been discussed or recommended by any of these.

While the Bhore Committee had more or less marked Indian systems of medicine and homeopathy (ISMH) as the obstacle to welfare and uplift, the Chopra report was ambitious in the opposite direction; it categorically stated that

[s]uch multiplicity of systems is only believed in and encouraged by people who have not clearly grasped the significance of the noble ideals as preached by the great Acharyas of Indian medicine and the savants of the Western medicine. The so-called "systems" merely represent different aspects and approaches to medical science as practised during different ages and in different parts of the world; anything of value emerging from these should be utilised for the benefit of humanity as a whole and without any reservation.

(Chopra et al, p. 7)

However, the report used the logic of failing rural health to urge development and formalization of ISMH 'away from everyday practice' (Berger p. 166), advocating, in addition to integration into healthcare systems, for a 'borrowing between traditions rather than a radical transformation of either' (Berger p. 167). Meanwhile, the report also, in tracing the histories of Ayurveda and Unani, reproduced earlier origin stories of Ayurveda as the primary source of Greek and modern medicine, and in its recommendations, proposed integrated teaching of Ayurvedic and Western medicine with no mention of Unani, which had been qualified as 'not strictly ... indigenous to India' (Chopra et al, p. 8). Importantly, it also called for a central register of 'authorized practitioners' (Berger, p. 168). The Committee suggested that this register be kept 'separate from that of the practitioners of Western medicine for the present. Later when the standard of education in the Colleges of Indian Medicine improves and the *non-institutionally qualified fade out*, the question may be reviewed' (Chopra et al. 1948, p. 193, italics mine). Finally, the Committee spoke of the importance of identifying and growing medicinal plants, along with registration and regulation of the same.

The Central Council for Research in Indian Medicine and Homeopathy, under the Ministry of Health and Family Welfare, reflects in an overview document put out in 1977 on the decade of development of indigenous medicine in the 1960s and 1970s. In its introductory paragraph, it talks of indigenous systems as 'Ayurveda, Siddha, Unani-Tibb, Nature Cure, Yoga and other traditional systems', but immediately focusses on 'Ayurveda, the science of life [that] has stood the greater test of time' (p. 1). This polemic is recognizable in several retrospective documents like this one, which position themselves somewhat between an objective historical account and a status report, providing evidence in the form of photographs of laboratories, practitioners at work, enumerations of institutions, practitioners, etc., perhaps responding to a pressure to prove its scientificity vis-à-vis biomedicine, as Sujatha and Abraham (2012) have also suggested while reflecting on state-supported institutions of ISM. Reflecting on the work of the Bhore and Chopra committees, this report speaks of the Central Research Institute set up at Jamnagar in Gujarat as 'the first milestone in the progress and development of Ayurveda' (p. 2), followed by a postgraduate training centre in 1956 and a full-fledged post-graduate training and research institute and an Ayurvedic college in 1962.[6] Such institutes were set up at Banaras Hindu University in 1962, and Ayurvedic dispensaries under the Central Government Health Scheme of GOI. With the Dave Committee of 1954 progressing towards preparing a model syllabus and recommending institutional teaching, the first Five-Year Plan saw the allocation of four million INR for research and development of Indian systems of medicine. A Central Board of Siddha was also set up in 1964–65; meanwhile integrated approaches to healing and therapeutics were being adopted by the teaching institutions, along with recommendations for standardization of curricula. A high-powered panel was set up by the Planning Commission in 1966 to study indigenous systems, which recommended research, education, training, and regulation of practice. Research institutes were set up with grants from the central government at Rajasthan, Ranikhet in UP, Madras, Thanjavur, Varanasi, and Aligarh Muslim University. 1969–70, says the report, 'can be said to be the Golden period in the history of development of Ayurveda and allied sciences' (p. 6), with, for one, government recognition of Indian systems of Medicine (ISM) following the Planning Panel recommendations, and the setting up of the Central Council – a precursor to several research institutions and schemes, drug and clinical research, and medicinal plant surveys. At this time, the Council claims to have 'collected about 1500 folklore claims' (p. 6), and 'published books containing simple remedies in Homoeopathy, Unani and Siddha for common ailments … besides technical reports and abstracts' (p. 6–7).

In this golden period, the approach seems to have been about taking stock of a vast and heterogeneous terrain, bringing the institutional and extra-institutional into view, in addition to doing 'intensive research' on specific diseases that showed 'encouraging results' (p. 7). Patents for

> 12 new processes ... [and] commercial exploitation of the patented drugs' were also being considered. 1972 saw the first scientific seminar that brought practitioners together across these traditions; in the previous year, the Central Council of Indian Medicine Act had been passed 'mainly to evolve uniform standards of education ... and to maintain a Central Register for these systems.
>
> (p. 10)

It is this legislation that precedes the most recent policy and law enactments in the 2020s. 1975 saw the 'bringing together [of] Teaching, Training and Research under one roof' (p. 10) with National Institutes for Homeopathy and Ayurveda, followed by a Central Research Institute for Yoga. During this period, the Drugs and Cosmetics Act was extended to cover indigenous medicines. Patents and the export of raw drugs were some of the other developments. The 'utility of ISM to rural population' was sought to be operationalized at this time through a 'six-point programme ... by the ... Department of Health'; this involved 'free medical aid in villages once a week ... making available simple and effective medical aid' (p. 12). Meanwhile, engagements with the governments of Iran, Afghanistan, and others were seen as routes to showcase Ayurveda and Unani.

While this account offers a promising present and future for indigenous medicine in the late 1970s, it is still a period when evidence-building, formalization, effectiveness, and global interest and appreciation continue to be parameters to build legitimacy for these fields. Each of these efforts is visible in the report.

Vocabularies and presence

Sujatha V. and Leena Abraham (2012), in their comprehensive exploration of indigenous systems of medicine in contemporary India, engage with the multiple labels attributed to a heterogeneous set of practices by the colonial as well as independent state, and in global documents. While we see both monikers – Indian and indigenous – being used in policy documents in independent India, the authors locate these vocabularies and terminologies in terms of disciplinary formations that have explored the field. In so doing, they trace 'an interesting division of labour between British historians looking at colonial influence, West European Sanskritists focusing on the Indological approach and North American anthropologists carrying out ethnographic studies' (p. 12). This division of labour also divides, or rather categorizes, the space and material being studied, and introduces specific lenses for the study. Complementary and alternative medicine (CAM) as a term is more visible in 'medical sociology ... in the West' (p. 4), the authors note. Traditional Medicine (TM), Asian medicine, and Indian medicine, are some of the terms used in anthropological literature. As they explore the historical approaches to this set of practices – sociological, civilizational, therapeutic – Sujatha and Abraham speak of medical pluralism, first introduced into medical anthropology by Leslie (1976), as one of the rationales that came into play for health policies to pay more attention to indigenous systems than had previously been the case. Leslie, whose foundational work has largely been on syncretism in modern Ayurveda, spoke of the 'Asian model' where traditions of biomedicine and Ayurveda were of different worldviews, both moral and epistemological, but were accessed in a cosmopolitan or 'syncretic' manner by village practitioners studied in the 1950's anthropological literature (1992). This multi-pronged practitioner approach is not presented as a rationale to deny 'systems' status to non-biomedical approaches, however. Mukharji suggests that 'medical pluralism repositions the patient – rather than the state – at the centre of medical history' (2009, p. 16), and thus finds it not entirely useful in medical historiography. Sujatha and Abraham, however, refer to medical pluralism as a social reality as well as a state position particularly on rural therapeutics. Ritu Priya (2012) in the same collection, further explores this idea to differentiate between undemocratic pluralism – a situation of marginal state support – and a more democratic pluralism that could support 'lay people's choices' (2012, p. 105) and increase infrastructure, rather than, as she notes, simply move AYUSH physicians from stand-alone AYUSH facilities to the public health system. Such a move, she suggests, only weakens the AYUSH structure without bringing real plurality of access to the public health system. We may, as we look at the Ayush ministry in the next section, following Ritu Priya, think about the tokenism and symbolism that seems to be even more visible in several of the newer formations. Moreover, as Sujatha V. and Abraham note, medical pluralism falters in accommodating 'indigenous systems that lie on the borderland between therapy and ritual and those enmeshed in the living conditions of the socially disprivileged ... [like] the *dai*' (2012, p. 25). We will, in the next section, look at more recent consolidations of what constitutes the indigenous – in policy, politics, and law. It is useful, however, as we close this discussion, to explore the histories of Preventive and Social Medicine (PSM), now referred to as Community Medicine, a bit further.

The community in Community Medicine

Medical practitioners trained in and writing histories of PSM in India mostly propose an origin story for the discipline relating to, as we have seen, the Bhore Committee recommendations on community-based primary and preventive health care, which strongly recommended a 3-month training period preparing medical graduates to become 'social physicians' (Park 2015, p. 873). Although PSM was thus seen as applicable to '"healthy" people' (Thakur et al 2001, p. 2), this version suggests that good PSM practitioners are likely to emerge only through a more integrated dynamic between medical colleges and healthcare systems – a connection that developed with the *Re-orientation of Medical Education* scheme in 1977. Some practitioners maintain that Community Medicine comprises public health as well as family medicine, and thus the clinical task is as important in primary preventive healthcare for community medicine physicians (Shewade et al 2014). Community physicians are expected to manage primary healthcare facilities, provide clinical services, orient medical students to primary healthcare, and train postgraduates of various specialities, as well as train medical and paramedical staff in the healthcare system. Research is another component of the mandate. In all of these roles, the community as the basis of training and service is expected to be paramount.

While the shift from PSM to community medicine has several contexts, including WHO's exhortation towards country-specific naming, Community Medicine in India seemed to take on more administrative and planning aspects than academic social medicine had, which focused on people in environments, and the conditions required to maintain optimum health among them. Specialties like epidemiology, maternal and child health, IEC, and health system management training within PSM make sense in this respect.

In reflecting on the current loss of direction in Community Medicine, practitioners focus on the primary role, i.e., clinical service, having been lost along the way, with the discipline having become merely academic – a charge that has been laid at the door of general biomedical training as well (Shewade et al. 2014). This is a useful critical impulse in medical training, as it keeps alive the question of holding the community at the centre of both clinical service and health management. Community Medicine departments have tried, on paper, to keep this impulse alive. By not taking 'the primary role of a community physician seriously' (Shewade et al. 2014, p. 30), however, medical practitioners lament the loss of commitment by practitioners who would rather stay within urban-centric super-specializations and approach public health in universalist ways. Some of this critique was also reflected in people's health movements that spoke primarily of lack of access as the cause of disease, particularly in Marxian frameworks, a phenomenon seen in Chile, Cuba, Nicaragua, and other Latin American countries (Porter, 2006). While this lament in the Indian context appears to be more of a pointer at a moral failure, and thus a comedown for a 'noble profession' than a professional and ethical one, it points to a larger question – that of responsibility and accountability to the community, and on whom that responsibility rests. For practitioners of biomedicine who are held 'outside' of the community in some way, particularly when they are implicitly seen as urban and the community as rural, this indictment is particularly significant, especially in the context of calls to synthesize with indigenous medicine. Also, the call to integration between preventive and curative, which is the primary impulse in Community Medicine, fails completely as the *practice* of community medicine remains aspirational, the seat of ideal scenario-building; in this scenario, the community-rural-vulnerable-indigenous hyphen[7] continues to languish.

There is another anchor for Community Medicine in India – the global focus on public health itself, one that begins with colonial ideas of tropical medicine and hygiene; this is evident even in the naming of the earliest institutions like the All India Institute of Hygiene & Public Health, set up in Calcutta in 1934. While this accompanied the developments in theories around disease causation from miasma to germ theory, as I discussed in Chapter 4, Dorothy Porter speaks of the global story of social medicine as a discipline that may have, in the 19th century, emerged in the discourse of health and social reform regarding 'the political role of medicine in creating egalitarian societies' (Porter 2006, p. 1667). While this translated in Latin American social medicine to a focus on socio-political transformations that impacted national health policy, Anglo-American contexts saw the rise of 'life-style medicine' – an approach that put down causation of disease – particularly chronic disease – to individual behaviours. This 'risk' approach took over global agendas on the management of health, with both social medicine and public health agendas becoming more medicalized, focusing on *'lifestyles* … [that] created major risks rather than *life conditions'* (Porter 2006, p. 1669). This medicalization approach remained different from the ALAMES (Latin American Social Medicine Association) position that helped produce social medicine curricula that took the social structural approach to disease causation; this approach, however, remains somewhat confined to the particular region.

So, Community Medicine in India has two paths – community responsibility and public health management. The latter goes with the dream of 'development as planning' which was the motto of the first prime minister of independent India – Jawaharlal Nehru. The former takes on the possibility of building indigenous therapeutic cultures. With Nehruvian agendas taking centre-stage in independent India, public health management took precedence, while community responsibility continued to hover as a moral goal. As Shewade et al. suggest, health systems planning became the career path for community physicians trained in primary healthcare (2014, p. 31). It is much later, in the contemporary era, with the emergence of a political class that directly pits majoritarianism as a valid, relevant, and successful approach against Nehruvianism, that a translation of indigeneity via majoritarian agendas cuts free of the hyphen, the substitutability with rurality or vulnerability, except in its symbolic form. It begins to occupy, perhaps in the performance of a surface synthesis, a systemic place of its own, no longer in contradiction with modernity. In independent India today, there is no real staging of an encounter with Western medicine; therefore, the staging is within, in a challenge to Nehruvian ideas of modernity, as a symbol of nationalist pride, and as a route to a place in the league of nations. I will examine this further in the next sections.

Other vocabularies of community

It is useful, at this point, to flag other vocabularies of community – poverty, rurality, access – that the Bhore model sought to foreground. Somewhat akin to the Latin American approach, this vocabulary, embedded in socialist understandings, sought to highlight poverty and literacy as the greatest barriers to health access, and gave rise to a slew of mobilizations of civil society as people's health movements globally focusing on rights of access, universal health coverage, gender justice, rational drug use, confronting the commercialization of healthcare, and the right to generic and low-cost medication, activating the 1981 WHO definition of Health for All into the slogan 'Health for All – Now!' in 2000. The *Jan Swasthya Abhiyan* (JSA), as the formal version of this network of nearly 20 collectives in India is known, has gone on to critique 'iniquitous globalization' (http://phmindia.org/about-us/) after the entry of the World Bank (WB) into the health sector in India. Critiques of WB functioning have pointed to the imperialist approach of its 1993 report titled 'Investment in Health', which criticizes 'need-based' countries for spending on tertiary care rather than basic health, among other criticisms – an attitude that scarcely respects the autonomy and internal mechanisms of these governments, as well as an attitude that diverts attention from the impact of structural adjustment policies on the economic well-being of people in these countries. The WB, following its report, prescribes the actual separation of preventive and curative work at the primary health care level, suggests the institution of 'user fees' to recover costs, and the transfer of curative medicine to the private sector. The WB also advised the setting up of vertical disease management programmes for malaria, tuberculosis, AIDS, leprosy, and blindness – all designed via target approaches that have been shown to have either failed or failed to produce expected outcomes (Ravindran 2007). Overall, the prescription to redistribute funds efficiently as an answer to a resource crunch recalls an old WB strategy – global managerialism (Murphy 2007).

Critiques of WB policies also offer a nod to indigeneity as a counter to the bank's ethnocentrism, but the primary thrust in these, and in the work of JSA, has been to recognize but leave to community the development of indigenous medicine and folk traditions without further discussion. The 1985 Rockefeller report, 'Good Health at Low Cost' (Halstead et al. 1985) had earlier explored the differences in health outcomes among low-income countries, identified that a commitment to equity both within and outside of healthcare systems was essential to support primary preventive healthcare, and indicted governments for lack of political will to treat health as a social goal. In a reassessment conducted 25 years down the line, the Indian state of Tamil Nadu from the 1980s to 2005 was one among the newer study sites. The findings indicate clearly that inclusion of indigenous medicine practitioners in primary healthcare has helped increase the use of public healthcare in rural areas (Muraleedharan, Dash, and Gilson 2011). This is, of course, in addition to efforts towards social equity measures like gender equality, literacy, and so on. Other critiques of WB recommendations suggest that a strong national health policy that takes into account indigenous systems, that involves indigenous practitioners in policy formulation, that introduces traditional medicine in allopathic training, among other steps, would improve national health, in addition to protecting India from plunging into international debt, which would be the obvious outcome of following WB recommendations (Srinivasan 1995).

We see, then, that while there is a recognition of the presence and value of non-allopathic systems by both state and non-state actors, these vocabularies of community focus primarily on access, political commitments, rights, and health citizenship (Porter 2011). The connections between indigeneity and vulnerability are primary here, and this is the connection that gets disrupted in majoritarian discourse.

Ayush and planning documents on ISM

It is in this context that we might look at the recent spate of legislations and policies around indigenous systems of medicine in India. The National Commission for Indian System of Medicine Bill was introduced by the Ministry of Ayush in the Rajya Sabha, the upper house of Parliament, on 7 January 2019. It was proposed to replace the Indian Medicine Central Council Act 1970 and is meant to regulate education and practice of Ayurveda, Unani, Siddha, and Sowa-Rigpa. Like earlier legislation, it also proposed to improve the quality of education in these systems, prevent malpractice, and provide for research on drugs. The Bill has similarities with the Indian Medicine Central Council (Amendment) Bill of 2005 which had also proposed the dissolving of the Central Council and its reconstitution by an interim Board of Governors, with members from states with registered Ayurveda, Siddha, and Unani practitioners. This bill was withdrawn in 2019, prior to the introduction of the current Bill which was then passed into law in September 2020.

Like the Midwifery Bill of 2020 and the earlier National Medical Commission Act of 2018, the Act provides for sharp centralization of regulation, with a proposed National Council of 29 members, all to be appointed by the Central Government, as opposed to the earlier mode of members being elected from among practitioners from the states. Like the Midwifery Bill, inspection and monitoring are to be conducted by an external agency on the grounds of removing the contradiction that the regulated conduct their own regulations, but leaving room for interference and undermining of practitioner autonomy. While the Bill did go to a Parliamentary Standing Committee for inputs, the latter's recommendations were limited to technicalities, including proposing more members from Ayurveda to be represented on the Council on account of their listed numbers, more state representation, a Board of Yoga and Naturopathy, and fee regulation. Civil society representation on the Commission, one of the questions asked of the Ayush Ministry, failed to find its way into the final recommendations. About the question of *dai* practitioners, the question was neither asked nor answered. The Committee was of the view that '[w]ith an increase in non-communicable diseases and chronic ailments, there has been a shift towards adopting lifestyle changes and growing emphasis on alternative systems of medicine. In such a scenario, India has the potential to emerge as a global hub for medical tourism in AYUSH' (Standing Committee Recommendations, p. 84). Medical tourism and infrastructure to that end, therefore, were the final recommendations of the Committee.

At around the same time, the Ministry of Health and Family Welfare brought two bills to Parliament – the National Commission for Allied and Healthcare Professionals Bill that was introduced and passed in Parliament in March 2021, and the National Medical Commission Bill 2019. The 2019 Bill, which was passed into law in August 2019, repeals the Indian Medical Council Act 1956, and effectively also does away with the Medical Council of India (MCI), the apex body for the registration and licensing of allopathic practitioners. The proposed National Medical Council, as the new regulator for education and practice, is not an elected body as the MCI was, is not diverse in representation, and has an over-representation of practitioners with no community representation. The Allied and Healthcare Professionals Bill aligns more with the International System of Classification of Occupations (ISCO). Hailed as a way to increase employability among youth and as a patient-centric approach, this legislation is a logical culmination and formalization of task shifting, but somewhat different from what we have seen in the appointment of ASHAs. Recognition as professionals and the granting of degrees and diplomas mark these allied professionals as recognized outposts of allopathic institutionalized medicine. It might be surmised that this allows more scope for privatization if more training organizations/institutions are set up. All this legislation, some of it tabled and passed by voice vote on the same day in Parliament, has been enacted during the pandemic years.

It is alongside this fast-paced set of legislations, and within the discourse around indigenous medicine as a powerful metaphor for the nationalist, patriotic impulse, that parallel state-level legislations like the Rajya Ayush Vishwavidyalaya, Uttar Pradesh Adhiniyam, 2020 (The State Ayush University, Uttar Pradesh Act, 2020), proposing the setting up of a state Ayush university at Gorakhpur, are to be seen. Within the context of the pandemic, other processes, like the formal launching of 'inter-disciplinary studies involving AYUSH interventions for COVID 19 situation' (https://prsindia.org/files/covid19/notifications/5781.IND_AYUSH_COVID.pdf) are also underway. As is the Drugs (Fourth Amendment) Rules 2021 to amend the Drugs Rules 1945, that revises license fees to manufacture Ayurveda, Siddha, or Unani drugs, and introduces applications for good practice certificates (in keeping with quality control manoeuvres).

What is new here? Can we draw linear connections between majoritarian political formations and increased visibility to indigenous medical systems, as critical scholars and activists have been wont to do? The Mudaliar Committee was the first to recommend the use of indigenous doctors for vertical healthcare programs (Rudra et al. 2017). The Ministry of Ayush was set up in November 2014, upgraded from the Department of AYUSH – an acronym for what are called the seven traditional systems – Ayurveda, Yoga and Naturopathy, Unani, Siddha, Homeopathy. The department itself was renamed as such in 2003, earlier being known as the Department of Indian Systems of Medicine and Homeopathy within the Ministry of Health and Family Welfare, set up in 1995, in the ninth 5-year plan, which saw increased budgetary allocation towards this field. Earlier policies like the Indigenous Systems of Medicine and Homeopathy Policy 2002 governed the work in this period, alongside the National Health Policy 2002. The stated rationale for the attention paid to this is the increasing relevance of AYUSH, which is now recognized as a safe and cost-effective treatment option (https://www.nhp.gov.in/ayush_ms), thus encouraging 'a pluralistic approach in healthcare where every system is allowed to grow on the basis of evident strength' (ibid). The ministry has now been renamed Ayush, mobilizing the word rather than the acronym (Gazette of India notification, 13 April 2021); the front page of the ministry website describes it as 'traditional and non-conventional systems of health care and healing which include Ayurveda, Yoga, Naturopathy, Unani, Siddha, Sowa-Rigpa and Homeopathy etc' (https://main.ayush.gov.in/). The word indicates, in Sanskrit and northern Indian languages, a long life – a hint at the metaphors of immortality that are popularly associated with Ayurveda legend, as also with salutations to live long.[8] Orientalist visions of Eastern mysticism and spirituality are not far behind.

Health is a state subject in Indian governance systems; however, in September 2014, a centrally sponsored National Ayush Mission was announced as one of the flagship schemes of the Ministry of Ayush. This scheme was launched to provide AYUSH services through primary health centres, community health centres and district hospitals, to provide grant-in-aid to upgrade and strengthen state government hospitals, pharmacies, and laboratories, to introduce good agricultural practices to support medicinal plant cultivation, and to support the convergence of cultivation and marketing of drugs and infrastructure. The latest star in this kitty is the Ayush Health and Wellness Centres approved by the Union Cabinet in March 2020, with the aim of introducing holistic models of health, continuum of care, reduction of out-of-pocket expenditure, and dissemination of information to the 'needy public' (https://namayush.gov.in/content/about-hwc#v-pills-messages). These aims were to be achieved by 'transforming existing Sub Health Centres and Primary Health Centres to deliver Comprehensive Primary Health Care' (Operational guidelines 2020, p. 16). Much along the lines of integrating primary health care with other levels as proposed in Bhore and other committees, but with Ayush now front and centre, the Ayush HWCs include community mobilization for preventive care, linkages with non-governmental organizations, and digitization. A 12-part service delivery framework is discussed, including maternal and childbirth care. Continuum of care is proposed through population enumeration, community screening, and risk assessment including a 44-page *Prakriti* questionnaire called *Prakriti* genetic screening, intended to identify the nature (translates as *prakriti*) of the individual and classify them using precepts of Ayurveda, Yoga, herbal gardens, diagnostic, and prescription services. Taking on the language of social determinants of health and partly global concerns around adolescent risk, the operational guidelines for Ayush HWCs speak of 'tobacco, alcohol and substance abuse, action against gender violence, [and] social evils' as among the seven priority areas demanding coordinated action and intersectoral convergence. Here too, as in other parts of the Ayushman Bharat flagship scheme of the central government, target-based incentivization is in place for the health officers. In conjunction with the digitization attached to all of these screening and clinical services, what we also have is an emerging data bank of a variety of individual behaviours and practices; the *Prakriti* screening questionnaire, for instance, includes questions on whether marriages have been inter-caste, inter-regional, inter-religious, among a host of other questions on physical characteristics, which are deemed to be important in Ayurveda practice.[9]

The 2002 National Policy on Indian Systems of Medicine (ISM) and Homeopathy emerged in a different context from the present, although also seeking integration of Indian systems with modern medicine. Actively placing itself within the critique of biomedicine inasmuch as chemical-based drugs are concerned, as well as the emergence of newer lifestyle diseases, the 2002 policy speaks of the existence but relative invisibility, as well as the unorganized character, of infrastructure, institutions, and practitioners of traditional medicine. Following the directive of the first National Health Policy in 1983, as well as the setting up of the Central Council for Health and Family Welfare in the 1980s, the policy sought to increase expenditure on, improve the quality of education in, and create sustainable growth systems for medicinal plants. The policy also took note of the need to protect intellectual property of ISM; it actively refers to the TRIPS agreement to which India is a signatory.

Payyappallimana (2010) delineates the several views of integration that operate in policy. One is the utilitarian view which attempts to validate and include aspects of traditional medicine (TM). A syncretic view brings together both to form a new system. Complementary medicine is a view that sees TM as supportive. Co-evolution, or Needham's view, sees different knowledge systems evolving simultaneously and discretely. A trans-cultural and transdisciplinary perspective recognizes the situated character of knowledge. TM is sometimes romanticized as 'good old ancient wisdom'. Payyappallimana avers that the utilitarian view is most in practice. According to Payyappallimana, India displays more of an 'inclusive' than 'integrated' system, since full official recognition, incorporation into national drug policy, availability of therapies at all hospitals and clinics, health insurance, and research and education, are not fully available.

The Ayush Mission differs in tone, claims, and objectives from the ISM & H policy 2002. While the 2002 policy aims for collaboration with allopathic institutions in specific illness constellations and is more tentative on these issues, Ayush has embraced the wellness discourse – in the form of Yoga, medicine gardens, *panchkarma* practices, etc. Strangely, this seems to be accompanied by some degree of deskilling in the new policy; while the operational guidelines are peppered with Ayurveda vocabulary, treatment infrastructure or specific Ayurveda treatment modalities are merely hinted at, most of the spelled-out interventions being in the domain of Yoga. At the same time, there is no mention of 'folk health traditions related to birth attendants, herbal healers, bone setters, Visha healers etc' that the 2002 policy speaks of selectively identifying and validating (section 16.8). What we have instead is moralizing presented as care services – for instance, 'staying away from electronic gadgets' is listed as a blanket strategy in child and adolescent healthcare guidelines. Overall, what emerges most visibly and strongly are screening tools like the *Prakriti* questionnaire, proposed on a community scale, and placed within natal kinship and caste endogamous structures. The sections on prevention and promotion of self-care read almost as a pointer to a prescribed 'way of life' via *Prakriti* ('a comprehensive understanding of psycho somatic constitution of an individual based on physical, psychological and social identity by using validated methods and tools'), *Dinacharya* (daily routine 'to be followed to stay connected to the rhythms of nature'), *Ritucharya* (seasonal routine), dietetics, and Yoga (p. 10 of operational guidelines, clause 4.1 on preventive and promotive measures for self-care).

One of the impulses we are seeing here, perhaps, is an effort to codify a vast array of heterogeneous practices. Although the Ayush vocabulary is no longer one of validation of indigenous systems with respect to allopathy standards, as the 2002 policy implicitly suggests, the model of categorization and classification is very much in place, as is the impulse to scale up. Seen along with the Pradhan Mantri Jan Arogya Yojana (PM-JAY) – presented as a universal health insurance scheme, and the second component within Ayushman Bharat, the strategy of universal interpellation, if not coverage, seems to have been activated.

Apart from the blitzkrieg of performance of culture-specific governance that is visible, however, what is the epistemic shift that has been achieved? Madhulika Banerjee, writing in the immediate context of the Indian Systems of Medicine and Homeopathy 2002 policy, brings up the many dilemmas at the heart of synthesis, development, and finding a place in the league of nations for India. Delineating what she calls the 'pharmaceutical episteme', Banerjee traces how the 'commercialisation, standardisation and professionalisation, already the main foci of transformation in the post-colonial civil society, were and continue to be taken up for the developmental agenda of the state' (2002, pp. 1136–7). The pharmaceutical episteme is defined by Banerjee as an episteme 'that focused on retaining Ayurveda's usefulness as a mere supplier of new pharmaceuticals and … dismissing its worldview on the body, health and disease' (p. 1136). This is the chief marker of Ayurveda's modernization project, Banerjee notes. Marking the Chopra Committee as the reference point for the standardizing impulse, as also for 'hastening specialisation in the traditional medical systems' (p. 1137), Banerjee points to how mass-scale commercial production becomes the recognized way to produce and commodify Ayurvedic medicines, and how this domain – of mass production and quality control – becomes the over-developed domain of what goes by Ayurveda. Girija notes this as well, in charting the making of modern Ayurveda in Kerala, as a movement begun in the 20th century, with Ayurvedic drug exhibitions and so on (2021). We have seen the impulses towards this in the Indigenous Drugs Committee meetings at the beginning of the 20th century. It stands to reason that this primacy to large-scale drug manufacturers comprehensively decentres the individual traditional practitioner for whom pre-preparation of a medicine itself would be considered against protocol. Of these large manufacturers, companies like *Dabur* or *Himalaya* have actually seen growth in cosmetics and personal care products that are plant-based and that claim to be based in or allied to Ayurveda, and multiple other FMCG manufacturers have introduced products from natural toothpaste to cooking oils and *kadhas* (drinks prepared as immunity boosters) in the pandemic years. The statistic that Ayurvedic products had less than 1% of the FMCG market in 2020 (Malviya, 2020) perhaps only indicates the potential of the sector. Even in the domain of Ayurvedic medicines, then, it is this section that seems the fastest growing. What Banerjee highlights as the 'Ayurveda touch' from the Udupa Committee report of 1959 is telling here; it is the 'salve of the "natural"' (p. 1144) that is being sold rather than an alternate knowledge model. The precisely and well-moulded tablet, then, is bound to upstage the *goli* (the oral medicine moulded by hand), and the ideology of mass production is what will reach the new, ecologically conscious consumer who wants the salve in the familiarity of neat packaging. Quality control, good agricultural practice in the growing of medicinal plants, that we see in the Ayush HWC discourse, also makes sense here.

Banerjee's primary evaluation of the 2002 policy yields a recognition of treating ISM & H at par with modern biomedicine – a shift from earlier positions. There is also a move towards medical pluralism. However, the attention to lesser, unregistered practitioners, and their participation in quality control, which would be required for this to sustain, seemed unclear at the time of Banerjee's analysis. The 'systems' question that the Chopra Committee had so comprehensively debunked also continues to be the framework of analysis; the encounter framework, in other words, although discredited, continues as a reference point. The idea of alternative knowledge models seems to find life only when embedded in a system of production, language, and institutions that have a recognizable, homogenous face. This might be the reason why TRIPS and patents – a marking of territory – are the shared framework, and why deforestation and over-exploitation of the land for large-scale manufacture become a concern; these manufacturers then either move to less-exploited terrain (from Karnataka to Chhattisgarh, for example, where unexploited forest cover is huge and labour costs are also a fraction) or to 'green commitments' offering incentives or 'partnerships' with medicinal plant growers (Hellwig 2015, https://ayushherbs.com/, Kulkarni 2013). State mechanisms continue to talk of IEC and 'community participation' (Roy et al. 2018). In Uttarakhand, this included declaring bio-diverse Uttarakhand a 'herbal state'. A state project collaborating with the Global Environment Facility and UNDP titled 'Mainstreaming Conservation and Sustainable Use of Medicinal Plant Diversity in Three Indian States' (Roy et al. 2018) involved training the community and school students to identify and classify medicinal plants, to encourage the use of 'good agricultural practices' to grow and 'harvest' medicinal and aromatic plants (MAPs) as a source of livelihood and income. Even traditional healers (named as *Vaidyas* – it is unclear whether this naming is local) were involved in helping identify MAPs, their use, and economic value, but it is unclear what their returns in terms of recognition as knowledge producers were. All of these exercises plug into the SDG slogan of 'Leave no one behind', pay homage to Alma Ata, and embrace the wellness paradigm.

Wellness

Is it this attention that we might trace, in part, in the discourse of Ayurveda and wellness in today's Ayush policy? Is there a shift from seeking validation to seeking collaboration? Is this true integration at work – bringing the bodily practices prescribed by Ayurveda to the healthcare system to ensure better preventive mechanisms alongside the curative aspects of biomedicine – the dream but failure of the 2002 policy? Have the Chopra Committee recommendations finally found fruition? Most of the rhetoric emerging from the current political leadership does seem to use integration as word wizardry in the various backronyms it uses – like LaQshya, mentioned above; such backronyms have become a ubiquitous feature of policy language in the past few years. But rhetoric apart, is there perhaps a new kind of West-facing Orientalism at work here? And is this where, along with marginality and vulnerability, the *dai* disappears?

Traditional medicine (TM) or complementary medicine (CAM) has been part of the WHO's overall health strategies since 1977, when its Traditional Medicine Programme was established. Over the years, attention to national programmes and policy development, research, safety and efficacy management, and promotion of respect for different knowledge traditions and their pharmacopoeia has been endorsed by the WHO. The *WHO Traditional Medicine (TM) Strategy 2014–2023* builds on some of these positions, most recently on an earlier *WHO TM Strategy 2002–2005*, which recommended that member states

> integrate TM within national health care systems, where feasible ... promote the safety, efficacy and quality of TM ... increase the availability and afford-ability of TM, with an emphasis on access for poor populations ... [and] promote therapeutically sound use of appropriate TM by practitioners and consumers.
>
> (WHO 2013, p. 11)

The Delhi Declaration on Traditional Medicine in 2013, mooted at the international conference organized by the GOI in collaboration with the WHO, listed nine items for cooperation, collaboration, and mutual support across member states, includ-ing 'common TM reference documents, encouraging sustainable development and resource augmentation of medicinal plants, and exchanging perspectives, experi-ences and experts' (WHO 2013, p. 65). The difficulty of evaluating TM advertising claims, as also the enforcement of regulations, continues to be flagged, however, and the 2014–23 strategy suggests that member states evolve their own policies and regulations, strengthen quality assurance through education, and 'promote uni-versal health coverage by integrating T&CM services into health service delivery and self-health care ... and ... ensuring users are able to make informed choices about self-health care' (WHO 2013, p. 12). '[H]arnessing the potential contribu-tion of TM to health, wellness and people-centred health care' (WHO 2013, p. 11) remains one of the core goals of the strategy. Both these documents, however, indicate that financial support from the WHO will be practically impossible.

The WHO's commitment to integration is consolidated in the 2014–23 strategy document. In addition, there is the push towards quality control, institutionalized and regulated education, and 'self-health care'. From the 1990s, when the first pro-gress reports were being prepared, to the latest strategy document, however, men-tion of traditional birth attendants, herbalists, or bone setters, is conspicuous by its disappearance. Mention of India is in terms of 'two categories of TM practitioners' (WHO 2013, p. 29) – registered Ayurveda, Yoga, Naturopathy, Unani, Siddha, and Homeopathy practitioners, and village-based Ayush community health workers. In the definition of TM, then, the *dai* is nowhere to be found.

How does wellness travel? Payyappallimana and Fadeeva's (2018) exploration of sustainability experiences across underserved and other communities across contexts may provide some clues. Regional Centres of Expertise (RCE) Network – a platform that is part of the UN Decade on Education for Sustainable Development, meant to record local solutions developed for local challenges, provided the premise of the exploration. The medicinal plant diversity project across the three biodiversity-rich Indian states of Arunachal Pradesh, Chhattisgarh, and Uttarakhand (Roy et al., 2018) under the community health theme of the RCE has been referred to above. In RCE

Grand Rapids, Michigan, the Health and Wellness Program aims at holistic healthcare, nutrition, focus on immunization, and healthcare screening – a broad, non-specific, prevention-centred interpretation of wellness that includes community-based solutions, wellness visits, and is focused on that red herring – *lifestyle*. These are embedded in the SDGs. While there are references to 'environmental health disparities ... that cannot be pursued in isolation' (p. 23), the Health and Wellness impact team here focuses on awareness of local nutrition, avoidance of junk and fast foods, local community gardens, etc. This local community model is cautiously lauded for not being integrated into any state-based model. Place-based strategies include learning to communicate with healthcare delivery professionals. Individuals are encouraged to take responsibility for their own wellness. In the Ayush policies, we have seen a focus on bodily practices through Yoga, and prescribed lifestyle shifts meant to bring greater alignment with environments, as a route to wellness.

If wellness is best achieved in place, how do we understand the varieties of wellness tourism that are in place in India and that are being actively promoted in policy? Promoters of wellness tourism hail India as a 'historical wellness destination', offering goals ranging from 'rest and relaxation to specific goals of detox' (Vasudevan 2021, p. 98), 'sought by people who do not have a medical condition ... and the primary motivation for the trip is to ensure lasting health' (p. 99). The Ministry of Tourism defines wellness tourism thus

> The potential of wellness systems, developed through centuries of wisdom of this ancient civilization ... is being done by positioning India as a centre of Ayurveda, Yoga, Siddha, Naturopathy etc together with the spiritual philosophy that has been integral to the *Indian way of life*.
> (https://tourism.gov.in/wellness-tourism#skipCont, italics mine)

It mentions guidelines for accreditation of wellness centres developed by the National Board for Accreditation of Hospitals and Healthcare Services (NABH) in consultation with Ayush. While medical tourism depends on privatization and outsourcing of healthcare by states, wellness tourism is seen as one of the active elements of the Ayush ministry's work. The study cited here also finds that Ayurveda and Yoga are the commonest keywords used to promote and brand wellness tourism destinations. 'Ayurveda touch' indicated by the Udupa Committee is of course very much in evidence here, as also sanitized Hindi-Hindu cultural vocabulary.[10] Wellness, then, may or may not be about sustainability and staying in place; it might well be about a package, offering a well-earned comma in an otherwise 'productive' life, and one that the Ayush avatar of indigeneity is uniquely positioned to provide. The hyphen is now this – indigenous-privileged-caste-Hindu-nation. Indigeneity is now a self-determined identity, not an ascribed one.

Kerala Ayurveda occupies a much earlier place in the history of wellness tourism in India. Known and trusted for Ayurvedic treatments, both the 120-year-old globally renowned Kottakkal Arya Vaidya Sala at Malappuram, and other centres, blur the boundaries between medical and wellness tourism. Abraham suggests that Kerala Ayurveda is known more for its treatments and medicinal products than cosmetic and other products (Abraham 2013). It is, perhaps, the most unapologetic apostle of caste Hindu cultural practices, from its website to its language. Girija and Abraham, among others, have spoken of the heterogeneous set of *naattuvaid-yam* practices from which Kerala Ayurveda emerges as a codified, recognizable, sanitized system, built on the erasure of a series of practitioners and practices – of *bhootavidyam, mantravadam,* and others (Abraham 2013). Naturalized as a way of life, immediately recognizable as Indian rather than Hindu, or rather with the two having been neatly merged, the imagery around this curated version of Ayurveda accompanying the image of the brass lamps, the sages at work on palmyra leaves, as depicted in the advertisements, has achieved brand status. The ancientness of the tradition, the age of the company, the civilizational permanence and stability, all come through in the images. The neatly arranged and uniformly sized packaging stands in for quality control. The images of oil treatments listed in textual sani-tized Malayalam edged with Sanskrit, with descriptions and diseases listed below, offer the right mix of the exotic and expert domains, translated via biomedicine for the comfort of the tourist. The efficacy of the treatments is delivered in legend and is not the issue here; standardization, accreditation, and state approval are. And so we arrive at wellness as a self-healthcare package within individual reach. While the nuances of this in globalization discourse can be explored much further, the endorsement via TM strategy documents of the WHO are the final stamp of approval for these entities. What counts as TM/CM obviously is determined by these standardization and accreditation processes; it is the practices that make it in, that will be allowed to be part of the wellness package. The early exhortation of the Chopra Committee may be recalled here – 'once the ... *non-institutionally qualified fade out'*.

A way of life?

It would be useful to briefly revisit the Health and Wellness Centres to better understand better the 'fading out of the non-institutionally qualified'. The Ayush HWC operational guidelines prescribe the structure and look for the HWCs, down to illustrations prescribed for the walls, the herbal garden, the Yoga *sthal* (space/place), the courtyard, and the integrated picture of the community. In a combina-tion of the Ayush physician, the ASHA, the Yoga instructor, the *safai karmachari* (the cleaning person), and the docile community, the HWCs, all looking the same and thus instantly recognizable, branded, somehow multiply across the country's digital map to more than 12,500. In some ways, the Ayush Health and Wellness Centre recreates the idyllic village.

What is this idyll? Is the community space a flat one? Gandhi's iconic specta-cles, with the slogan of the Swachh Bharat Mission, appear on the websites of both of Ayush and the Ministry of Health and Family Welfare. This logo was launched in September 2014, with the slogan *'ek kadam swachhata ki aur'* (a step towards cleanliness) with the then urban development minister M. Venkaiah Naidu stating that 'For the Mahatma, cleanliness and India were like his two eyes through which he envisioned a clean India' (Naidu 2014). Critical scholarship has remarked on this visual framing, reading the spectacles as a superficial rendering of Gandhi's philosophy of honesty, self-reflection, and cleanliness, or as a form of surveillance (Jeffrey 2015, Rodrigues and Niemann 2017). While Gandhi's position against untouchability, sitting as it does alongside his acceptance of caste-based occupations, has been critiqued, it is the literal lifting of the trope of sanitation from his polemics set in the backdrop of his vision of a just community into the rhetoric of hygiene seemingly separated from the caste question, and as community vigilantism, that is relevant for my purposes. This is the kind of rhetoric that builds a case for a 'way of life' that is ahistorical, structurally flat, and most importantly, anchored in the lives of the socially dominant. It takes Gandhi's idea of cleaning toilets being a dignified occupation like any other, circumvents the material, historical, and symbolic association of pollution with the caste-based occupation of sewage disposal, in fact, avoids the discussion of sewage disposal altogether (Joshi and Khattri 2019), and travels straight into the dream of the clean equal community rather than the caste-riven community structures that are our reality, then and now. The vigilantism that it encourages – the taking of pictures of women defecating in the open – is a good, if morbid, example of the consequences of such sleight of hand.[11] More insidiously, the decoupling of sanitation from sanitation work. *Swachh* is a word that carries connotations of cleanliness, *purity*, colour, as also integrity of purpose, particularly in the context of its recent usage, and is a more Sanskritized word that has been brought into common usage in place of words like *saaf* or *saaf-suthra* which would reflect more closely the material cleanliness in question here. The decoupling succeeds both in invisibilizing the caste oppression linked with sanitation work, and centring and making standard the privileged-caste and middle-class narratives of hygiene and health. It erases, quite comprehensively, the histories of caste oppression. In primary healthcare, it establishes a dominant identity for indigenous therapeutics.

Yoga and indigeneity

Yoga is officially classified within allied forms of health knowledge, that 'have been adapted as health applications' (Payyappallimana 2010, p. 59), rather than as traditional medicine per se according to global classifications. It has, however, become front and centre at Ayush, more coherently so in the last few years, with the ministry indicating a 'Common Yoga Protocol' for all Yoga classes to follow across the country, 'for the masses to reap all the benefits of Yoga' (https://yoga.ayush.gov.in/), mass *Surya Namaskara* and other *asana* videos, international Yoga conferences, and of course the International Day of Yoga. There are, therefore, both inward and outward looking aspects to this exercise.

In his speech at the UN General Assembly in September 2014, the current Indian Prime Minister Narendra Modi proposed an International Yoga Day, stating that 'Yoga is an invaluable gift of India's ancient tradition. It embodies unity of mind and body ... By changing our lifestyle and creating consciousness, it can help in well being'. The UN subsequently declared 21st June as International Yoga Day, with a record number of 175 countries co-sponsoring the India-led resolution, adopted without a vote under the agenda of Global Health and Foreign Policy. Subsequently, starting in 2015, International Yoga Day has been celebrated with spectacular media attention, with events led in India by the prime minister, and across the world, breaking Guinness World Book records.

It is useful to see the discourse around Yoga in the present alongside the rubric of integration. While standardization, accreditation, and regulation on the terms of modern biomedicine have been the thorn in the flesh of Ayurveda and other indigenous systems of medicine, Yoga, drawn into the fold, seems to have done the work, not of the dominant utilitarian view of integration Payyappallimana speaks of, but of positioning India as the *maker* of the standard in this practice, thus implicitly suggesting trans-cultural synergy; and this is bound to have ripple effects in other aspects of traditionality. The 'viral' images of the PM leading Yoga sessions on International Yoga Day in 2017 in a rain-drenched *Ambedkar Sabha Sthal* in Lucknow, Uttar Pradesh, do something to the question of who validates whom. And yet, this is not a romanticized view of the East; the East is now literally within the homes of the West, asking for a change of lifestyle and offering a well-packaged way to do it.

Is this India-led though? Gautam and Droogan speak of the contexts within which Yoga is being amplified today, as 'already ... a global and globalised cultural export seen as being quintessentially Indian and that has become big business both in India and throughout the world' (2018, p. 7). Some of the earliest large-scale movements that took Yoga to the West were the *Hare Krishna* movements in the 1960s (Rochford, 2007). If the counter-cultures of the 60s were about recognizing the dangers of excess in Western lifestyles, a danger that Gandhi states unambiguously in his *Hind Swaraj* as the problem with doctors, lawyers, and railways – symbols of Western modernity – today this has reappeared as the dangers of unsustainable development. The entire discourse of the SDGs rests on this. With a 'good narrative strategy' (p. 6) to respond to this perceived lifestyle in place, then, the current amplification of Yoga internationally by the Indian government may be seen in context.

How may we read this narrative strategy? Apart from the metaphors of 'timelessness, holism' (p. 1), inclusiveness and tolerance associated with Hinduism in the broadly speaking western world, the 'soft power' Gautam and Droogan speak of has other contexts and components. The authors define one of these, cultural nationalism, thus – 'Like other postcolonial nations, India has experienced the steady rise of various cultural nationalisms, each of which emphasises the adoption of politically active identities characterised by a commitment to tradition' (p. 2). These identities may emerge in the context of an experience of threat to previously dominant ways of being in the pace of modernity and globalization; they may be aggravated in the face of rights-based movements that have used the language of modernity to articulate needs. The ideologies of perceived threat and resentment may have emerged as 'a political response to modernity that appropriates and modernises heritage and tradition in order to make them more compatible with the unique pressures of modern politics and nation building' (p. 3). For the political class, this presents an opportunity to mobilize, at home, aspects of resentment to promote a 'way of life' that must not be dislodged, and in the world, a 'way of life' that can be an exemplar. This is what might be called soft Hindutva cultural nationalism – 'an innovative blend of exclusivist Hindutva (traditionally associated with the Hindu right) with the democratic state-focused cultural nationalism utilised by Nehru and the Congress party for decades immediately prior to and after independence' (p. 4). Wellness as a prescription may well operate through this discourse – as *a way of life* that always was, and whose recovery is the best route both to self-care and to lead the world. Gandhi's voice reappears in an eerie new format here; *swaraj* – the call to self-discipline in order to attain freedom, slides into bodily practices associated with masculinist organizational training in Hindutva organizations. *Dinacharya, Ritucharya*, make more sense in this framework.

The idea of Hindutva as a way of life is not new. Justice Verma, offering a judgement in 1995 on the use of the term in elections, had made this statement, albeit innocent of its present connotations – a judgement received with jubilation in the then BJP manifesto. The judgement provoked criticism, particularly in the context of Savarkar's definition of Hindutva as a racial, territorial attribute that conflated Hinduness with the land one lived on, from the Himalayas to the ocean. Today, with the centrality given to Yoga, its promotion on the international stage as India's gift to the world, its discourse entirely populated and linked with the idea of ancient protocol, and the hypervisibilizing of its religious elements – mantra chanting and Hindu imagery – it is this 'way of life' argument that is consolidated. As I have mentioned earlier, this bleeds into other components of Ayush as well. In this soil, Ayurveda imagery that could earlier be read patronizingly as 'local', now makes absolute global sense in this regime of soft power. I would further suggest this is a staging – of soft power – that allows more virulent forms to flourish under the table while not needing to be the official line.

Larger-than-life phenomena like Baba Ramdev, a self-styled Yoga guru cum godman and co-founder of the company Patanjali that manufactures Ayurvedic products, also flourish in this climate. Showcasing a quasi-subaltern roughshod masculinity, extreme bodily agility as a marker of virility, glamourizing conservative *swadeshi* positions on gender and sexuality,[12] alongside a near-caricatural challenge to 'foreign' commodities in the FMCG market, claiming authentic *Bharatiyata*,[13] appealing to an anti-intellectualism that is the bedrock of Hindutva politics, Ramdev is outside of the institution yet amazingly successful and singular. Ramdev represents, according to Tripathy, 'the resurgence of the margin' (2019, p. 420). Banerjee avers that 'Patanjali is more an economic than a cultural rupture' (Banerjee 2002, p. 421), staying within the pharmaceutical episteme of mass production and standardization. I would suggest, following Tripathy, that Ramdev is a measure of the success of the global pharma-wellness framework, 'creat[ing] Ayurveda as a moral discourse where Ayurveda is not just an economic imperative, but also a cultural and national urge' (Tripathy 2019, p. 423).

While it is tempting to further examine the Ramdev phenomenon, it is not the focus of this discussion; I would, however, draw one point about Yoga in the wellness discourse that Ramdev particularly manifests, and that is the aspect of somatic nationalism (Alter 1994, Chakraborty 2007). The bodily practice that

Yoga represents, in today's climate, aligns intuitively with bodily disciplinary exercises that have, since the 1920s, spoken of racial regeneration as a prelude to *Swaraj* or self-determination. We might usefully recall here Foucault's arguments around technologies of the self. Longkumer suggests that this somatic nationalism is 'forged not by its steely traditional militancy, but by its liquidity according to the nature of its host' (Longkumer 2018, p. 417), as the author explores the spread of Patanjali beyond the 'cow belt' to Nagaland, one of the states on the northeastern border. The 'way of life' argument, then, is sufficiently flexible to allow local experimentation, while still retaining its goals of assimilation. It is this very fluidity, its extra-institutional character, that the indigenous wellness discourse, and Yoga within it, supports; a fluidity that nonetheless holds up racial and caste purity – through language, control of 'excess', and elimination of vulnerability. In this framing, the indigenous is physically invulnerable, originally pure, and a source of textual knowledge. Caste privilege is a natural qualifier here. The bone-setter, the *dai*, or the street *fakir*, are necessarily abjected in this new framing.

The uneven nature of the indigenous

What happens, then, to Unani, Siddha, and to the varieties of practitioners that have constituted the realm of the indigenous, but are barely visible in Ayush? In the movement around, if not towards integration, are alternate expert domains being created using somatic nationalism? Lambert and Mukharji have spoken extensively of bone setters and other practitioners who practice rather than have a practitioner identity; these practices may therefore entirely escape the net of regulation. Unani and Siddha continue to retain specific kinds of 'locality'; this is sometimes performed and marginalized in the public eye, as was evident in the early pandemic period, when 'immunity packages' from Siddha were being offered by the Tamil Nadu government and ridiculed on national television by anchors who put together a mishmash of corporatized Ayurveda pill-pushing campaigns, including Patanjali's, to compare it with.

What of the *dai*? In her administratively visible form, she has been comprehensively rejected, first by institutional settings, and then through the community health worker or ASHA. She continues to persist as the dreaded, undomesticated figure who still has access, and some degree of power, over community. Metaphorically, however, she has been recast as a niche participant in natural childbirth, alongside classist niche articulations of feminine traditions that are barely short of Orientalist. In childbirth villages emerging within the domain of international private medical tourism in Kerala, for instance, story upon story of 'natural birthing' experiences speak of the compassionate and caring midwife in a 'home-like environment', a counter to the 'production line' – an obvious reference to institutional deliveries. The midwife here is the modern biomedical actor – the product of modern midwifery training, with a dash of care thrown in; the indigenous is Ayurveda – the 'ancient Indian wellness program ... [that brings] Abhyangam, or full body massage ... with curative and therapeutic oils ... [that] will vary as per ... body constitution' (https://birthvillage.in/ayurveda/). Also indigenous is the habitat, the 'village' – the *aab-o-hawa* of old Unani fame, but without a trace of that practice. This is the habitat the non-resident Indian comes to birth in, the indigenous she returns to, for an authentic home experience. There is but a nearly forgettable hint at the one who will, who has always, remove[d] the afterbirth – 'the *chechi* [sister] who came in to clean up late in the night after I created a bloody mess!' (ibid). With no place in the dominant indigenous, however, she does not 'make it' into traditional or complementary medicine, into institutional or natural childbirth. We will find out, I suppose, if the privileged-caste familial birth attendant manages to achieve a place in the indigenous sun, sometime down the line.

Notes

1 Sir Joseph Bhore, who headed the committee, was deeply influenced by the welfare model in the UK of the time, and stressed on preventive health work. By the time of the later committees and monitoring, compartmentalization of health work was more evident, with family planning becoming a more visible and separate programme. Institutional deliveries and birth control then became primary targets.

2 This connection emerged clearly during conversations on deskilling and the generation of multiple tasks in this exercise, with China Mills.

3 Task shifting has sometimes been used interchangeably with task sharing (Deller et al 2015), as related but distinct (Orkin et al 2021). The Concepts and Opportunities to Advance Task Shifting and Task Sharing (COATS) Framework suggested that 'task shifting concerns delegation, while task sharing focuses on collaboration between different workers' (Orkin et al 2021, p. 4). The binary of expertise and experience, however, that I am concerned with here, persists.

4 'Community volunteers, referred to as Community Health Nutrition Sanitation Mobilisers (CHNSMs) or in local language Bal Parivar Mitra (BPMS) meaning "friend of families with young children" were selected and assigned the task of reaching the "at risk families" at least once a fortnight' (Chaudhary 2012, p. 1183).

5 With a first edition being put out in 1970 by a local publisher who almost functioned like a university press for the Medical College in Jabalpur, Park's textbook of preventive and social medicine has shaped community medicine discourse in medical colleges in India over several generations. The time of its first author, who was trained in London's School of Hygiene and Tropical Medicine, and also advisor to the WHO, to ICMR, and an international presence, is significant for independent India's foray into community medicine. It is therefore to be expected that even later editions of the text have continued to focus on the 'socialist secular' of the Indian medical establishment and societal fabric as the way to think of community.

6 Jamnagar is today significant in the setting up of a WHO Global Centre for Traditional Medicine (WHO GCTM) in April 2022, amid the pandemic, under the Ayush ministry – a step that is expected 'to position AYUSH systems across the globe' and 'provide leadership on global health matters pertaining to traditional medicine' (https://pib.gov.in /PressReleasePage.aspx?PRID=1804289), a claim endorsed by the present WHO director, Tedros Adhanom Ghebreyesus. Jamnagar's history as the home of the world's first Ayurvedic college was highlighted by the Indian prime minister during the inaugural event. This claim to formal training may be challenged easily enough. The website of the Ayurveda college at Tripunithara suggests that Thiruvananthapuram is said to have hosted the first ever study centre for Ayurveda under government control in 1889, formal Ayurvedic education was started in the princely state of Cochin in 1926 at Tripunithara, and separate courses for Ayurveda were started here in 1936 (https://ayurvedacollege.ac .in/a-short-history-of-the-college/). Other such claims may be available. More impor-

tant, however, is the attention that K.P. Girija draws to the historically heterogeneous field of practice and transmission of knowledge that was a constituent feature of what might be called Ayurveda.

As a perhaps non-trivial aside, Gujarat has in the present few decades become hyper-visible for a model of development that is capitalist-friendly, spectacular technology-enabled, and yet culturally appropriate. It is also the state from where the present PM launched, and honed, his political career.

7 I use the hyphen here, unlike the borderlands idea proposed by Anzaldua (1987) or the mixed identity location that Stavans (1999) refers to, as a limited resource to indicate the ways in which each of these terms – community, rurality, and indigeneity, act as placeholders for each other in the biomedical as well as healthcare and health planning discourse.

8 *Ayushmanabhava* – a greeting familiarized in popular culture from the 1990s televised version of Mahabharata, a war epic of ancient India.

9 At the time of writing, there has been a further change in nomenclature of these centres, to Ayushman Arogya Mandirs, proposing a purported integration of comprehensive primary health care with the celebrated PM-JAY health insurance scheme that offers a 'health insurance cover of Rs. 5 lakhs per year to over 10 crore poor and vulnerable families for seeking secondary and tertiary care' (https://ab-hwc.nhp.gov.in/).While a detailed analysis of this move is beyond the scope of this discussion,we can see the connections in vocabulary between normativised majoritarian impulses, dominant indigenous vocabulary, and corporatized healthcare.

10 Consider, for instance, recent translations of COVID protocol – like *Raksha kavach* (safety shield) – using religio-cultural tropes for advocacy.

11 In 2016, several districts in Uttar Pradesh officially adopted the policy of garlanding, ringing a bell, or beating plates, in addition to photographing people, including women, who seem to be going to relieve themselves with a 'lota' – a vessel with water. This policy of 'disturbing and shaming' 'offenders', was offered to school students and other members of community; 'offenders' could be fined or jailed. This was part of the mission of declaring villages open-defecation-free, under the Swachh Bharat Mission. Toilets are to be constructed by individual households at their own expense, with a claim to Rs 12000 that can be made to the government thereafter. For details see https://www.hindustantimes.com/india/name-and-shame-up-to-photograph-people-defecating-in-the-open/story-YqBr8wJFx6pzkjzOaovqsI.html.

12 https://www.deccanchronicle.com/131211/news-current-affairs/article/homosexuality-disease-yoga-can-cure-it-ramdev. This was after the unfavourable Supreme Court verdict on Sec 377 of the IPC.

13 This is a term now set up in direct opposition to Indianness, to stand in for the nation as opposed to the colony. More recent developments around naming may be referred for this. https://indianexpress.com/article/world/india-bharat-row-united-nations-name-change-policy-8928441/.

References

Books and articles

Abraham, L. (2013, Autumn). From Vaidyam to Kerala Ayurveda. *The Newsletter, 65,* 32.

Alavi, S. (2008). *Islam and healing: Loss and recovery of an Indo-Muslim medical tradition, 1600–1900.* London: Palgrave Macmillan.

Alcoff, L., & Dalmiya, V. (1993). Are old wives' tales justified? In L. Alcoff & E. Potter (Eds.), *Feminist epistemologies* (pp. 217–244). New York and London: Routledge.

Alter, J. S. (1994). Celibacy, sexuality, and the transformation of gender into nationalism in North India. *The Journal of Asian Studies, 53*(1), 45–66.

266 *Indigenous therapeutics in the present*

Anzaldúa, G. (1987). Borderlands:The New Mestiza. San Francisco: Aunt Lute Books.
Arnold, D. (1993). *Colonizing the body: State medicine and epidemic disease in nineteenth-century India.* Berkeley and Los Angeles: University of California Press.
Azher, S. (2017). Professional niche differentiation: Understanding Dai (Traditional Midwife) survival in rural Rajasthan. *ASIANetwork Exchange: A Journal for Asian Studies in the Liberal Arts, 24*(1), 132–150.
Bajpai, V., & Saraya, A. (2013). NRHM-The panacea for rural health in India: A critique. *Indian Journal of Public Health Research & Development, 4*(1), 241.
Banerjee, M. (2002, March 23–29). Public policy and ayurveda: Modernising a great tradition. *Economic and Political Weekly, 37* (12), 1136–1146.
Berger, R. (2013). *Ayurveda made modern: Political histories of indigenous medicine in Northern India, 1900–1955.* New York: Palgrave Macmillan.
Bhatia, K. (2014). Community health worker programs in India: A rights-based review. *Perspectives in Public Health, 134*(5), 276–282.
Campbell, C., & Scott, K. (2011). Retreat from Alma Ata? The WHO's report on task shifting to community health workers for AIDS care in poor countries. *Global Public Health, 6*(2), 125–138.
Chakraborty, C. (2007). The Hindu ascetic as fitness instructor: Reviving faith in Yoga. *The International Journal of the History of Sport, 24*(9), 1172–1186.
Chawla, J. (2002). Hawa, gola and mother-in-law's big toe. In S. Rozario & G. Samuel (Eds.), *The Daughters of Hariti: Childbirth and female healers in South and Southeast Asia* (pp. 147–162). London: Routledge.
Chawla, J. (2019). *Towards a Female Shastra.* Ernakulam: Matrika.
Chatterjee, P. (2000). Development planning and the Indian state. In Z. Hasan (Ed.), *Politics and the State in India* (pp. 120–125). New Delhi: Sage Publications.
Chaudhary, D. N. (2012). Reducing malnutrition: An analysis of the Integrated Child Development Services (ICDS) scheme. In S. C. Vir (Ed.), *Public health and nutrition in developing countries* (Part I and II, pp.1154–1194). New Delhi, Cambridge, Oxford and Philadelphia: WPI India.
Chopra, R. N. (1965). Problems and prospects of a pharmacological career in India. *Annual Review of Pharmacology, 5*(1), 1–9.
Chopra, R. N., et al. (1948). *Report of the committee on indigenous systems of medicine* (Vol. I, Report and Recommendations).* New Delhi: Ministry of Health, Government of India.
Committee, H. A. (1946). *Report of the health and survey development committee Vol. I. Government of India.* New Delhi: Manager of Publications.
Dalmiya, V. (2002). Why should a knower care? *Hypatia, 17*(1), 34–52.
Deleuze, G., Guattari, F. (1987). Massumi, B. (translator and contributor). *A thousand plateaus: Capitalism and schizophrenia.* Minneapolis, London: University of Minnesota Press.
Deller, B., Tripathi, V., Stender, S., Otolorin, E., Johnson, P., & Carr, C. (2015). Task shifting in maternal and newborn health care: Key components from policy to implementation. *International Journal of Gynecology & Obstetrics, 130*(S2), S25–S31.
Department of Family Welfare, Ministry of Health and Family Welfare, Government of India. (2000). *National population policy 2000.* New Delhi: Government of India.
Fraser, N. (2021). Rethinking the public sphere: A contribution to the critique of actually existing democracy. In M. Mitrašinović & V. Mehta (Eds.), *Public space reader* (pp. 34–41). New York and Oxon: Routledge.
Garnham, N. (2007). Habermas and the public sphere. *Global Media and Communication, 3*(2), 201–214.
Gautam, A., & Droogan, J. (2018). Yoga soft power: How flexible is the posture? *The Journal of International Communication, 24*(1), 18–36.
Girija, K. P. (2021). *Mapping the history of Ayurveda: Culture, hegemony and the rhetoric of diversity.* London and New York: Routledge.

Ghosh, A. (2006). *Power in print: Popular publishing and the politics of language and culture in a colonial society, 1778–1905.* New Delhi: Oxford University Press.

Ghoshal, R. (2014, October 18). Death of a Dai: Development-modernity's 'success' story. *Economic & Political Weekly, 49*(42), 27–29.

Gopal, M. (2017). Traditional knowledge and feminist dilemmas: Experience of the midwives of the barber caste in South Tamil Nādu. In S. Krishna & G. Chadha (Eds.), *Feminists and science: Critiques and changing perspectives in India* (Vol. 2, pp. 23–45). New Delhi: Sage Publications & Stree.

Halstead, S. B., Walsh, J. A., & Warren, K. S. (1985, October). *Good health at low cost: Proceedings of a conference.* New York: The Rockefeller Foundation.

Harrison, M., & Pati, B. (2009). Social history of health and medicine: Colonial India. In B. Pati & M. Harrison (Eds.), *The social history of health and medicine in colonial India* (pp. 1–14). London and New York: Routledge.

Jeffrey, R. (2015). Clean India! Symbols, policies and tensions. *South Asia: Journal of South Asian Studies, 38*(4), 807–819.

Joshi, P. C., & Khattri, P. (2019). On Gandhi and Sanitation. *Journal of the Anthropological Survey of India, 68*(2), 210–224.

King, C. R. (1994). *One language, two scripts: The Hindi movement in nineteenth century India.* Bombay: Oxford University Press.

Kohli, C., Kishore, J., Sharma, S., & Nayak, H. (2015, July–September). Knowledge and practice of accredited social health activists for maternal healthcare delivery in Delhi. *Journal of Family Medicine and Primary Care, 4*(3), 359–363.

Kumar, R. (2016). Bachelor of public health course to upgrade the competencies of health assistants. *Indian Journal of Public Health, 60*(3), 169–170.

Lambert, H. (2013). Wrestling with tradition: Towards a subaltern therapeutics of bonesetting and vessel treatment in north India. In D. Hardiman & P. B. Mukharji (Eds.), *Medical marginality in South Asia: Situating subaltern therapeutics* (pp. 109–125). London and New York: Routledge.

Lang, S. (2005, December). Drop the demon dai: Maternal mortality and the state in Colonial Madras, 1840–1875. *Social History of Medicine, 18*(3), 357–378.

Legg, S. (2009). Of scales, networks and assemblages: The League of Nations apparatus and the scalar sovereignty of the Government of India. *Transactions of the Institute of British Geographers, 34*(2), 234–253.

Legg, S. (2016). Dyarchy: Democracy, autocracy, and the scalar sovereignty of interwar India. *Comparative Studies of South Asia, Africa and the Middle East, 36*(1), 44–65.

Leslie, C. M. (Ed.). (1976). *Asian medical systems: A comparative study.* Berkeley, Los Angeles and London: University of California Press.

Leslie, C. M., Leslie, C. M., & Young, A. (Eds.). (1992). *Paths to Asian medical knowledge* (No. 32). Berkeley, Los Angeles and London: University of California Press.

Longkumer, A. (2018). 'Nagas can't sit lotus style': Baba Ramdev, Patanjali, and Neo-Hindutva. *Contemporary South Asia, 26*(4), 400–420.

Malhotra, A. (2003). Of dais and midwives: 'Middle-class' interventions in the management of women's reproductive health—a study from Colonial Punjab. *Indian Journal of Gender Studies, 10*(2), 229–259.

Mayra, K., Padmadas, S. S., & Matthews, Z. (2021) Challenges and needed reforms in midwifery and nursing regulatory systems in India: Implications for education and practice. *PLoS One, 16*(5), e0251331.

Ministry of Health and Family Welfare. (2018). *Guidelines on midwifery services in India: 2018.* New Delhi: Government of India.

Mukharji, P. B. (2009). *Nationalizing the body: The medical market, print and Daktari medicine.* London and New York: Anthem Press.

Mukharji, P. B. (2013). Chandshir Chikitsa: A nomadology of subaltern medicine. In D. Hardiman & P. B. Mukharji (Eds.), *Medical marginality in South Asia: Situating subaltern therapeutics* (pp. 85–108). London and New York: Routledge.

Muraleedharan, V., Dash, U., & Gilson, L. (2011). Tamil Nādu 1980s-2005: A success story in India. In D. Balabanova, M. McKee, & A. Mills (Eds.), *'Good health at low cost' 25 years on. What makes a successful health system?* London: London School of Hygiene & Tropical Medicine.

Murphy, J. (2007). *The world bank and global managerialism* (1st ed.). London: Routledge.

Nandan, D. (2005). National rural health mission-" Rhetoric or Reality". *Indian Journal of Public Health, 49*(3), 168–192.

Nandi, S., & Schneider, H. (2014). Addressing the social determinants of health: A case study from the Mitanin (community health worker) programme in India. *Health Policy and Planning, 29*(Suppl. 2), ii71–ii81.

Nordfeldt, C., & Roalkvam, S. (2010). Choosing vaccination: Negotiating child protection and good citizenship in modern India. *Forum for Development Studies, 37*(3), 327–347Orkin, A. M., Rao, S., Venugopal, J. et al (2021). Conceptual framework for task shifting and task sharing: An international Delphi study. *Human Resources for Health 19,* 61.

Olding, M., Boyd, J., Kerr, T., & McNeil, R. (2021, February). "And we just have to keep going": Task shifting and the production of burnout among overdose response workers with lived experience. *Social Science & Medicine, 270,* 113631.

Park, K. (2015). *Park's textbook of preventive and social medicine* (23rd ed.). Jabalpur: Banarsidas Bhanot Publishers.

Payyappallimana, U. (2010). Role of traditional medicine in primary health care: an overview of perspectives and challenges. *Yokohama Journal of Social Sciences, 14*(6), 58–77.

Payyappallimana, U., & Fadeeva, Z. (2018). Ensure healthy lives and promote well-being for all: Experiences of community health, hygiene, sanitation and nutrition. In *Innovation in local and global learning systems for sustainability: Learning contributions of the regional centres of expertise on education for sustainable development* (pp. 8–19). Tokyo, Japan: United Nations University Institute for the Advanced Study of Sustainability.

Pinto, S. (2008). *Where there is no midwife: Birth and loss in rural India.* New York and Oxford: Berghahn Books.

Porter, D. (2006). How did social medicine evolve, and where is it heading? *PLoS Med, 3*(10), e399.

Porter, D. (2011). Health citizenship: Essays in social medicine and biomedical politics. United States: University of California, Medical Humanities Consortium. San Fransisco.

Ramasubban, R. (2022). Imperial health in British India 1857–1900. In M. Macleod & M. Lewis (Eds.), *Disease, medicine & empire: Perspectives on the medicine and the experience of European expansion.* London: Routledge.

Ravindran, T. K. S. (2007, July–September). World Bank and India's health sector. *Medico Friend Circle Bulletin, 323–324,* 1–7.

Rao, K. D., Sundararaman, T., Bhatnagar, A. Gupta, G., Kokho, P., & Jain, K. (2013). Which doctor for primary health care? Quality of care and non–physician clinicians in India. *Social Science & Medicine, 84,* 30–34.

Ritu Priya. (2012). AYUSH and public health: Democratic pluralism and the quality of health services. In V. Sujatha & L. Abraham (Eds.), *Medical pluralism in contemporary India* (pp. 103–129). Hyderabad: Orient Blackswan.

Rochford, E. B. (2007). *Hare Krishna transformed.* New York and London: New York University Press.

Rodrigues, U. M., & Niemann, M. (2017). Social media as a platform for incessant political communication: a case study of Modi's "clean India" campaign. *International Journal of Communication, 11,* 23.

Roy, S., Mir, R. A., Gangwar, A. K., & Gangwar, R. (2018). Herbs for health: Communicating for conservation, cultivation and sustainable utilisation of medicinal and aromatic plants. In U. Payyappallimana & Z. Fadeeva (Eds.), *Innovation in local and global learning systems for sustainability. Ensure healthy lives and promote well-being for all, experiences of community health, hygiene, sanitation and nutrition* (pp. 62–71). Tokyo, Japan: Learning Contributions of the Regional Centres of Expertise on Education for Sustainable Development, UNU-IAS.

Rudra, S., Kalra, A., Kumar, A., & Joe, W. (2017) Utilization of alternative systems of medicine as health care services in India: Evidence on AYUSH care from NSS 2014. *PLoS One, 12*(5), e0176916.

Sadgopal, M. (2009, April 18–24). Can maternity services open up to the indigenous traditions of midwifery? *Economic and Political Weekly, 44*(16), 52–59.

Scott, K., George, A. S., & Ved, R. R. (2019). Taking stock of 10 years of published research on the ASHA programme: Examining India's national community health worker programme from a health systems perspective. *Health Research Policy and Systems, 17*(1), 1–17.

Scott, K., & Shanker, S. (2010). Tying their hands? Institutional obstacles to the success of the ASHA community health worker programme in rural north India. *AIDS Care: Psychological and Socio-medical Aspects of AIDS/HIV, 22*(Suppl. 2), 1606–1612.

Shewade, H. D., Jeyashree, K., & Chinnakali, P. (2014). Reviving community medicine in India: the need to perform our primary role. *International Journal of Medicine and Public Health, 4*(1), 29–32.

Sivaramakrishnan, K. (2006). *Old potions, new bottles: Recasting Indigenous medicine in Colonial Punjab (1850–1945)* (New Perspectives in South Asian History, number 12). Hyderabad: Orient Longman.

Spencer, H.R. (1927). *The history of British Midwifery from 1650 to 1800, the Fitz-Patrick lectures for 1927, delivered before the Royal College of Physicians of London.* London: John Bale, Sons & Danielsson, Ltd.

Srinivasan, P. (1995). National health policy for traditional medicine in India. In *World Health Forum 1995, 16* (2), 190–193.

Srivastava, A., Gope, R., Nair, N., Rath, S., Rath, S., Sinha, R., ... Bhattacharyya, S. (2015). Are village health sanitation and nutrition committees fulfilling their roles for decentralised health planning and action? A mixed methods study from rural eastern India. *BMC Public Health, 16*(1), 1–12.

Stavans, I. (1999). On separate ground. In M. Agosin (Ed.), *Passion, memory, and identity,* (pp. 1–16). Albuquerque: University of New Mexico Press.

Stock, T. (2007). *Task shifting to tackle health worker shortages* (WHO/HSS/2007.03). Retrieved from https://chwcentral.org/wp-content/uploads/2013/07/Task-shifting-to-tackle-health-worker-shortages.pdf

Sujatha, V., & Abraham, L. (Eds.). (2012). *Medical pluralism in contemporary India.* Hyderabad: Orient Blackswan.

Thakur, H. P., Pandit D. D., & Subramanian P. (2001). History of preventive and social medicine in India. *Journal of Postgraduate Medicine, 47(*4), 283–285.

Thakur, R., Sinha, A. K., & Pathak, R. K. (2017). Transition in local home birth practices in Mashobra block of Inner Himalayas, Himachal Pradesh: Assessing role and status of traditional birth attendants. *The Oriental Anthropologist, 17*(1), 171–183.

Tripathy, J. (2019). Consuming indigeneity: Baba Ramdev, Patanjali Ayurveda and the Swadeshi project of development. *Journal of Developing Societies, 35*(3), 412–430.

Unnithan-Kumar, M. (2002). Midwives among others: Knowledges of healing and the politics of emotions in Rajasthan, Northwest India. In S. Rozario & G. Samuel (Eds.), *The Daughters of Hariti: Childbirth and female healers in South and Southeast Asia* (pp. 109–129). London: Routledge.

Vasudevan, S. (2021). Heal the world: Wellness tourism and market readiness in Post Corona travel. In C. Cobanoglu, E. G. Kucukaltan, M. Tuna, A. Basoda, & S. Dogan (Eds.), *Advances in managing tourism across continents* (pp. 98–108). University of South Florida M3 Publishing.

Government and other committee reports

Bhore, J. (1946). Report of the Health Survey and Development Committee. New Delhi and Calcutta: Survey. Manager of Publications.

Department of AYUSH. (2002). *National policy on Indian systems of medicine & homoeopathy-2002.* New Delhi: Ministry of Health & Family Welfare, Government of India

Department-related parliamentary standing committee on Health and family welfare. *Report on The national commission for indian system of medicine Bill, 2019* (115th report). Rajya Sabha Secretariat, New Delhi: Parliament of India.

Ministry of Ayush. Government of India. (2020). *Ayushman Bharat. AYUSH health and wellness centres. Operational guidelines.* New Delhi. Retrieved from https://namayush .gov.in/sites/default/files/doc/AYUSH_HWCs_Operational_Guideline_English.pdf

Ministry of Ayush, Government of India. Notification. (2021, April 13). *Gazette of India.*

World Health Organization. (2013). *WHO traditional medicine strategy: 2014–2023.* World Health Organization.

Newspaper and online reports

Chishti, S. (2017, January 3). Why, 22 years on, the SC's 'Hindutva judgment' remains elephant in room. *The Indian Express.* Retrieved from https://indianexpress.com/article /explained/gujarat-riot-nhrc-religion-elections-vote-bank-supreme-court-why-22-years -on-the-scs-hindutva-judgment-remains-elephant-in-room-4456258/

Hellwig, C. (2015, June 29). *Deforestation impacting pharmaceutical industry. Global risk insights: Know your world.* Retrieved from https://globalriskinsights.com/2015/06/ deforestation-impacting-pharmaceutical-industry/

Kulkarni, M. (2013, January 20). Ayurvedic medicine makers go North. *Business Standard.* Retrieved from https://www.business-standard.com/article/sme/ayurvedic-medicine -makers-go-north-111060700093_1.html

Malviya, S. (2020, September 22). Ayurvedic products less than 1 per cent of India's FMCG market: Kantar Worldpanel. *The Economic Times.* Retrieved from https://economictimes .indiatimes.com/industry/healthcare/biotech/healthcare/ayurvedic-products-less-than-1-per -cent-of-indias-fmcg-market-kantar-worldpanel/articleshow/78256231.cms?from=mdr.

PTI. (2014, December 11). UN declares June 21 as 'international day of yoga'. *The Economic Times.* Retrieved from https://economictimes.indiatimes.com/news/politics-and-nation/ un-declares-june-21-as-international-day-of-yoga/articleshow/45481256.cms

TNN (2014, September 26). Gandhi's vision captured in Swachh Bharat Logo. *The Times of India.*

Archival references

From Wellcome Trust Collections, London, UK –

Whitbread family. *Whitbread Family Receipt Book: 1700-1811?* [Manuscript Receipt Book containing culinary, medical, cosmetic, household and a few veterinary … receipts, in several different hands, including diseases of pregnancy, labour and miscarriage]. (MS. 8745).

British Library, UK -

Salient features in the decade of development of indigenous systems of medicine. (1977). New Delhi: Central Council for Research in Indian Medicine and Homoeopathy, Ministary [sic] of Health and Family Planning, Govt. of India. (Asia, Pacific & Africa T 32699, UIN: BLL01009294302).

Index

278   *Index*

Zandu Pharmacy 112
Zaroori Itilaa Awaam Ko 106
zenana: as category 180; education 179,
190, 197, 229; hospitals 125, 141, 173,
187; women 126, 138, 143, 164, 183,
185, 186; woman 87, 140, 143, 145,
151, 154, 164, 165, 173, 181, 183, 185,
186, 212